2007
YEAR BOOK OF
VASCULAR SURGERY®

The 2007 Year Book Series

Year Book of Allergy, Asthma, and Clinical Immunology™: Drs Rosenwasser, Boguniewicz, Milgrom, Routes, and Weber

Year Book of Anesthesiology and Pain Management™: Drs Chestnut, Abram, Black, Gravlee, Lee, Mathru, and Roizen

Year Book of Cardiology®: Drs Gersh, Cheitlin, Elliott, Graham, Sundt, and Waldo

Year Book of Critical Care Medicine®: Drs Dellinger, Parrillo, Balk, Bekes, Dorman, and Dries

Year Book of Dentistry®: Drs McIntyre, Belvedere, Buhite, Davis, Henderson, Johnson, Jureyda, Ohrbach, Olin, Scott, Spencer, and Zakariasen

Year Book of Dermatology and Dermatologic Surgery™: Drs Thiers and Lang

Year Book of Diagnostic Radiology®: Drs Osborn, Birdwell, Dalinka, Gardiner, Levy, Elster, Oestreich, and Rosado de Christenson

Year Book of Emergency Medicine®: Drs Hamilton, Handly, Quintana, Werner, and Bruno

Year Book of Endocrinology®: Drs Mazzaferri, Bessesen, Clarke, Howard, Kennedy, Leahy, Meikle, Molitch, Rogol, and Schteingart

Year Book of Family Practice®: Drs Bowman, Apgar, Dexter, Neill, Scherger, and Zink

Year Book of Gastroenterology™: Drs Lichtenstein, Burke, Campbell, Dempsey, Drebin, Jaffe, Katzka, Kochman, Morris, Rombeau, Shah, and Stein

Year Book of Hand and Upper Limb Surgery®: Drs Chang and Steinmann

Year Book of Medicine®: Drs Barkin, Berney, Frishman, Garrick, Loehrer, Mazzaferri, Phillips, and Snydman

Year Book of Neonatal and Perinatal Medicine®: Drs Fanaroff, Ehrenkranz, and Stevenson

Year Book of Neurology and Neurosurgery®: Drs Kim and Verma

Year Book of Nuclear Medicine®: Drs Coleman, Blaufox, Royal, Strauss, and Zubal

Year Book of Obstetrics, Gynecology, and Women's Health®: Dr Shulman

Year Book of Oncology®: Drs Loehrer, Arceci, Glatstein, Gordon, Hanna, Morrow, and Thigpen

Year Book of Ophthalmology®: Drs Rapuano, Cohen, Eagle, Flanders, Hammersmith, Myers, Nelson, Penne, Sergott, Shields, Tipperman, and Vander

Year Book of Orthopedics®: Drs Morrey, Beauchamp, Peterson, Swiontkowski, Trigg, and Yaszemski

Year Book of Otolaryngology-Head and Neck Surgery®: Drs Paparella, Gapany, and Keefe

Year Book of Pathology and Laboratory Medicine®: Drs Raab, Parwani, Bejarano, and Bissell

Year Book of Pediatrics®: Dr Stockman

Year Book of Plastic and Aesthetic Surgery™: Drs Miller, Bartlett, Garner, McKinney, Ruberg, Salisbury, and Smith

Year Book of Psychiatry and Applied Mental Health®: Drs Talbott, Ballenger, Buckley, Frances, Jensen, and Markowitz,

Year Book of Pulmonary Disease®: Drs Phillips, Barker, Lewis, Maurer, Tanoue, and Willsie

Year Book of Rheumatology, Arthritis, and Musculoskeletal Disease™: Drs Panush, Furst, Hadler, Hochberg, Lahita, and Paget

Year Book of Sports Medicine®: Drs Shephard, Pierrynowski, Cantu, Feldman, McCrory, Nieman, Rowland, Jankowski, and Shrier

Year Book of Surgery®: Drs Copeland, Bland, Cerfolio, Daly, Eberlein, Fahey, Mozingo, Pruett, and Seeger

Year Book of Urology®: Drs Andriole and Coplen

Year Book of Vascular Surgery®: Dr Moneta

2007

The Year Book of VASCULAR SURGERY®

Editor-in-Chief

Gregory L. Moneta, MD

Professor and Chief of Vascular Surgery, Oregon Health and Science University; and Chief of Vascular Surgery, Oregon Health and Science University Hospital and Portland VA Hospital, Portland, Oregon

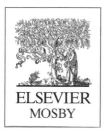

ELSEVIER
MOSBY

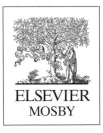

ELSEVIER
MOSBY

Vice President, Continuity Publishing: John A. Schrefer
Associate Developmental Editor: Ruth Malwitz
Production Manager, Electronic Year Books: Thomas C. Pohlman
Senior Issue Manager: Pat Costigan
Illustrations and Permissions Coordinator: Dawn Vohsen

Printed in the United States of America
Composition by Thomas Technology Solutions, Inc.
Printing/binding by Sheridan Books, Inc

Editorial Office:
Elsevier
Suite 1800
1600 John F. Kennedy Blvd
Philadelphia, PA 19103-2899

International Standard Serial Number: 0749-4041
International Standard Book Number: 0-323-04644-4
                              978-0-323-04644-2

Contributors

Scott A. Berceli, MD, PhD
Associate Professor of Surgery, University of Florida, and Chief of Vascular Surgery, Malcom Randall VA Medical Center, Gainesville, Florida

Mark K. Eskandari, MD
Associate Professor of Surgery and Radiology, Northwestern University Feinberg School of Medicine; and Attending Surgeon, Northwestern Memorial Hospital, Chicago, Illinois

Peter K. Henke, MD
Associate Professor of Surgery and Chief of Vascular Surgery, Ann Arbor Veterans Affairs Medical Center, University of Michigan, Ann Arbor, Michigan

Karthikeshwar Kasirajan, MD
Assistant Professor of Surgery, Department of Surgery, Division of Vascular Surgery, Emory University Hospital; and Atlanta VA Medical Center, Atlanta, Georgia

C. Keith Ozaki, MD
Associate Professor of Surgery, University of Florida College of Medicine; and Chief, Surgical Service, North Florida/South Georgia Veterans Health System, Gainesville, Florida

Joseph D. Raffetto, MD, MS
Assistant Professor of Surgery, Boston University; and Chief of Vascular Surgery, VA Boston Healthcare System, West Roxbury, Massachusetts

Table of Contents

Journals Represented

Journals represented in this YEAR BOOK are listed below.

Acta Paediatrica
American Journal of Cardiology
American Journal of Epidemiology
American Journal of Kidney Diseases
American Journal of Medicine
American Journal of Neuroradiology
American Journal of Physiology Heart and Circulation Physiology
American Journal of Roentgenology
Anesthesia and Analgesia
Annals of Internal Medicine
Annals of Rheumatic Diseases
Annals of Surgery
Annals of Thoracic Surgery
Annals of Vascular Surgery
Archives of Surgery
British Journal of Surgery
British Medical Journal
Canadian Medical Association Journal
Cardiovascular Pathology
Chest
Circulation
Critical Care Medicine
Dermatologic Surgery
Diabetes Care
European Journal of Radiology
European Journal of Vascular and Endovascular Surgery
International Journal of Cardiology
Journal of Bone and Joint Surgery (American Volume)
Journal of Bone and Joint Surgery (British Volume)
Journal of Clinical Investigation
Journal of Clinical Pathology
Journal of Neurology, Neurosurgery and Psychiatry
Journal of Neurosurgery
Journal of Orthopaedic Trauma
Journal of Pediatric Surgery
Journal of Rheumatology
Journal of Surgical Research
Journal of Thoracic and Cardiovascular Surgery
Journal of Ultrasound in Medicine
Journal of Vascular Surgery
Journal of Vascular and Interventional Radiology: JVIR
Journal of the American College of Cardiology
Journal of the American College of Surgeons
Journal of the American Geriatrics Society
Journal of the American Medical Association
Kidney International
Lancet
Medical Journal of Australia
Medicine

Medicine and Science in Sports and Exercise
Nephrology, Dialysis, Transplantation
Neurology
New England Journal of Medicine
Plastic and Reconstructive Surgery
Radiology
Radiotherapy and Oncology
Stroke
Surgery
Thrombosis Research
Vascular Medicine
Vascular and Endovascular Surgery

STANDARD ABBREVIATIONS

The following terms are abbreviated in this edition: acquired immunodeficiency syndrome (AIDS), cardiopulmonary resuscitation (CPR), central nervous system (CNS), cerebrospinal fluid (CSF), computed tomography (CT), deoxyribonucleic acid (DNA), electrocardiography (ECG), health maintenance organization (HMO), human immunodeficiency virus (HIV), intensive care unit (ICU), intramuscular (IM), intravenous (IV), magnetic resonance (MR) imaging (MRI), ribonucleic acid (RNA), and ultrasound (US).

NOTE

The YEAR BOOK OF VASCULAR SURGERY® is a literature survey service providing abstracts of articles published in the professional literature. Every effort is made to assure the accuracy of the information presented in these pages. Neither the editors nor the publisher of the YEAR BOOK OF VASCULAR SURGERY® can be responsible for errors in the original materials. The editors' comments are their own opinions. Mention of specific products within this publication does not constitute endorsement.

To facilitate the use of the YEAR BOOK OF VASCULAR SURGERY® as a reference tool, all illustrations and tables included in this publication are now identified as they appear in the original article. This change is meant to help the reader recognize that any illustration or table appearing in the YEAR BOOK OF VASCULAR SURGERY® may be only one of many in the original article. For this reason, figure and table numbers will often appear to be out of sequence within the YEAR BOOK OF VASCULAR SURGERY®.

Introduction

Each year, the YEAR BOOK OF VASCULAR SURGERY serves as a depository of outstanding articles pertinent to vascular disease. The goal is to provide a broad overview of important papers from the previous year. There is no attempt to focus only on the technical aspects of vascular procedures. What separates vascular surgeons from many physicians interested in vascular disorders is their willingness to be vascular specialists, evaluate their patients personally, talk to their families, and follow their patients over time. This is crucial to maintaining vascular surgery as a viable specialty. One needs to only look at the current difficulties of our interventonal radiology and cardiac surgical colleagues to understand this evolving medical paradigm. The goal is for the YEAR BOOK OF VASCULAR SURGERY to help vascular surgeons develop and maintain a broad knowledge base with respect to vascular disease. Knowledge, technical skill, a willingness to change, and dedication to long-term care of patients combine to make vascular surgery a thriving and growing specialty. It has been estimated there are about 8 available jobs for every finishing vascular surgical resident. It is a good time to be a vascular surgeon.

Vascular disease affects people of all ages and affects all organs of the body. Every physician will care for at least some patients with vascular disorders. Articles pertinent to vascular disease are therefore published in hundreds of journals and many languages. Each year as editor of the YEAR BOOK, I am charged with selecting the articles to be included in the YEAR BOOK OF VASCULAR SURGERY. Whereas I serve as the point person of the selection process, selection of articles to be included in the YEAR BOOK actually involves hundreds of individuals. Every article in the YEAR BOOK has been published in a peer-reviewed journal. Dozens of editorial boards and journal editors have therefore, in a sense, participated in the selection process for the YEAR BOOK. Authors themselves participate in the selection process by virtue of which journals they choose to submit their work. I pay more attention to articles published in so-called "major" journals, assuming authors have submitted their best work to these journals. There is therefore perhaps overrepresentation in the YEAR BOOK of articles published in *The New England Journal of Medicine, Circulation, Stroke, Journal of Vascular Surgery,* and the *European Journal of Vascular and Endovascular Surgery*. However, interesting work is not restricted to just "major" journals, and articles from many journals are included in the YEAR BOOK. Good work is also not restricted to publications in English, but I am not multilingual. I am sure I miss many non-English publications each year that may be of exceptional value. I encourage authors who publish in languages other than English to send me copies of their work along with a letter (in English) explaining why their article is important. Such correspondence will be taken seriously and the article considered for inclusion in the YEAR BOOK.

Vascular surgery is technically demanding. Certainly the techniques are changing, but technical excellence is still required to achieve excellent results. Both endovascular and open surgical techniques are featured throughout the YEAR BOOK, and there continues to be a section focusing primarily on new and innovative techniques.

However, as I emphasized above, my bias is that vascular surgeons must be more than technicians. This bias is reflected in the articles selected for the YEAR BOOK. I am not a bench scientist, but basic research is featured prominently in the YEAR BOOK. Basic research in the long run is perhaps the most important research. "Basic" is defined somewhat loosely for purposes of the YEAR BOOK. Among other topics, there are articles in this year's YEAR BOOK on molecular signaling mechanisms (a couple; not many!), endothelial cell biology, plaque composition, aspirin resistance, and gene expression in various disease states. Practicing surgeons are not expected to understand the details of bench research, but they should be aware of topics of interest in basic research as they relate to vascular disease. Basic research will profoundly change how we practice and therefore is included rather prominently in the YEAR BOOK.

Imaging is crucial to diagnosis and treatment of vascular disease. Clearly, ultrasound remains one of the cornerstones of the diagnostic vascular laboratory. Ultrasound techniques will be routinely used to quantify and characterize plaque composition. Every year, there are more and more articles on ultrasound-determined plaque composition and potential selection of patients for arterial interventions, particularly carotid interventions. Several of these articles are featured in this year's YEAR BOOK. The days of using stenosis alone to determine who should have a carotid intervention are hopefully drawing to a close. No one will regret the passing of those days where we had to do 20 interventions in asymptomatic patients to save 1 stroke over 5 years.

Computed tomography (CT) and magnetic resonance (MR) imaging studies are assuming an ever-increasing role in noninvasive vascular diagnosis. The vascular surgeon must be familiar with all forms of vascular imaging to make proper choices for his or her patients. Formal training in CT and MR imaging will someday be a part of vascular surgical training. It has to be. If vascular surgeons are to remain independent, they cannot rely on others to make decisions for intervention. There is a lot about imaging throughout the YEAR BOOK OF VASCULAR SURGERY.

Some people belittle randomized clinical trials, especially if the results do not conform to their beliefs. Certainly, not all randomized trials are definitive. For the most part, however, randomized trials remain the standard for determining clinical efficacy. Randomized trials are featured heavily in the YEAR BOOK. This year's YEAR BOOK includes trials examining β-blocker therapy to reduce perioperative mortality, coronary artery bypass grafting versus stents for treatment of coronary artery disease, intensive lipid lowering in patients with stable coronary artery disease, treatment of *Chlamydia pneumonia* following acute coronary syndromes, open versus endovascular treatment of popliteal artery aneurysms, adjunctive treatment of ischemic stroke, duplex surveillance of infrainguinal vein grafts, endovascular versus open repair of abdominal aortic aneurysm in both standard and high-risk patients, use of cilostazol for treatment of intracranial artery stenosis, surgery versus conservative treatment of varicose veins, and a comparison of multiple stab phlebectomies versus transilluminated power phlebectomy for removal of varicose veins. And there are others.

Aortic endografting remains a major topic in the vascular surgical world, but the focus is shifting to the thoracic aorta. There are still many YEAR BOOK abstracts that focus on defining the details of endograft treatment of abdominal aortic aneurysms, but there also many exploring thoracic aortic endografting as well. At the VEITH Symposium last fall, it seemed there were an enormous number of talks on thoracic endografts. I think, however, it is fair to say interest is high but progress is slow.

The availability of thoracic endografts has stimulated a resurgence of interest in the old DeBakey procedures of isolation of the thoracic aorta through performance of multiple bypasses to the visceral aortic branches. De-branching procedures of the aorta are, however, a procedure of interest for the short term while technology catches up with imagination and creativity. The thoracic aorta is proving to be a tougher opponent than the abdominal aorta. Arch configuration, issues of sizing, varying disease processes, and those pesky branches to major organs all are combining to slow progress. On the other hand, we have learned from the abdominal aortic experience. The issues complicating endografting of the thoracic aorta are being defined. The problems are primarily engineering, and engineering issues can and will be solved. There are some very clever surgeons and some very smart engineers out there.

Renal artery stents are now well established in clinical practice, although there is still little solid prospective data to support their use. There are, however, ongoing prospective trials of renal artery stents. Superior mesenteric artery (SMA) stenting is following a similar course of renal artery stents. More and more reports of SMA stents are appearing. The results of SMA stents parallel those of endovascular intervention of renal arteries. SMA stents can be placed with high rates of technical success. Morbidity is less than with open surgery, but durability also is less. Mesenteric vascular disease is, however, much less common than renal artery stenosis. It is, in fact, sufficiently uncommon that it is very unlikely we will ever have prospective randomized data for SMA stents. Readers of the YEAR BOOK should study the SMA stent articles carefully. There are unlikely to be any substantially different ones in the next 5 years.

I have once again included in the YEAR BOOK a number of articles on percutaneous interventions directed toward the carotid and superficial femoral arteries (SFAs). There have been no groundbreaking publications this year in these areas by the time the YEAR BOOK went into production. Large numbers of SFAs are being treated and retreated in the name of minimally invasive therapy. I remain somewhat skeptical about the ethics and efficacy of SFA interventions for moderate distance claudication. I have now seen several patients with intermittent claudication converted to amputees after a percutaneous SFA procedure that went badly. I am afraid there will be more.

Carotid stents continue to be placed in large numbers. There are now articles appearing providing some guidance as to what plaques and arteries may be associated with greater risks with carotid stenting. There are also articles highlighted in this year's YEAR BOOK indicating the results of carotid endarterectomy are improving and so-called high-risk patients may not be such "high risk" in all cases. The definition of "high risk" is sufficiently nebulous and contentious that eventually there may be panels of physicians to decide who actually is "high risk." One thing totally clear to me is that it is unethical for a patient to be declared high risk for a carotid intervention without ever having been seen by a vascular surgeon.

It is my pleasure to acknowledge the Associate Editors of the YEAR BOOK. These individuals are selected by me each year to participate in writing the "comments" that accompany each abstract in the YEAR BOOK. I try to choose younger academic vascular surgeons as associate editors. These individuals come to my attention either through recommendations of more senior surgeons or through my awareness of their publications. They are the future leaders of our specialty. I respect their productivity, intelligence, and dedication. I have, however, been a bit provincial in my choices of associate editors in that most are US surgeons. In future editions of the YEAR BOOK, there will be more associate editors from outside the US. This is needed to reflect the ever-increasing volume of work emanating from outside the United States.

I also wish to thank my office staff for transcribing the comments that accompany each abstract. As always, my thanks to Jenna Bowker for keeping this all organized and running so smoothly throughout the year.

I also thank my current vascular surgical partners at Oregon Health and Science University (Gregory Landry, Timothy Liem, and Erica Mitchell) for putting up with the time required for my academic pursuits. Finally, a grateful good-bye to 2 longstanding vascular surgical partners who retired this year, Richard Yeager and Lloyd Taylor Jr. I practiced vascular surgery with them for 18 years. Dr Yeager spent his entire academic career at the Portland VA Hospital. Early in my career, he helped me through some difficult cases and complications that could have easily destroyed the confidence of a young surgeon. Dr Taylor has served as mentor, partner, and surgical and life advisor for my entire time in Portland. He views the world differently than most and perhaps with more clarity than most. I will miss these men more than they can ever understand.

I hope everyone enjoys this book. I learn a great deal each year putting the YEAR BOOK together. I certainly hope the readers find it worth their effort to pick it up once in a while. I welcome any comments on how the whole process can be improved.

Gregory L. Moneta, MD

1 Basic Considerations

C-Reactive Protein, Interleukin-6, and Soluble Adhesion Molecules as Predictors of Progressive Peripheral Atherosclerosis in the General Population: Edinburgh Artery Study
Tzoulaki I, Murray GD, Lee AJ, et al (Univ of Edinburgh, Scotland; Univ of Aberdeen, Scotland; Univ of Glasgow, Scotland)
Circulation 112:976-983, 2005   1–1

Background.—The relationship between levels of circulating inflammatory markers and risk of progressive atherosclerosis is relatively undetermined. We therefore studied inflammatory markers as predictors of peripheral atherosclerotic progression, measured by the ankle-brachial index (ABI) at 3 consecutive time points over 12 years.

Method and Results.—The Edinburgh Artery Study is a population cohort study of 1592 men and women aged 55 to 74 years. C-reactive protein (CRP), interleukin-6 (IL-6), intercellular adhesion molecule-1 (ICAM-1), vascular adhesion molecule-1 (VCAM-1), and E-selectin were measured at baseline. Valid ABI measurements were obtained on 1582, 1081, and 813 participants at baseline and 5-year and 12-year follow-up examinations, respectively. At baseline, a significant trend was found between higher plasma levels of CRP ($P \leq 0.05$) and increasing severity of peripheral arterial disease (PAD), after adjustment for baseline cardiovascular risk factors. IL-6 at baseline ($P \leq 0.001$) was associated with progressive atherosclerosis at 5 years (ABI change from baseline), and CRP ($P \leq 0.01$), IL-6 ($P \leq 0.001$), and ICAM-1 ($P \leq 0.01$) were associated with changes at 12 years, independently of baseline ABI, cardiovascular risk factors, and baseline cardiovascular disease. Only IL-6 independently predicted ABI change at 5 years ($P \leq 0.01$) and 12 years ($P \leq 0.05$) in analyses of all inflammatory markers simultaneously and adjusted for baseline ABI, cardiovascular risk factors, and cardiovascular disease at baseline.

Conclusions.—These findings suggest that CRP, IL-6, and ICAM-1 are molecular markers associated with atherosclerosis and its progression. IL-6 showed more consistent results and stronger independent predictive value than other inflammatory markers. The changes in the ABI measured at 5 and 12 years in this population, while statistically significant given the large numbers of patients, are unlikely to be clinically significant. The changes in ABI over time vary between a mean of 0.04 and a mean of 0.07. Clinical care will obviously not be influenced by this study. The main value of this study is to implicate a likely relationship between inflammation and *progression* of *peripheral* arterial disease.

G. L. Moneta, MD

Trends in Serum Lipids and Lipoproteins of Adults, 1960-2002
Carroll MD, Lacher DA, Sorlie PD, et al (Centers for Disease Control and Prevention, Hyattsville, Md; NIH, Bethesda, Md; Univ of Texas, Dallas)
JAMA 294:1773-1781, 2005   1–2

Context.—Serum total and low-density lipoprotein (LDL) cholesterol contribute significantly to atherosclerosis and its clinical sequelae. Previous analyses of data from the National Health and Nutrition Examination Surveys (NHANES) showed that mean levels of total cholesterol of US adults had declined from 1960-1962 to 1988-1994, and mean levels of LDL cholesterol (available beginning in 1976) had declined between 1976-1980 and 1988-1994.

Objective.—To examine trends in serum lipid levels among US adults between 1960 and 2002, with a particular focus on changes since the 1988-1994 NHANES survey.

Design, Setting, and Participants.—Blood lipid measurements taken from 6098 to 15 719 adults who were examined in 5 distinct cross-sectional surveys of the US population during 1960-1962, 1971-1974, 1976-1980, 1988-1994, and 1999-2002.

Main Outcome Measures.—Mean serum total cholesterol, LDL cholesterol, high-density lipoprotein (HDL) cholesterol, and geometric mean serum triglyceride levels, and the percentage of adults with a serum total cholesterol level of at least 240 mg/dL ($\geq$6.22 mmol/L).

Results.—Between 1988-1994 and 1999-2002, total serum cholesterol level of adults aged 20 years or older decreased from 206 mg/dL (5.34 mmol/L) to 203 mg/dL (5.26 mmol/L) (P=.009) and LDL cholesterol levels decreased from 129 mg/dL (3.34 mmol/L) to 123 mg/dL (3.19 mmol/L) (P<.001). Greater and significant decreases were observed in men 60 years or older and in women 50 years or older. The percentage of adults with a total cholesterol level of at least 240 mg/dL ($\geq$6.22 mmol/L) decreased from 20% during 1988-1994 to 17% during 1999-2002 (P<.001). There was no change in mean HDL cholesterol levels and a nonsignificant increase in geometric mean serum triglyceride levels (P = .06).

Conclusions.—The decrease in total cholesterol level observed during 1960-1994 and LDL cholesterol level observed during 1976-1994 has continued during 1999-2002 in men 60 to 74 years and women 50 to 74 years. The target value of no more than 17% of US adults with a total cholesterol level of at least 240 mg/dL ($\geq$6.22 mmol/L), an objective of *Healthy People 2010*, has been attained. The increase in the proportion of adults using lipid-lowering medication, particularly in older age groups, likely contributed to the decreases in total and LDL cholesterol levels observed. The increased prevalence of obesity in the US population may have contributed to the increase in mean serum triglyceride levels.

▶ The data indicate continued and sustained progress in reducing cholesterol levels in the US population. Now only 17% of the US adult population has a total cholesterol level $\geq$ 240 mg/dL. Clearly, there is still room for improvement. Further efforts to reduce cholesterol levels in patients at particularly high risk of coronary disease and other forms of vascular disease are needed.

G. L. Moneta, MD

Effect of C-reactive protein on gene expression in vascular endothelial cells
Wang Q, Zhu X, Xu Q, et al (Morehouse School of Medicine, Atlanta, Ga)
Am J Physiol Heart Circ Physiol 288:H1539-H1545, 2005   1–3

C-reactive protein (CRP) is significantly associated with the risk of ischemic cardiovascular disease in epidemiological studies. To explore if CRP has a functional role, we investigated its effect on the gene expression profile of vascular endothelial cells. Human vascular endothelial cells (human umbilical vein endothelial cells and human aortic endothelial cells) were incubated with CRP at various concentrations (0–10 µg/ml). Microarray analysis showed that a total of 11 genes increased (IL-8, core promoter element binding protein, activin A, monocyte chemoattractant protein 1, Exostoses 1, Cbp/p300-interacting transactivator with Glu/Asp-rich COOH-terminal domain 2, plasminogen activator inhibitor 1, fibronectin-1, gravin, connexin43, and sortilin-related receptor-1) and 6 genes decreased (methionine adenosyltransferase 2A, tryptophan-rich basic protein, reticulocalbin 1, membrane-associated RING-CH protein VI, cytoplasmic dynein1, and annexin A_1) by more than twofold for their mRNA levels. IL-8 was the most significantly upregulated gene (13.6-fold), which demonstrated a clear dose- and time-dependent pattern revealed by quantitative real-time PCR. Cell adhesion assay showed that CRP enhanced the monocyte adhesion to endothelial cell monolayer by 2-fold ($P < 0.01$), which was partially blocked by an anti-IL-8 antibody (34.2% inhibition, $P < 0.01$). Inhibition of ERK MAPK pathway using U0126 prevented CRP-induced IL-8 upregulation, and Western blot analysis revealed a rapid activation of ERK1/2 after CRP stimulation. These data showed that CRP can significantly influence gene expressions in vascular endothelium. The CRP-responsive genes suggested that CRP may have a broad functional role in cell growth and differentiation, vascular remodeling and solid tumor development.

▶ We are all aware of CRP as a marker of cardiovascular risk. It is, however, unclear whether CRP itself induces changes detrimental to the vascular system or whether it is merely a byproduct of other biochemical abnormalities that eventually result in increased atherosclerotic risk. These data here suggest that there are genes responsive to CRP levels. Many of the genes in this study shown to be responsive to CRP have broad functional roles in cell differentiation, cell growth, and vascular remodeling. These data do not rule out CRP as primarily a byproduct of some of these processes. It does, however, indicate CRP itself possesses some biological activity that may affect features of the vascular wall and, by inference, atherosclerosis.

G. L. Moneta, MD

Plaque Rupture After Short Periods of Fat Feeding in the Apolipoprotein E–Knockout Mouse: Model Characterization and Effects of Pravastatin Treatment
Johnson J, Carson K, Williams H, et al (Univ of Bristol, England)
Circulation 111:1422-1430, 2005   1–4

Background.—These studies examined the early time course of plaque development and destabilization in the brachiocephalic artery of the apolipoprotein E–knockout mouse, the effects of pravastatin thereon, and the effects of pravastatin on established unstable plaques.

Method and Results.—Male apolipoprotein E–knockout mice were fed a high-fat, cholesterol-enriched diet from the age of 8 weeks. Animals were euthanized at 1-week intervals between 4 and 9 weeks of fat feeding. Acutely ruptured plaques were observed in the brachiocephalic arteries of 3% of animals up to and including 7 weeks of fat feeding but in 62% of animals after 8 weeks, which suggests that there is a sharp increase in the number of plaque ruptures at 8 weeks. These acute plaque ruptures then appear to heal and form buried fibrous caps; after 9 weeks of fat feeding, mice had 1.05 ± 0.15 buried fibrous caps at a single site in the brachiocephalic artery. Pravastatin (40 mg/kg of body weight per day for 9 weeks; resultant plasma concentration 16 ± 4 nmol/L) had no effect on plasma cholesterol concentration in fat-fed apolipoprotein E–knockout mice but reduced the number of buried fibrous caps by 43% ($P<0.0001$). In longer-term experiments, the delay of pravastatin treatment until unstable plaques had developed reduced the incidence of acute plaque rupture by 36% ($P<0.0001$).

Conclusions.—Plaque rupture occurs at high frequency in the brachiocephalic arteries of male apolipoprotein E–knockout mice after 8 weeks of fat feeding. Pravastatin treatment inhibits early plaque rupture and is also effective when begun after unstable plaques have developed.

▶ Translational differences between apolipoprotein E mice and human beings do exist, but these elegant experiments still support the notion that "statins" are a true vascular panacea: they decrease the frequency of plaque rupture as well as animal death, all without significantly lowering plasma lipid concentrations. These agents have clinical trial data also suggesting a significant benefit to their use in all patients with peripheral arterial disease. Even more exciting is the recent clinical trial showing that high-dose statin therapy can cause plaque regression in coronary arteries. Sooner or later, statins may well be in the drinking water.

P. K. Henke, MD

Inflammation and Endothelial Function: Direct Vascular Effects of Human C-Reactive Protein on Nitric Oxide Bioavailability
Clapp BR, Hirschfield GM, Storry C, et al (BHF Labs, London; Royal Free Campus, London; Inst of Child Health, London; et al)
Circulation 111:1530-1536, 2005   1–5

Background.—Circulating concentrations of the sensitive inflammatory marker C-reactive protein (CRP) predict future cardiovascular events, and CRP is elevated during sepsis and inflammation, when vascular reactivity may be modulated. We therefore investigated the direct effect of CRP on vascular reactivity.

Method and Results.—The effects of isolated, pure human CRP on vasoreactivity and protein expression were studied in vascular rings and cells in vitro, and effects on blood pressure were studied in rats in vivo. The temporal relationship between changes in CRP concentration and brachial flow-mediated dilation was also studied in humans after vaccination with *Salmonella typhi* capsular polysaccharide, a model of inflammatory endothelial dysfunction. In contrast to some previous reports, highly purified and well-characterized human CRP specifically induced hyporeactivity to phenylephrine in rings of human internal mammary artery and rat aorta that was mediated through physiological antagonism by nitric oxide (NO). CRP did not alter endothelial NO synthase protein expression but increased protein expression of GTP cyclohydrolase-1, the rate-limiting enzyme in the synthesis of tetrahydrobiopterin, the NO synthase cofactor. In the vaccine model of inflammatory endothelial dysfunction in humans, increased CRP concentration coincided with the resolution rather than the development of endothelial dysfunction, consistent with the vitro findings; however, administration of human CRP to rats had no effect on blood pressure.

Conclusions.—Pure human CRP has specific, direct effects on vascular function in vitro via increased NO production; however, further clarification of the effect, if any, of CRP on vascular reactivity in humans in vivo will require clinical studies using specific inhibitors of CRP.

▶ Elevated CRP levels are highly correlated with late cardiovascular events, but whether they are simply a marker of inflammation or are directly involved in the process has not been well established. Prior in vitro studies suggest that CRP may have some direct negative vascular inflammatory effects. This carefully done study evaluated the effect of CRP on human arteries in vitro and (counterintuitively) shows that CRP increases endothelial-dependant relaxation and decreases the intensity of constriction caused by adrenergic agents. This was also correlated in vivo with a small human cohort. Because these findings were counterintuitive, the controls on this study were thorough and well done. The jury is still out on the subject of how much direct effect CRP has on atherogenesis in vivo. My vote is that CRP is primarily a cardiovascular risk marker and not a direct vascular toxin.

P. K. Henke, MD

Identification of a homocysteine receptor in the peripheral endothelium and its role in proliferation

Chen H, Fitzgerald R, Brown AT, et al (Central Arkansas Veterans Healthcare System, Little Rock; Univ of Arkansas, Little Rock)

J Vasc Surg 41:853-860, 2005   1–6

Background.—Homocysteine, a risk factor for atherosclerosis, increases intimal hyperplasia after carotid endarterectomy with associated smooth muscle cell proliferation and modulation of cytokines. The N-methyl-D-aspartate receptor (NMDAr), a glutamate-gated ion channel receptor, is associated with homocysteine-induced cerebrovascular injury; however, the receptor has not been identified in peripheral vascular cells, nor has any interaction with homocysteine been clarified. Our objectives were first, to identify NMDAr in rat carotid artery and rat aorta endothelial cells (RAEC); and second, to determine whether homocysteine activates NMDAr in the endothelium.

Methods.—NR1 and NR2A, two NMDAr subunits, were probed in rat carotid arteries by immunohistochemistry. RNA was isolated from RAECs, and expression of all NMDAr subunits (NR1, 2A, 2B, 2C, and 2D) were examined by RT-PCR and sequencing. For receptor protein expression, RAEC were incubated with different homocysteine concentrations and incubation times and also were treated with 50 µM homocysteine and/or preincubated with 50 µM dizocilpine MK-801, an NMDAr inhibitor.

Results.—Both NR1 and NR2A were expressed in rat carotid arteries. All NMDAr subunits were expressed in the RAECs, and there was 92% to 100% similarity compared with rat NMDAr from the National Center for Biotechnology Information (NCBI) GenBank. Homocysteine upregulated NR1 expression and increased cell proliferation. RAEC pretreatment with MK-801 reduced homocysteine-mediated cell proliferation.

Conclusion.—This study is the first to show that NMDAr exists in the peripheral vasculature, and that homocysteine may act via NMDAr to increase intimal hyperplasia.

Clinical Relevance.—Our objectives included the identification of a homocysteine receptor in the peripheral vasculature. The possible inhibition of a homocysteine receptor to prevent intimal hyperplasia rather than treat established stenosis would make a significant clinical impact. This will open further avenues of study in determining the role of homocysteine in the pathogenesis of intimal hyperplasia.

▶ This team continues to work at understanding the link between hyperhomocystinemia and vascular disease, now looking more mechanistically into previous in vivo observations. Here, they discover the NMDAr (an ion channel receptor) in RAECs, and experiments using an NMDAr inhibitor suggest that homocysteine acts via NMDAr to promote cell proliferation. It would also be interesting to examine it in a co-culture system that included smooth muscle cells and endothelial cells. The study is relevant not only for prevention of occlusive peripheral vascular lesions but also in multiple other organ systems in which NMDAr resides.

C. K. Ozaki, MD

Impaired Progenitor Cell Activity in Age-Related Endothelial Dysfunction

Heiss C, Keymel S, Niesler U, et al (Heinrich-Heine-Univ, Düsseldorf, Germany)

J Am Coll Cardiol 45:1441-1448, 2005   1–7

Objectives.—We investigated whether human age-related endothelial dysfunction is accompanied by quantitative and qualitative alterations of the endothelial progenitor cell (EPC) pool.

Background.—Circulating progenitor cells with an endothelial phenotype contribute to the regeneration and repair of the vessel wall. An association between the loss of endothelial integrity and EPC modification may provide a background to study the mechanistic nature of such age-related vascular changes.

Methods.—In 20 old and young healthy individuals (61 ± 2 years and 25 ± 1 year, respectively) without major cardiovascular risk factors, endothelial function, defined by flow-mediated dilation of the brachial artery via ultrasound, as well as the number and function of EPCs isolated from peripheral blood, were determined.

Results.—Older subjects had significantly impaired endothelium-dependent dilation of brachial artery (flow-mediated dilation [FMD] 5.2 ± 0.5% vs. 7.1 ± 0.6%; $p < 0.05$). Endothelium-independent dilation after glycerol trinitrate (GTN) was not different, but the FMD/GTN ratio was significantly lower in old subjects (49 ± 4% vs. 37 ± 3%; $p < 0.05$), suggesting endothelial dysfunction. There were no differences in the numbers of circulating EPCs, defined as CD34/KDR or CD133/KDR double-positive cells in peripheral blood. In contrast, lower survival (39 ± 6 cells/mm^2 vs. 65 ± 11 cells/mm^2; $p < 0.05$), migration (80 ± 12 vs. 157 ± 16 cells/mm^2; $p < 0.01$), and proliferation (0.20 ± 0.04 cpm vs. 0.44 ± 0.07 cpm; $p < 0.05$) implicate functional impairment of EPCs from old subjects. The FMD correlated univariately with EPC migration ($r = 0.52$, $p < 0.05$) and EPC proliferation ($r = 0.49$, $p < 0.05$). Multivariate analysis showed that both functional features represent independent predictors of endothelial function.

Conclusions.—Maintenance of vascular homeostasis by EPCs may be attenuated with age based on functional deficits rather than depletion of CD34/KDR or CD133/KDR cells.

▶ Age is a dominant vascular disease risk factor. Specific mechanisms for this are unclear. The authors correlate human endothelial function (flow-mediated brachial artery reactivity) with the quantity and quality of circulating EPCs, using chronological age as a variable. "Healthy" older individuals demonstrated endothelial dysfunction, but the numbers of circulating EPCs were similar to younger control subjects. However, the older EPCs were qualitatively different (eg, shorter survival and less proliferation and migration). It remains unclear whether these changes in EPC phenotype are due to environmental factors or preprogrammed events.

C. K. Ozaki, MD

Blockade of Interleukin-12 Function by Protein Vaccination Attenuates Atherosclerosis

Hauer AD, Uyttenhove C, de Vos P, et al (Leiden Univ, The Netherlands; Ludwig Inst for Cancer Research, Brussels, Belgium; Université de Louvain, Belgium)
Circulation 112:1054-1062, 2005   1–8

Background.—Interleukin-12 (IL-12) has been identified as a key inducer of a type 1 T-helper cell cytokine pattern, which is thought to contribute to the development of atherosclerosis. We sought to study the role of IL-12 in atherosclerosis by inhibition of IL-12 using a newly developed vaccination technique that fully blocks the action of IL-12.

Method and Results.—LDL receptor–deficient (LDLr$^{-/-}$) mice were vaccinated against IL-12 by 5 intramuscular injections of IL-12-PADRE complex in combination with adjuvant oil-in-water emulsion (low dose)/MPL/QS21 every 2 weeks. Two weeks thereafter, atherogenesis was initiated in the carotid artery by perivascular placement of silicone elastomer collars. IL-12 vaccination resulted in the induction of anti–IL-12 antibodies that functionally blocked the action of IL-12 as determined in an IL-12 bioassay. Blockade of IL-12 by vaccination of LDLr$^{-/-}$ mice resulted in significantly reduced (68.5%; $P<0.01$) atherogenesis compared with control mice without a change in serum cholesterol levels. IL-12 vaccination also resulted in a significant decrease in intima/media ratios (66.7%; $P<0.01$) and in the degree of stenosis (57.8%; $P<0.01$). On IL-12 vaccination, smooth muscle cell and collagen content in the neointima increased 2.8-fold ($P<0.01$) and 4.2-fold ($P<0.01$), respectively.

Conclusions.—Functional blockade of endogenous IL-12 by vaccination resulted in a significant 68.5% reduction in atherogenesis in LDLr$^{-/-}$ mice. Vaccination against IL-12 also improved plaque stability, from which we conclude that the blockade of IL-12 by vaccination may be considered a promising new strategy in the treatment of atherosclerosis.

▶ IL-12 favors pro-atherosclerotic events. This group sought to modify the pro-inflammatory type 1 T-helper cell cytokine pattern using a novel anti–IL-12 vaccination strategy (generation of anti–IL-12 antibodies) in an effort to abrogate atherogenesis. The approach seems to attenuate lesion size and may lead to more stable plaque morphological features. The murine perivascular carotid artery cuff model tested, however, may differ substantially from the long-term chain of events in human atherosclerosis. Unknown is the impact on response to pathogens, especially as the antibody also probably interacts with the p40 subunit of IL-23. If successful, this could be a very economical way to not only lower the atherosclerotic disease burden but also treat other conditions.

C. K. Ozaki, MD

Intensive Treatment With Atorvastatin Reduces Inflammation in Mononuclear Cells and Human Atherosclerotic Lesions in One Month
Martín-Ventura JL, Blanco-Colio LM, Gómez-Hernández A, et al (Autónoma Univ, Madrid; Complutense Univ, Madrid; Pfizer, Madrid)
Stroke 36:1796-1800, 2005   1–9

Background and Purpose.—To investigate the effect of short-term high-dose atorvastatin on blood and plaque inflammation in patients with carotid stenosis.

Methods.—Twenty patients undergoing carotid endarterectomy without previous statin treatment were randomized to receive either atorvastatin 80 mg/d (n=11) or no statins (n=9) for 1 month. We studied inflammatory mediators in plasma (enzyme-linked immunosorbent assay), peripheral blood mononuclear cells (PBMCs; quantitative RT-PCR and EMSA) and plaques (immunohistochemistry and Southwestern histochemistry).

Results.—Atorvastatin significantly decreased total and low-density lipoprotein cholesterol and prostaglandin E_2 plasma levels. PBMCs from treated patients showed impaired NF-κB activation and MCP-1 and COX-2 mRNA expression. Carotid atherosclerotic plaques demonstrated a significant reduction in macrophage infiltration, activated NF-κB, and COX-2 and MCP-1 expression.

Conclusions.—Intensive treatment with atorvastatin decreases inflammatory activity of PBMCs and carotid atherosclerotic plaques in 1 month. These data strongly suggest that the antiinflammatory effect of high doses of statins in humans can be seen very early.

▶ The lipid independent mechanisms of statin cardiovascular protection are not well understood. This small human study suggests rapid local and systemic anti-inflammatory effects for high-dose atorvastatin. Twenty patients were randomly assigned to receive atorvastatin or no statins for 1 month before endarterectomy. At the time of endarterectomy, peripheral blood monocytes and the excised plaque were examined for inflammatory end points. The atorvastatin group demonstrated decreased monocyte and plaque inflammatory activity. This article gives insights into potential mechanisms for the observation of decreased perioperative stroke and mortality around the time of carotid endarterectomy with statin use that was seen by the Johns Hopkins group.[1]

C. K. Ozaki, MD

Reference

1. McGirt MJ, Perler BA, Brooke BS, et al: 3-Hydroxy-3-methylglutaryl coenzyme A reductase inhibitors reduce the risk of perioperative stroke and mortality after carotid endarterectomy. *J Vasc Surg* 42:829-836, 2005.

The Thromboxane A$_2$ Receptor Antagonist S18886 Prevents Enhanced Atherogenesis Caused by Diabetes Mellitus

Zuccollo A, Shi C, Mastroianni R, et al (Boston Univ; Institut de Recherches Internationales Servier, Courbevoie, France; Institut de Recherches Servier, Croissy, France; et al)

Circulation 112:3001-3008, 2005   1–10

Background.—S18886 is an orally active thromboxane A$_2$ (TXA$_2$) receptor (TP) antagonist in clinical development for use in secondary prevention of thrombotic events in cardiovascular disease. We previously showed that S18886 inhibits atherosclerosis in apolipoprotein E–deficient (apoE$^{-/-}$) mice by a mechanism independent of platelet-derived TXA$_2$. Atherosclerosis is accelerated by diabetes and is associated with increased TXA$_2$ and other eicosanoids that stimulate TP. The purpose of this study was to determine whether S18886 lessens the enhanced atherogenesis in diabetic apoE$^{-/-}$ mice.

Method and Results.—Diabetes mellitus was induced in apoE$^{-/-}$ mice with streptozotocin and was treated or not with S18886 (5 mg · kg^{-1} · d^{-1}). After 6 weeks, aortic lesion area was increased >4-fold by diabetes in apoE$^{-/-}$ mice, associated with similar increases in serum glucose and cholesterol. S18886 largely prevented the diabetes-related increase in lesion area without affecting the hyperglycemia or hypercholesterolemia. S18886 prevented deterioration of endothelial function and endothelial nitric oxide synthase expression, as well as increases in intimal markers of inflammation associated with diabetes. In human aortic endothelial cells in culture, S18886 also prevented the induction of vascular cell adhesion molecule-1 and prevented the decrease in endothelial nitric oxide synthase expression caused by high glucose.

Conclusions.—The TP antagonist inhibits inflammation and accelerated atherogenesis caused by diabetes, most likely by counteracting effects on endothelial function and adhesion molecule expression of eicosanoids stimulated by the diabetic milieu.

▶ This intriguing study of an orally active eicosanoid receptor antagonist shows that TXA$_2$ inhibition significantly decreases vascular injury in diabetic and hypercholesterolemic mice. The data are rigorously analyzed, and the experiments are well controlled. The mechanism of action is multifactoral but is primarily by inhibiting endothelial dysfunction. Whether this agent stimulates circulating endothelial progenitor cell release to heal damaged endothelium is not answered. If this agent is safe and goes to human trials, it might significantly alter vascular disease care for patients with diabetes, independent of glucose homeostasis.

P. K. Henke, MD

Circulating Endothelial Progenitor Cells and Cardiovascular Outcomes
Werner N, Kosiol S, Schiegl T, et al (Univ of Saarland, Hojmburg–Saar, Germany)
N Engl J Med 353:999-1007, 2005   1–11

Background.—Endothelial progenitor cells derived from bone marrow are believed to support the integrity of the vascular endothelium. The number and function of endothelial progenitor cells correlate inversely with cardiovascular risk factors, but the prognostic value associated with circulating endothelial progenitor cells has not been defined.

Methods.—The number of endothelial progenitor cells positive for CD34 and kinase insert domain receptor (KDR) was determined with the use of flow cytometry in 519 patients with coronary artery disease as confirmed on angiography. After 12 months, we evaluated the association between baseline levels of endothelial progenitor cells and death from cardiovascular causes, the occurrence of a first major cardiovascular event (myocardial infarction, hospitalization, revascularization, or death from cardiovascular causes), revascularization, hospitalization, and death from all causes.

Results.—A total of 43 participants died, 23 from cardiovascular causes. A first major cardiovascular event occurred in 214 patients. The cumulative event-free survival rate increased stepwise across three increasing baseline levels of endothelial progenitor cells in an analysis of death from cardiovascular causes, a first major cardiovascular event, revascularization, and hospitalization. After adjustment for age, sex, vascular risk factors, and other relevant variables, increased levels of endothelial progenitor cells were associated with a reduced risk of death from cardiovascular causes (hazard ratio, 0.31; 95 percent confidence interval, 0.16 to 0.63; P=0.001), a first major cardiovascular event (hazard ratio, 0.74; 95 percent confidence interval, 0.62 to 0.89; P=0.002), revascularization (hazard ratio, 0.77; 95 percent confidence interval, 0.62 to 0.95; P=0.02), and hospitalization (hazard ratio, 0.76; 95 percent confidence interval, 0.63 to 0.94; P=0.01). Endothelial progenitor-cell levels were not predictive of myocardial infarction or of death from all causes.

Conclusions.—The level of circulating CD34+KDR+ endothelial progenitor cells predicts the occurrence of cardiovascular events and death from cardiovascular causes and may help to identify patients at increased cardiovascular risk (Fig 1).

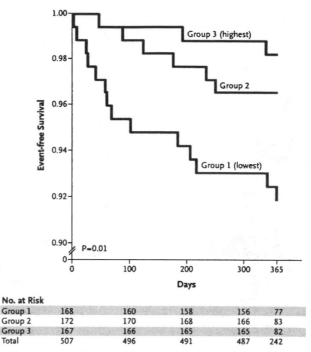

No. at Risk					
Group 1	168	160	158	156	77
Group 2	172	170	168	166	83
Group 3	167	166	165	165	82
Total	507	496	491	487	242

FIGURE 1.—Cumulative event-free survival in an analysis of death from cardiovascular causes at 12 months, according to levels of circulating CD34+KDR+ endothelial progenitor cells at the time of enrollment. (Reprinted by permission of *The New England Journal of Medicine* from Werner N, Kosiol S, Schiegl T, et al: Circulating endothelial progenitor cells and cardiovascular outcomes. *N Engl J Med* 353:999-1007. Copyright 2005, Massachusetts Medical Society. All rights reserved.)

▶ The role of endothelial progenitor cells and rejuvenation of vascular endothelium is currently an area of intensive investigation. It appears that these immature cells may modify the pathogenesis of atherosclerotic disease. Measurement of endothelial progenitor cells may also improve risk stratification in patients with cardiovascular disease.

G. L. Moneta, MD

Trajectories of Growth among Children Who Have Coronary Events as Adults

Barker DJP, Osmond C, Forsén TJ, et al (Univ of Southampton, England; Natl Public Health Inst, Helsinki)
N Engl J Med 353:1802-1809, 2005
1–12

Background.—Low birth weight is a risk factor for coronary heart disease. It is uncertain how postnatal growth affects disease risk.

Methods.—We studied 8760 people born in Helsinki from 1934 through 1944. Childhood growth had been recorded. A total of 357 men and 87 women had been admitted to the hospital with coronary heart disease or had

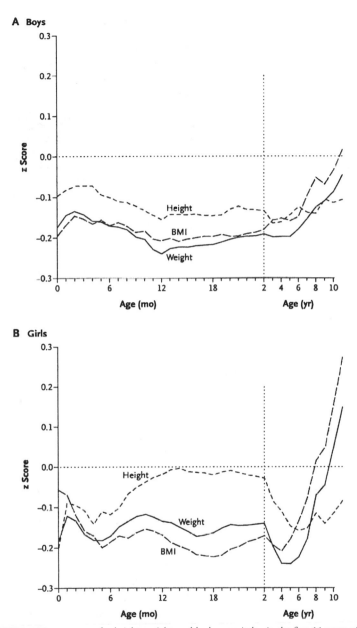

FIGURE 1.—Mean z scores for height, weight, and body-mass index in the first 11 years after birth among boys and girls who had coronary heart disease as adults. The mean values for all boys and all girls are set at 0, with deviations from the mean expressed as standard deviations (z scores). (Reprinted by permission of *The New England Journal of Medicine* from Barker DJP, Osmond C, Forsén TJ, et al: Trajectories of growth among children who have coronary events as adults. *N Engl J Med* 353:1802-1809. Copyright 2005, Massachusetts Medical Society. All rights reserved.)

died from the disease. Coronary risk factors were measured in a subset of 2003 people.

Results.—The mean body size of children who had coronary events as adults was below average at birth. At two years of age the children were thin; subsequently, their body-mass index (BMI) increased relative to that of other children and had reached average values by 11 years of age. In simultaneous regressions, the hazard ratios associated with a 1 SD increase in BMI were 0.76 (95 percent confidence interval, 0.66 to 0.87; P<0.001) at 2 years and 1.14 (95 percent confidence interval, 1.00 to 1.31; P=0.05) at 11 years among the boys. The corresponding figures for the girls were 0.62 (95 percent confidence interval, 0.46 to 0.82; P=0.001) and 1.35 (95 percent confidence interval, 1.02 to 1.78; P=0.04). Low BMI at 2 years of age and increased BMI from 2 to 11 years of age were also associated with raised fasting insulin concentrations (P<0.001 for both).

Conclusions.—On average, adults who had a coronary event had been small at birth and thin at two years of age and thereafter put on weight rapidly. This pattern of growth during childhood was associated with insulin resistance in later life. The risk of coronary events was more strongly related to the tempo of childhood gain in BMI than to the BMI attained at any particular age (Fig 1).

▶ There is increasing evidence that poor prenatal and early childhood nutrition can increase the risk of late coronary heart disease. The results of this study suggest that the tempo of early weight gain in childhood is also a risk factor for coronary disease later in life, possibly through the development of insulin resistance. Fetal undernutrition may result in "metabolic settings" that promote insulin resistance and place the individual at increased risk of development of atherosclerosis.

G. L. Moneta, MD

Secondary prevention of macrovascular events in patients with type 2 diabetes in the PROactive Study (PROspective pioglitAzone Clinical Trial In macroVascular Events): a randomised controlled trial
Dormandy JA, for the PROactive investigators (St Georges Hosp, London; et al)
Lancet 366:1279-1289, 2005   1–13

Background.—Patients with type 2 diabetes are at high risk of fatal and non-fatal myocardial infarction and stroke. There is indirect evidence that agonists of peroxisome proliferator-activated receptor γ (PPAR γ) could reduce macrovascular complications. Our aim, therefore, was to ascertain whether pioglitazone reduces macrovascular morbidity and mortality in high-risk patients with type 2 diabetes.

Methods.—We did a prospective, randomised controlled trial in 5238 patients with type 2 diabetes who had evidence of macrovascular disease. We recruited patients from primary-care practices and hospitals. We assigned patients to oral pioglitazone titrated from 15 mg to 45 mg (n=2605) or matching placebo (n=2633), to be taken in addition to their glucose-lowering drugs and other medications. Our primary endpoint was the composite of all-cause mortality, non-fatal myocardial infarction (including silent myocardial infarction), stroke, acute coronary syndrome, endovascular or surgical intervention in the coronary or leg arteries, and amputation above the ankle. Analysis was by intention to treat. This study is registered as an International Standard Randomised Controlled Trial, number ISRCTN NCT00174993.

Findings.—Two patients were lost to follow-up, but were included in analyses. The average time of observation was 34.5 months. 514 of 2605 patients in the pioglitazone group and 572 of 2633 patients in the placebo group had at least one event in the primary composite endpoint (HR 0.90, 95% CI 0.80–1.02, p=0.095). The main secondary endpoint was the composite of all-cause mortality, non-fatal myocardial infarction, and stroke. 301 patients in the pioglitazone group and 358 in the placebo group reached this endpoint (0.84, 0.72–0.98, p=0.027). Overall safety and tolerability was good with no change in the safety profile of pioglitazone identified. 6% (149 of 2065) and 4% (108 of 2633) of those in the pioglitazone and placebo groups, respectively, were admitted to hospital with heart failure; mortality rates from heart failure did not differ between groups.

Interpretation.—Pioglitazone reduces the composite of all-cause mortality, non-fatal myocardial infarction, and stroke in patients with type 2 diabetes who have a high risk of macrovascular events.

▶ Pioglitazone reduces levels of inflammatory markers such as C-reactive protein. These effects are independent of its effect on glycemic control. Detailed analysis of the data indicates the drug had no effect on leg revascularization or the need for amputation. Evidence is beginning to be accumulated showing that systemic markers of inflammation are perhaps more important in predicting coronary events than events secondary to peripheral vascular disease. If this proves to be true, then the results of this study would make sense, in that one of the primary effects of this drug is to lower markers of systemic inflammation.

G. L. Moneta, MD

Efficacy and Safety of Edifoligide, an E2F Transcription Factor Decoy, for Prevention of Vein Graft Failure Following Coronary Artery Bypass Graft Surgery: PREVENT IV: A Randomized Controlled Trial
Alexander JH, for the PREVENT IV Investigators (Duke Univ, Durham, NC; Louisiana State Univ, New Orleans; Corgentech, South San Francisco; et al)
JAMA 294:2446-2454, 2005   1–14

Context.—Coronary artery bypass graft (CABG) surgery with autologous vein grafting is commonly performed. Progressive neointimal hyperplasia, however, contributes to considerable vein graft failure. Edifoligide is an oligonucleotide decoy that binds to and inhibits E2F transcription factors and thus may prevent neointimal hyperplasia and vein graft failure.

Objective.—To assess the efficacy and safety of pretreating vein grafts with edifoligide for patients undergoing CABG surgery.

Design, Setting, and Participants.—A phase 3 randomized, double-blind, placebo-controlled trial of 3014 patients undergoing primary CABG surgery with at least 2 planned saphenous vein grafts and without concomitant valve surgery, who were enrolled between August 2002 and October 2003 at 107 US sites.

Intervention.—Vein grafts were treated ex vivo with either edifoligide or placebo in a pressure-mediated delivery system. The first 2400 patients enrolled were scheduled for 12- to 18-month follow-up angiography.

Main Outcome Measures.—The primary efficacy end point was angiographic vein graft failure ($\geq 75\%$ vein graft stenosis) occurring 12 to 18 months after CABG surgery. Other end points included other angiographic variables, adverse events through 30 days, and major adverse cardiac events.

Results.—A total of 1920 patients (80%) either died (n = 91) or underwent follow-up angiography (n = 1829). Edifoligide had no effect on the primary end point of per patient vein graft failure (436 [45.2%] of 965 patients in the edifoligide group vs 442 [46.3%] of 955 patients in the placebo group; odds ratio, 0.96 [95% confidence interval {CI}, 0.80-1.14]; $P = .66$), on any secondary angiographic end point, or on the incidence of major adverse cardiac events at 1 year (101 [6.7%] of 1508 patients in the edifoligide group vs 121 [8.1%] of 1506 patients in the placebo group; hazard ratio, 0.83 [95% CI, 0.64-1.08]; $P = .16$).

Conclusions.—Failure of at least 1 vein graft is quite common within 12 to 18 months after CABG surgery. Edifoligide is no more effective than placebo in preventing these events. Longer-term follow-up and additional research are needed to determine whether edifoligide has delayed beneficial effects, to understand the mechanisms and clinical consequences of vein graft failure, and to improve the durability of CABG surgery.

▶ This study, along with Prevent III, which also failed to show a benefit of the E2F decoy in preventing vein graft failure for peripheral artery reconstructions, provides conclusive evidence as to the ineffectiveness of the E2F decoy in preventing neointimal hyperplasia. It is now known, however, that the E2F family of transcription factors contains at least 8 unique E2F transcription factors.[1] Some of the transcription factors inhibit neointimal hyperplasia while others appear to promote neointimal hyperplasia. Edifoligide inhibits the entire E2F family; therefore, failure of the apparent "shotgun" approach used in Prevent III and IV seems logical in retrospect. Further research in this area will need to focus on the effects of specific E2F transcription factor decoys.

G. L. Moneta, MD

Reference

1. Maiti B, Jing L, de Bruin A, et al: Cloning and characterization of mouse *E2F8*, a novel mammalian *E2F* family member capable of blocking cellular proliferation. *J Biol Chem* 280:18211-18220, 2005.

Sirolimus-Eluting and Paclitaxel-Eluting Stents for Coronary Revascularization

Windecker S, Remondino A, Eberli FR, et al (Univ Hosp Bern, Switzerland; Univ Hosp Zurich; Univ of Bristol, England)
N Engl J Med 353:653-662, 2005   1–15

Background.—Sirolimus-eluting stents and paclitaxel-eluting stents, as compared with bare-metal stents, reduce the risk of restenosis. It is unclear whether there are differences in safety and efficacy between the two types of drug-eluting stents.

Methods.—We conducted a randomized, controlled, single-blind trial comparing sirolimus-eluting stents with paclitaxel-eluting stents in 1012 patients undergoing percutaneous coronary intervention. The primary end point was a composite of major adverse cardiac events (death from cardiac causes, myocardial infarction, and ischemia-driven revascularization of the

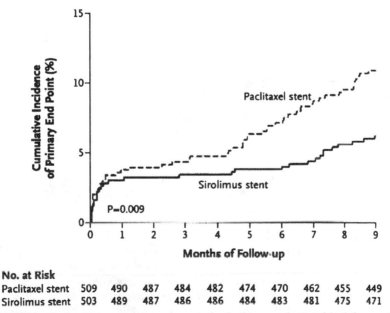

No. at Risk

Paclitaxel stent	509	490	487	484	482	474	470	462	455	449
Sirolimus stent	503	489	487	486	486	484	483	481	475	471

FIGURE 1.—Kaplan–Meier cumulative-event curves for the primary end point of death from cardiac causes, myocardial infarction, or ischemia-driven revascularization of the target lesion. (Reprinted by permission of *The New England Journal of Medicine* from Windecker S, Remondino A, Eberli FR, et al: Sirolimus-eluting and paclitaxel-eluting stents for coronary revascularization. *N Engl J Med* 353:653-662. Copyright 2005, Massachusetts Medical Society. All rights reserved.)

target lesion) by nine months. Follow-up angiography was completed in 540 of 1012 patients (53.4 percent).

Results.—The two groups had similar baseline clinical and angiographic characteristics. The rate of major adverse cardiac events at nine months was 6.2 percent in the sirolimus-stent group and 10.8 percent in the paclitaxel-stent group (hazard ratio, 0.56; 95 percent confidence interval, 0.36 to 0.86; P=0.009). The difference was driven by a lower rate of target-lesion revascularization in the sirolimus-stent group than in the paclitaxel-stent group (4.8 percent vs. 8.3 percent; hazard ratio, 0.56; 95 percent confidence interval, 0.34 to 0.93; P=0.03). Rates of death from cardiac causes were 0.6 percent in the sirolimus-stent group and 1.6 percent in the paclitaxel-stent group (P=0.15); the rates of myocardial infarction were 2.8 percent and 3.5 percent, respectively (P=0.49); and the rates of angiographic restenosis were 6.6 percent and 11.7 percent, respectively (P=0.02).

Conclusions.—As compared with paclitaxel-eluting stents, the use of sirolimus-eluting stents results in fewer major adverse cardiac events, primarily by decreasing the rates of clinical and angiographic restenosis (Fig 1).

▶ This article, along with currently available data from randomized clinical trials and registries (see Table 1 in the original article), suggests that sirolimus-eluting stents have clinical and angiographic advantages over paclitaxel-eluting stents for coronary revascularization. This whole field will likely need to be re-examined as the technology evolves. Currently, there are trials under way involving second-generation drug-eluting stents with different stent platforms, stent struts, drugs, and polymers.

G. L. Moneta, MD

Strut Position, Blood Flow, and Drug Deposition: Implications for Single and Overlapping Drug-Eluting Stents
Balakrishnan B, Tzafriri AR, Seifert P, et al (Massachusetts Inst of Technology, Cambridge; Harvard Med School, Boston)
Circulation 111:2958-2965, 2005   1–16

Background.—The intricacies of stent design, local pharmacology, tissue biology, and rheology preclude an intuitive understanding of drug distribution and deposition from drug-eluting stents (DES).

Method and Results.—A coupled computational fluid dynamics and mass transfer model was applied to predict drug deposition for single and overlapping DES. Drug deposition appeared not only beneath regions of arterial contact with the strut but surprisingly also beneath standing drug pools created by strut disruption of flow. These regions correlated with areas of drug-induced fibrin deposition surrounding DES struts in porcine coronary arteries. Fibrin deposition immediately distal to individual isolated drug-eluting struts was twice as great as in the proximal area and for the stent as a whole was greater in distal segments than proximal segments. Adjacent and overlapping stent struts increased computed arterial drug deposition by far less than the sum of their combined drug load. In addition, drug eluted from the abluminal stent strut surface accounted for only 11% of total deposition, whereas, remarkably, drug eluted from the adluminal surface accounted for 43% of total deposition. Thus, local blood flow alterations and location of drug elution on the strut were far more important in determining arterial wall drug deposition and distribution than were drug load or arterial wall contact with coated strut surfaces.

Conclusions.—Simulations that coupled strut configurations with flow dynamics correlated with in vivo effects and revealed that drug deposition occurs less via contact between drug coating and the arterial wall than via flow-mediated deposition of blood-solubilized drug.

▶ Antiproliferative DESs have revolutionized coronary arterial interventions for occlusive disease. The Achilles' heal is potential stent thrombosis if patients stop receiving anti-platelet therapy. Drug deposition is not uniform from these stents. For those readers with a strong mathematical and bioengineering background, this is a very interesting and well-written report. However, for the clinical practitioner, DESs will likely undergo further improvements with regard to how blood flow and stent apposition determine drug release. This might be more important in the peripheral circulation (infrainguinal), where DESs have not been as successful as in the coronary circulation.

P. K. Henke, MD

Leisure Time, Occupational, and Commuting Physical Activity and the Risk of Stroke

Hu G, Sarti C, Jousilahti P, et al (Natl Public Health Inst, Helsinki; Univ of Helsinki; Univ of Kuopio, Finland; et al)
Stroke 36:1994-1999, 2005   1–17

Background and Purpose.—The role of physical activity, especially that of occupational and commuting physical activity, in the prediction of stroke risk is not properly established. We assessed the relationship of different types of physical activity with total and type-specific stroke risk.

Methods.—We prospectively followed 47 721 Finnish subjects 25 to 64 years of age without a history of coronary heart disease, stroke, or cancer at baseline. Hazard ratios (HRs) for incident stroke were estimated for different levels of leisure time, occupational, and commuting physical activity.

Results.—During a mean follow-up of 19.0 years, 2863 incident stroke events were ascertained. The multivariate-adjusted (age, sex, area, study year, body mass index, systolic blood pressure, cholesterol, education, smoking, alcohol consumption, diabetes, and other 2 types of physical activity) HRs associated with low, moderate, and high leisure time physical activity were 1.00, 0.86, and 0.74 ($P_{trend}<0.001$) for total stroke, 1.00, 0.87, and 0.46 ($P_{trend}=0.011$) for subarachnoid hemorrhage, 1.00, 0.77, and 0.63 ($P_{trend}=0.024$) for intracerebral hemorrhage, and 1.00, 0.87, and 0.80 ($P_{trend}=0.001$) for ischemic stroke, respectively. The multivariate-adjusted

HRs associated with none, 1 to 29, and ≥30 minutes of active commuting were 1.00, 0.92, and 0.89 (P_{trend}=0.043) for total stroke, and 1.00, 0.93, and 0.86 (P_{trend}=0.028) for ischemic stroke, respectively. Occupational activity had a modest association with ischemic stroke in the multivariate analysis (P_{trend}=0.046).

Conclusions.—A high level of leisure time physical activity reduces the risk of all subtypes of stroke. Daily active commuting also reduces the risk of ischemic stroke.

▶ Of all studies investigating the effects of physical activity and stroke, this study has the largest sample size and the largest portion of women. The results must be taken seriously. The study is, however, limited by the use of the self-reported assessment of physical activity. It is likely patients overreport their physical activity. In addition, no data exist on possible changes in physical activity during follow-up. These limitations, however, would tend to lead to an underestimation of the association between physical activity and stroke.

G. L. Moneta, MD

Association Between Alcohol Consumption and Subclinical Carotid Atherosclerosis: The Study of Health in Pomerania

Schminke U, Luedemann J, Berger K, et al (Ernst Moritz Arndt Univ, Greifswald, Germany; Hanse-Hosp, Stralsund, Germany; Univ of Muenster, Germany; et al)
Stroke 36:1746-1752, 2005

1–18

Background and Purpose.—Epidemiologic studies have shown a J-shaped association between alcohol consumption and vascular diseases. However, only few studies have reported on the association between alcohol intake and subclinical atherosclerosis. The aim of the study was to investigate the relation between alcohol intake and carotid intima-media thickness (IMT) in participants of the population-based Study of Health in Pomerania.

Methods.—In 1230 men and 1190 women, the mean IMT of the right and left common carotid arteries was measured by B-mode ultrasonography. Alcohol consumption was assessed with a computer-assisted face-to-face interview.

Results.—In men, carotid IMT as a function of alcohol intake was depicted as a J-shaped curve with a nadir for the alcohol intake category of 61 to 80 g/d. Linear regression models controlled for age, diabetes, systolic blood pressure, leisure time physical activity, food frequency patterns, smoking status, and education revealed a significant inverse association between IMT and alcohol intake ≤80 g/d in men (β=−0.009, P<0.02), which became insignificant after further controlling for HDL cholesterol and fibrinogen (β=−0.007, P=NS). In women, neither a J-shaped relation nor significant differences in IMT between the drinking and nondrinking groups were found.

Conclusions.—Alcohol consumption is inversely correlated with carotid IMT in men but not in women. However, the total daily level of alcohol intake that shows a maximum protective effect against atherosclerosis is above the threshold where severe alcohol related comorbidity and organ damage have been reported.

► Alcohol is generally regarded as protective against atherosclerosis, but, apparently, more alcohol is not more protective and may increase subclinical atherosclerosis. There really can be too much of a good thing!

G. L. Moneta, MD

Association of a Functional Polymorphism in the Clopidogrel Target Receptor Gene, *P2Y12*, and the Risk for Ischemic Cerebrovascular Events in Patients With Peripheral Artery Disease
Ziegler S, Schillinger M, Funk M, et al (Med Univ of Vienna)
Stroke 36:1394-1399, 2005   1–19

Background and Purpose.—There is considerable variability in the antiplatelet effects of the thienopyridine agent "clopidogrel." We tested for an association of gene sequence variations in *P2Y12* and occurrence of neurological adverse events in patients with symptomatic peripheral artery disease (PAD) during clopidogrel treatment.

Methods.—We studied 137 patients undergoing antiplatelet therapy with clopidogrel and 336 patients with aspirin for the occurrence of neurological events (ischemic stroke and/or carotid revascularization). Prevalence of 2 previously described exonic polymorphisms of the *P2Y12* gene, 34C>T and 52G>T, was determined by polymerase chain reaction.

Results.—Genotype frequencies for mutated, heterozygous, and wild-type alleles for the 34C>T and the 52G>T polymorphisms were 9% (n=40), 44% (n=210), and 47% (n=223), and 4% (n=17), 27% (n=127), and 70% (n=329), respectively. During the median follow-up of 21 months, neurological events occurred in 8% of patients. In patients with aspirin therapy, neither polymorphism was associated with neurological events. However, in clopidogrel patients, carriers of at least one 34T allele had a 4.02-fold increased adjusted risk for neurological events compared with carriers of only 34C alleles (95% confidence interval, 1.08 to 14.9). Neither polymorphism was associated with all-cause mortality.

Conclusions.—In PAD patients, clopidogrel response variability exists, which may result in increased risk for cerebrovascular events. Sequence alterations of the target receptor gene represent one possible mechanism for clopidogrel failure. Whether identification of the 34C>T polymorphism as a contributor to this process could serve as risk stratification tool, an indicator for higher clopidogrel doses, or the use of alternate agents warrants further investigation.

▶ As with aspirin, significant interindividual variability of the antiplatelet effect of clopidogrel appears to exist. This study suggests that identification of the 34C>T polymorphism may serve as a predictor of the efficacy of clopidogrel to prevent neurologic events in patients with PAD. Patients receiving antiplatelet therapy because of neurologic events should probably be assessed for either aspirin or clopidogrel resistance, and their antiplatelet agent should be adjusted accordingly.

G. L. Moneta, MD

Screening for Aspirin Responsiveness After Transient Ischemic Attack and Stroke: Comparison of 2 Point-of-Care Platelet Function Tests With Optical Aggregometry
Harrison P, Segal H, Blasbery K, et al (Churchill Hosp, Oxford, England; Univ of Oxford, England)
Stroke 36:1001-1005, 2005   1–20

Background and Purpose.—Recent studies suggest that patients who do not respond to aspirin (ASA) therapy may be at increased risk of ischemic vascular events. The availability of simple to use point-of-care (POC) platelet function tests now potentially allows aspirin nonresponsiveness to be identified in routine clinical practice. However, there are very few data on whether the different tests produce consistent results. We therefore compared 2 POC tests (PFA-100 device and the Ultegra-RPFA [RPFA]) with conventional light transmission aggregometry (LTA).

Methods.—Platelet function was assessed by all 3 tests in 100 patients receiving low-dose ASA therapy after transient ischemic attack (TIA) or ischemic stroke.

Results.—The incidence of ASA nonresponsiveness was 17% by the RPFA and 22% by the PFA-100, compared with only 5% by LTA (ie, as defined with both arachidonic acid and ADP). Agreement between the RPFA and the PFA-100 and arachidonic acid induced LTA was poor ($\kappa=0.16$, 95% CI, -0.08 to 0.39, $P=0.11$; and $\kappa=0.09$ -0.12 to 0.30, $P=0.32$, respectively). Agreement between the 2 POC tests was also poor ($\kappa=0.14$, -0.08 to 0.36, $P=0.15$). Only 2% of patients were aspirin nonresponders by all 3 tests.

Conclusions.—The prevalence of apparent ASA nonresponsiveness was higher with both the POC tests than with LTA. However, agreement between the tests was poor and very few patients were ASA nonresponsive by all 3 tests. Aspirin nonresponsiveness is therefore highly test-specific and large prospective studies will be required to determine the prognostic value of each of the separate tests.

▶ ASA is a mainstay of contemporary cardiovascular risk reduction, although individuals with ASA resistance may derive less benefit. The diagnosis of ASA resistance has been hampered by lack of standardized, convenient testing. This work compares 3 platelet function tests—2 simple US Food and Drug Administration approved POC tests, and 1 conventional LTA—in 100 patients receiving low-dose ASA after TIA or stroke. The POC tests yielded substantially higher nonresponsiveness (resistance) rates, and the agreement between all 3 tests was strikingly poor. The results bring into question the current utility of any of these tests.

C. K. Ozaki, MD

Ankle-Brachial Index and Subclinical Cardiac and Carotid Disease: The Multi-Ethnic Study of Atherosclerosis

McDermott MM, Liu K, Criqui MH, et al (Northwestern Univ, Chicago; Univ of California at San Diego, La Jolla; Wake Forest Univ, Winston-Salem, NC; et al)
Am J Epidemiol 162:33-41, 2005   1–21

The authors studied associations between ankle-brachial index (ABI) and subclinical atherosclerosis in the Multi-Ethnic Study of Atherosclerosis. Participants included 3,458 women (average age = 62.6 years) and 3,112 men (average age = 62.8 years) who were free of clinically evident cardiovascular disease. Measurements included ABI, carotid artery intima-media thickness, and coronary artery calcium assessed with computed tomography. Five ABI categories were defined: <0.90 (definite peripheral arterial disease (PAD)), 0.90–0.99 (borderline ABI), 1.00–1.09 (low-normal ABI), 1.10–1.29 (normal ABI), and ≥1.30 (high ABI). Compared with that in men with normal ABI, significantly higher internal carotid artery intima-media thickness was observed in men with definite PAD (1.58 vs. 1.09; $p < 0.001$), borderline ABI (1.33 vs. 1.09; $p < 0.001$), and low-normal ABI (1.18 vs. 1.09; $p < 0.001$) after adjustment for confounders. Fully adjusted odds ratios for a coronary artery calcium score greater than 20 decreased across progressively higher ABI categories in both women (2.85 (definite PAD), 1.27 (borderline ABI), 1.11 (low-normal ABI), 1.00 (normal ABI; referent), and 0.78 (high ABI); p for trend = 0.0002) and men (3.26 (definite PAD), 1.72 (borderline ABI), 1.14 (low-normal ABI), 1.00 (normal ABI; referent), and 1.43 (high ABI); p for trend = 0.0002). These findings indicate excess coronary and carotid atherosclerosis at ABI values below 1.10 (men) and 1.00 (women) and may imply increased risk of cardiovascular events in persons with borderline and low-normal ABI.

▶ The data suggest that borderline and low-normal ABIs may not really be normal and that such patients are at higher risk of having increased degrees of coronary and carotid atherosclerosis. A truly normal ABI as a marker for a patient free of atherosclerosis may be slightly higher than previously suspected.

G. L. Moneta, MD

Heritability of Carotid Artery Atherosclerotic Lesions: An Ultrasound Study in 154 Families

Moskau S, Golla A, Grothe C, et al (Univ Hosp Bonn, Germany)

Stroke 36:5-8, 2005   1–22

Background and Purpose.—Ultrasound examination of the carotid arteries yields several quantitative measures that may serve as intermediate phenotypes in genetic studies. This study was undertaken to compare the heritabilities of 3 ultrasound measures: intima-media thickness (IMT), plaque score, and maximal stenosis.

Methods.—We studied 565 individuals from 154 families ascertained by an affected parent with carotid artery atherosclerosis. IMT, plaque score, and maximal stenosis of the carotid arteries were examined by B-mode ultrasound and analyzed quantitatively. Heritability estimates were obtained by variance component analysis as implemented in the program SOLAR (sequential oligogenic linkage analysis routines). Covariates were age, sex, weight, height, body mass index (BMI), arterial hypertension, diabetes mellitus, amount of nicotine consumed, and plasma levels of low-density lipoprotein (LDL) and high-density lipoprotein (HDL) cholesterol, LDL/HDL ratio, lipoprotein(a) [Lp(a)], triglycerides, factor VIII, factor XIII, fibrinogen, and von Willebrand factor (vWF).

Results.—After accounting for the covariables age, sex, hypertension, diabetes mellitus, and Lp(a), heritability of IMT was estimated as $h^2 = 0.61 \pm 0.17$ ($P = 0.001$). Variation of plaque score was influenced by age, sex, hypertension, diabetes mellitus, hypercholesterolemia, amount of nicotine consumed, factor VIII, and vWF. When these were considered, no significant heritability could be detected. Heritability of stenosis was estimated as $h^2 = 0.47 \pm 0.07$ ($P = 0.006$), with age, sex, BMI, hypertension, diabetes mellitus, amount of nicotine consumed, and LDL/HDL ratio as covariates.

Conclusions.—Among the 3 ultrasound measures studied, IMT had the highest heritability. IMT was strongly influenced by genetic determinants other than those influencing known risk factors. This makes IMT a promising candidate for use as an intermediate phenotype in genetic studies aiming to identify novel genes for atherosclerosis.

▶ Noninvasive measures of atherosclerosis to predict and improve stratification of late risk of cardiovascular events hold significant promise for reducing patient mortality. As elegantly shown in this population-based epidemiologic genetic study, the carotid IMT measure has the highest correlation to heritability as compared with carotid stenosis and carotid plaque area (matched for patient risk factors). This may be clinically useful. For example, young patients with an increased IMT, or their direct descendants, may be candidates for very aggressive lipid-lowering therapies to prevent later clinical disease. Unfortunately, carotid IMT examinations are no longer reimbursed by Centers for Medicare and Medicaid Services.

P. K. Henke, MD

Age-related changes in plaque composition: A study in patients suffering from carotid artery stenosis

van Oostrom O, Velema E, Schoneveld AH, et al (UMCU, Utrecht, The Netherlands; Interuniversity Cardiology Inst of The Netherlands; Antonius Hosp Nieuwegein, The Netherlands; et al)

Cardiovasc Pathol 14:126-134, 2005   1–23

Objective.—The extent of atherosclerotic plaque burden and the incidence of atherosclerosis-related cardiovascular events accelerate with increasing age. The composition of the plaque is associated with plaque thrombosis and acute coronary occlusion. Surprisingly, however, the relation between advancing age and atherosclerotic plaque composition is still unclear. In the present study, we investigated the association between plaque characteristics and advancing age in a population of patients with haemodynamically significant carotid artery stenosis.

Methods.—Patients ($N=383$), ages 39–89 years, underwent carotid endarterectomy (CEA). Morphometric analysis was performed on the dissected atherosclerotic plaques to study the prevalence of fibrous and atheromatous plaques. Picro sirius red, haematoxylin eosin, alfa actin and CD68 stainings were performed to investigate the extent of collagen, calcification, smooth muscle cells and macrophages in carotid plaques, respectively. The presence of metalloproteinases-2 and -9 was assessed by ELISA.

Results.—With aging, a decrease in fibrous plaques and an increase in atheromatous plaques were observed. This was accompanied by an age-associated decrease in smooth muscle cell content in carotid plaques. Macrophage content slightly increased with age. In addition, total matrix metalloprotease (MMP)-2 was negatively and MMP-9 positively related with age. Differences in plaque phenotype were most prominent for the youngest age quartile compared with older age quartiles.

Conclusions.—With increasing age, the morphology of atherosclerotic plaques from patients with carotid artery stenosis changes. Plaques become more atheromatous and contain less smooth muscle cells with increasing age. Local inflammation and MMP-9 levels slightly increased with age in plaques obtained from patients suffering from haemodynamically significant advanced atherosclerotic lesions.

▶ Numerous studies have evaluated the histomorphological features of plaques. This article adds to this literature by showing differences between carotid plaques in younger and older patients who underwent CEA. Not surprisingly, older plaques displayed evidence of increased MMP-9, which may contribute to plaque instability. Unfortunately, this article is not very rigorous in its analysis. Furthermore, it would have been more useful to compare asymptomatic and symptomatic plaque histomorphological features.

P. K. Henke, MD

Vitamin B$_{12}$, homocysteine and carotid plaque in the era of folic acid fortification of enriched cereal grain products

Robertson J, Iemolo F, Stabler SP, et al (McMaster Univ, Hamilton, Ont, Canada; Catania Univ, Italy; Univ of Western Ontario, London, Canada; et al)
CMAJ 172:1569-1573, 2005   1–24

Background.—The presence of carotid plaque is a strong predictor of cardiovascular events. High homocysteine levels, which are associated with plaque formation, can result from inadequate intake of folate and vitamin B$_{12}$. Folic acid fortification of enriched cereal grain products began in North America in 1996 and became mandatory in 1998, and vitamin B$_{12}$ has now become an important determinant of homocysteine levels. This study investigated the prevalence of low serum levels of vitamin B$_{12}$ and their relationship to homocysteine levels and carotid plaque area among patients referred for treatment of vascular disease in the years since folic acid fortification of enriched grain products was initiated.

Methods.—The study was conducted among 421 consecutive new patients with complete data. The patients were evaluated in a vascular disease prevention clinic between January 1998 and January 2002. They included 215 men and 206 women who ranged in age from 37 to 90 years (mean age, 66 years).

The total carotid plaque area was measured by US, and homocysteine and serum vitamin B$_{12}$ levels were determined. Most of the patients were taking medications for hypertension (67%) and dyslipidemia (62%).

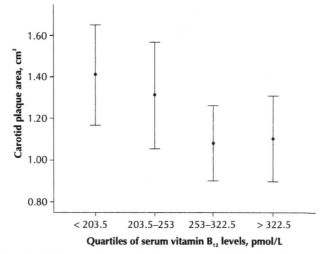

FIGURE 2.—Carotid plaque area by quartiles of serum vitamin B$_{12}$ levels. *Error bars* represent 95% confidence intervals. Carotid plaque area is significantly related to a median split of vitamin B$_{12}$ (p=0.012). (Reprinted from Robertson J, Iemolo F, Stabler SP, et al: Vitamin B$_{12}$, homocysteine and carotid plaque in the era of folic acid fortification of enriched cereal grain products. *CMAJ* 172:1569-1573, 2005. Copyright 2005, Canadian Medical Association.)

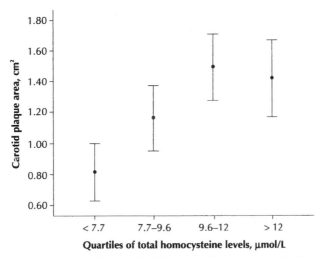

FIGURE 3.—Carotid plaque area by quartiles of plasma total homocysteine levels. Error bars represent 95% confidence intervals. (Reprinted from Robertson J, Iemolo F, Stabler SP, et al: Vitamin B$_{12}$, homocysteine and carotid plaque in the era of folic acid fortification of enriched cereal grain products. *CMAJ* 172:1569-1573, 2005. Copyright 2005, Canadian Medical Association.)

Results.—Vitamin B$_{12}$ deficiency was present in 73 patients (17%). The mean area of carotid plaque was significantly greater among the patients whose vitamin B$_{12}$ level was below the median of 253 pmol/L compared with patients whose vitamin B$_{12}$ level was above the median (Figs 2 and 3).

Conclusions.—Vitamin B$_{12}$ deficiency is a common finding among patients with vascular disease. In the setting of folic acid fortification, low serum levels of vitamin B$_{12}$ are a significant determinant of elevated homocysteine levels and increased carotid plaque area.

▶ Since folic acid fortification became widespread in the late 1990s, vitamin B$_{12}$ has become an important determinant of homocysteine levels. The authors found approximately 17% of their vascular patients had vitamin B$_{12}$ deficiency, and these patients exhibited significantly more carotid atherosclerotic disease.

Important next steps include studies in which the folate levels are actually measured, more details regarding interplay with medical therapies (eg, statins) that are known to impact atherosclerotic end points, inclusion of longitudinal clinical end points (perhaps a surrogate for plaque stability), and trial arms with active vitamin B$_{12}$ replacement. The current findings suggest that "folate therapy" for lowering homocysteine levels is no longer appropriate. The focus should now be on vitamin B$_{12}$.

C. K. Ozaki, MD

Presence of Intraplaque Hemorrhage Stimulates Progression of Carotid Atherosclerotic Plaques: A High-Resolution Magnetic Resonance Imaging Study

Takaya N, Yuan C, Chu B, et al (Univ of Washington, Seattle; Juntendo Univ, Tokyo; Mountain-Whisper-Light Statistical Consulting, Seattle)
Circulation 111:2768-2775, 2005   1–25

Background.—Previous studies suggest that erythrocyte membranes from intraplaque hemorrhage into the necrotic core are a source of free cholesterol and may become a driving force in the progression of atherosclerosis. We have shown that MRI can accurately identify carotid intraplaque hemorrhage and precisely measure plaque volume. We tested the hypothesis that hemorrhage into carotid atheroma stimulates plaque progression.

Method and Results.—Twenty-nine subjects (14 cases with intraplaque hemorrhage and 15 controls with comparably sized plaques without intraplaque hemorrhage at baseline) underwent serial carotid MRI examination with a multicontrast weighted protocol (T1, T2, proton density, and 3D time of flight) over a period of 18 months. The volumes of wall, lumen, lipid-rich necrotic core, calcification, and intraplaque hemorrhage were measured with a custom-designed image analysis tool. The percent change in wall volume (6.8% versus −0.15%; $P=0.009$) and lipid-rich necrotic core volume (28.4% versus −5.2%; $P=0.001$) was significantly higher in the hemorrhage group than in controls over the course of the study. Furthermore, those with intraplaque hemorrhage at baseline were much more likely to have new plaque hemorrhages at 18 months compared with controls (43% versus 0%; $P=0.006$).

Conclusions.—Hemorrhage into the carotid atherosclerotic plaque accelerated plaque progression in an 18-month period. Repeated bleeding into the plaque may produce a stimulus for the progression of atherosclerosis by increasing lipid core and plaque volume and creating new destabilizing factors.

▶ It is well accepted that plaque instability is important for the development of clinical atherosclerotic symptoms. Longitudinal specialized MRI scanning of the carotid artery was undertaken in a group of patients to delineate the occurrence of intraplaque hemorrhaging. Not surprisingly, those patients with necrotic cores and prior evidence of hemorrhaging into a plaque were more likely on follow-up scans to have recurrent hemorrhaging and increases in the degree of stenosis. This modality is preliminary and not powered to detect hard clinical end points, but it may be an exciting way to better assess specifically those patients who have moderate asymptomatic stenosis and who may benefit from a carotid intervention if their plaque is "unstable."

P. K. Henke, MD

Cilostazol Prevents the Progression of the Symptomatic Intracranial Arterial Stenosis: The Multicenter Double-Blind Placebo-Controlled Trial of Cilostazol in Symptomatic Intracranial Arterial Stenosis

Kwon SU, Cho Y-J, Koo J-S, et al (Univ of Ulsan, Seoul, Korea; Inje Univ, Gyeonggido, Korea; Eulji Univ, Seoul, Korea; et al)
Stroke 36:782-786, 2005   1–26

Background and Purpose.—Cilostazol, a phosphodiesterase inhibitor, has been reported to reduce restenosis rate after coronary angioplasty and stenting. This study was performed to investigate the effect of cilostazol on the progression of intracranial arterial stenosis (IAS).

Methods.—We randomized 135 patients with acute symptomatic stenosis in the M1 segment of middle cerebral artery or the basilar artery to either cilostazol 200 mg per day or placebo for 6 months. Aspirin 100 mg per day was also given to all patients. Patients with potential embolic sources in the heart or extracranial arteries were excluded. IAS was assessed by magnetic resonance angiogram (MRA) and transcranial Doppler (TCD) at the time of recruitment and 6 months later. The primary outcome was the progression of symptomatic IAS on MRA and secondary outcomes were clinical events and progression on TCD.

Results.—Thirty eight patients were prematurely terminated. Dropout rates and reasons for dropouts were similar between the cilostazol and placebo groups. There was no stroke recurrence in either cilostazol or placebo group, but there was 1 death and 2 coronary events in each group. In cilostazol group, 3 (6.7%) of 45 symptomatic IAS progressed and 11 (24.4%) regressed. In placebo group, 15 (28.8%) of symptomatic IAS progressed and 8 (15.4%) regressed. Progression of symptomatic IAS in cilostazol group was significantly lower than that in placebo group ($P=0.008$).

Conclusions.—Our study suggests that symptomatic IAS is a dynamic lesion and cilostazol may prevent its progression.

▶ Although this is a study of intracranial arterial lesions, the study is of interest in that it documents an effect of cilostazol on an established arterial stenosis associated with neurologic symptoms. The high frequency of progression and regression of intracranial lesions noted in this study suggests that IAS may behave much differently than extracranial carotid stenosis. Nevertheless, the idea that it may be possible to induce a relatively high rate of regression of an arterial lesion with the use of pharmacologic manipulation is of considerable interest.

G. L. Moneta, MD

Ethnicity and Peripheral Arterial Disease: The San Diego Population Study

Criqui MH, Vargas V, Denenberg JO, et al (Univ of California, San Diego, La Jolla)

Circulation 112:2703-2707, 2005

1–27

Background.—Previous studies have indicated higher rates of peripheral arterial disease (PAD) in blacks than in non-Hispanic whites (NHWs), with limited information available for Hispanics and Asians. The reason for the PAD excess in blacks is unclear.

Method and Results.—Ethnic-specific PAD prevalence rates were determined in a randomly selected defined population that included 4 ethnic groups; NHWs, blacks, Hispanics, and Asians. A total of 2343 participants aged 29 to 91 years were evaluated. There were 104 cases of PAD (4.4%). In weighted logistic models with NHWs as the reference group and containing demographic factors only, blacks had a higher PAD prevalence than NHWs (OR=2.30, $P<0.024$), whereas PAD rates in Hispanics and Asians, although somewhat lower, were not significantly different from NHWs. Blacks had significantly more diabetes and hypertension than NHWs and a significantly higher body mass index. Inclusion of these variables and other PAD risk factors in the model did not change the effect size for black ethnicity (OR=2.34, $P=0.048$). A model containing interaction terms for black ethnicity and each of the other risk factors revealed no significant interaction terms, which indicates no evidence that blacks were more "susceptible" than NHWs to cardiovascular disease risk factors.

Conclusions.—Black ethnicity was a strong and independent risk factor for PAD, which was not explained by higher levels of diabetes, hypertension, and body mass index. There was no evidence of a greater susceptibility of blacks to cardiovascular disease risk factors as a reason for their higher PAD prevalence. Thus, the excess risk of PAD in blacks remains unexplained and requires further study.

▶ The tendency has been to blame the higher incidence of PAD in black patients on an increased prevalence of diabetes, hypertension, and obesity. These data are intriguing in that they indicate no objective evidence to support those suppositions. There must be other factors that predispose black patients to a greater susceptibility to PAD.

G. L. Moneta, MD

Relationship Between HbA$_{1c}$ Level and Peripheral Arterial Disease

Muntner P, DeSalvo KB, Wildman RP, et al (Tulane Univ, New Orleans, La)

Diabetes Care 28:1981-1987, 2005

1–28

Objective.—Homeostatic glucose control may play an important role in the development of peripheral arterial disease among individuals without diabetes. We sought to evaluate the association of HbA$_{1c}$ (A1C) with peripheral arterial disease in a representative sample of the U.S. population with and without diabetes.

Research Design and Methods.—A cross-sectional study was conducted among 4,526 National Health and Nutrition Examination Survey 1999–2002 participants ≥40 years of age. Peripheral arterial disease was defined as an ankle-brachial index <0.9 ($n = 327$).

Results.—Among nondiabetic subjects, the age-standardized prevalence of peripheral arterial disease was 3.1, 4.8, 4.7, and 6.4% for participants with an A1C <5.3, 5.3–5.4, 5.5–5.6, and 5.7–6.0%, respectively (P trend <0.001). The prevalence of peripheral arterial disease was 7.5 and 8.8% for diabetic participants with A1C <7 and ≥7%, respectively. After multivariable adjustment and compared with nondiabetic participants with A1C <5.3%, the odds ratio (95% CI) of peripheral arterial disease for nondiabetic participants with an A1C of 5.3–5.4, 5.5–5.6, and 5.7–6.0% was 1.41 (0.85–2.32), 1.39 (0.70–2.75), and 1.57 (1.02–2.47), respectively, and it was 2.33 (1.15–4.70) and 2.74 (1.25–6.02) for diabetic participants with A1C <7 and ≥7%, respectively.

Conclusions.—An association exists between higher levels of A1C and peripheral arterial disease, even among patients without diabetes. Individuals with A1C levels ≥5.3% should be targeted for aggressive risk factor reduction, which may reduce the burden of subclinical cardiovascular disease even among those without diabetes.

▶ Higher levels of A1C in patients without diabetes may serve as a marker for an increased risk of subclinical cardiovascular disease. It may be that it's not so much diabetes but glucose control that contributes to the risk of atherosclerosis. Perhaps diabetes merely serves as one end of the spectrum of the adverse effects of increased glucose levels on atherosclerosis.

G. L. Moneta, MD

Autologous Transplantation of Granulocyte Colony–Stimulating Factor–Mobilized Peripheral Blood Mononuclear Cells Improves Critical Limb Ischemia in Diabetes

Huang P, Li S, Han M, et al (Chinese Academy of Med Sciences & Peking Union of Med College, Tianjin)
Diabetes Care 28:2155-2160, 2005   1–29

Objective.—To assess the application of autologous transplantation of granulocyte colony–stimulating factor (G-CSF)–mobilized peripheral blood mononuclear cells (PBMNCs) in the treatment of critical limb ischemia (CLI) of diabetic patients and to evaluate the safety, efficacy, and feasibility of this novel therapeutic approach.

Research Design and Methods.—Twenty-eight diabetic patients with CLI were enrolled and randomized to either the transplant group or the control group. In the transplant group, the patients received subcutaneous injections of recombinant human G-CSF (600 µg/day) for 5 days to mobilize stem/

progenitor cells, and their PBMNCs were collected and transplanted by multiple intramuscular injections into ischemic limbs. All of the patients were followed up after at least 3 months.

Results.—At the end of the 3-month follow-up, the main manifestations, including lower limb pain and ulcers, were significantly improved in the patients of the transplant group. Their laser Doppler blood perfusion of lower limbs increased from 0.44 ± 0.11 to 0.57 ± 0.14 perfusion units ($P < 0.001$). Mean ankle-brachial pressure index increased from 0.50 ± 0.21 to 0.63 ± 0.25 ($P < 0.001$). A total of 14 of 18 limb ulcers (77.8%) of transplanted patients were completely healed after cell transplantation, whereas only 38.9% of limb ulcers (7 of 18) were healed in the control patients ($P = 0.016$ vs. the transplant group). No adverse effects specifically due to cell transplantation were observed, and no lower limb amputation occurred in the transplanted patients. In contrast, five control patients had to receive a lower limb amputation ($P = 0.007$, transplant vs. control group). Angiographic scores were significantly improved in the transplant group when compared with the control group ($P = 0.003$).

Conclusions.—These results provide pilot evidence indicating that the autologous transplantation of G-CSF–mobilized PBMNCs represents a simple, safe, effective, and novel therapeutic approach for diabetic CLI.

▶ This is a new approach to therapeutic angiogenesis: transplanted stem cells are used to induce lower extremity angiogenesis. The results of this study are encouraging and should foster the design of larger trials to more fully assess the therapeutic potential of using stem cells as angiogenic mediators.

G. L. Moneta, MD

Skeletal muscle phenotype is associated with exercise tolerance in patients with peripheral arterial disease

Askew CD, Green S, Walker PJ, et al (Univ of Queensland, Brisbane, Australia; Queensland Univ of Technology, Australia; Victoria Univ, Australia; et al)
J Vasc Surg 41:802-807, 2005   1–30

Objective.—To better understand the association between skeletal muscle and exercise intolerance in peripheral arterial disease (PAD), we assessed treadmill-walking performance and gastrocnemius muscle phenotype in healthy control subjects and in patients with PAD. We hypothesized that gastrocnemius muscle characteristics would be altered in PAD compared with control subjects and that exercise tolerance in patients with PAD would be related to muscle phenotype.

Methods.—Sixteen patients with PAD and intermittent claudication and 13 healthy controls of the same age participated. Each subject completed a graded treadmill-walking test and underwent a resting muscle biopsy. Muscle biopsy samples were obtained from the medial gastrocnemius muscle of the most ischemic limb in PAD and a limb chosen at random in controls. Samples were analyzed for fiber type and cross-sectional area, capillary-to-fiber ratio, the number of capillaries in contact with each fiber type, and the optical density of glycogen within each fiber by using histochemical procedures. Total muscle glycogen content was determined biochemically.

Results.—Exercise capacity measured on the incremental walking test in the PAD group was only 30% to 40% of that observed in controls. The PAD group had a lower proportion of type I muscle fibers ($P < .05$), fewer capillaries per muscle fiber ($P < .05$), and tended to have smaller fiber areas ($P = .08$). The relative area of type I fibers, the capillary-to-fiber ratio, capillary contacts with type I and IIa fibers, and the optical density of glycogen in type I fibers were all positively correlated with exercise tolerance in the PAD group ($P < .05$) but not controls.

Conclusions.—These data suggest that muscle phenotype is altered in PAD and that such alterations are associated with the exercise intolerance in these patients. In light of these findings, therapies such as resistance training or electrical stimulation that target skeletal muscle in PAD may prove beneficial, and further investigation of such therapies is warranted.

▶ Symptoms of PAD relate not only to the hemodynamic magnitude of the occlusive lesions but also appear to depend on the skeletal muscle phenotype. In this study, biological end points such as capillary contacts of type I and IIa fibers and muscle glycogen content correlated with treadmill peak power in the PAD group. Thus, therapies directed at the muscle rather than the occlusive lesions may be of benefit. Unclear is whether the phenotype differences are genetically determined or the result of environmental factors such as chronic low-grade ischemia or disuse.

C. K. Ozaki, MD

Markers of Coagulation Activation, Endothelial Stimulation and Inflammation in Patients with Peripheral Arterial Disease
Cassar K, Bachoo P, Ford I, et al (Univ of Aberdeen, Scotland; Aberdeen Royal Infirmary, Scotland)
Eur J Vasc Endovasc Surg 29:171-176, 2005   1–31

Objectives.—Patients with peripheral arterial disease have a significantly increased risk of cardiovascular and cerebrovascular mortality. Studies have shown that some haemostatic and inflammatory markers are elevated in these patients but the effect of the severity of the disease has not been fully documented. The aim of this study was to assess the level of coagulation activation, endothelial stimulation and inflammation in patients with claudication and critical limb ischaemia (CLI) compared to healthy controls.

Design and Methods.—A prospective observational study was conducted amongst 202 subjects: 132 claudicants, 30 patients with critical ischaemia, and 40 controls. D-dimer (DD) and thrombin–antithrombin III (TAT) levels were measured using ELISA as markers of coagulation activation. von Willebrand factor (vWF) and high-sensitivity C-reactive protein (CRP) levels were measured as markers of endothelial and inflammatory stimulation.

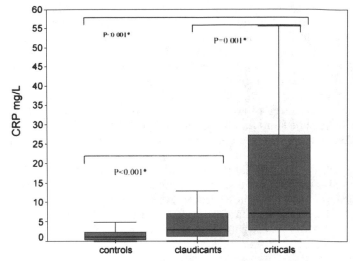

FIGURE 1.—Boxplots of C-reactive protein levels in controls, claudicants, and criticals. (*Bars*, median values; *whiskers*, smallest and largest values excluding extremes; *top of box+*, 75th percentile; *bottom of box*, 25th percentile). *Statistically significant difference. (Reprinted from Cassar K, Bachoo P, Ford I, et al: Markers of coagulation activation, endothelial stimulation and inflammation in patients with peripheral arterial disease. *Eur J Vasc Endovasc Surg* 29(2):171-176, 2005. Copyright 2005 by permission of the publisher.)

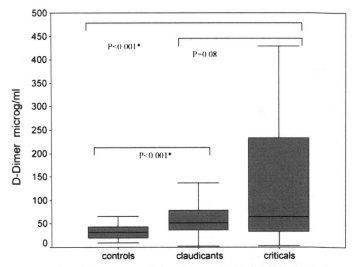

FIGURE 3.—Boxplots of C-reactive protein levels in controls, claudicants, and criticals. (*Bars*, median values; *whiskers*, smallest and largest values excluding extremes; *top of box+*, 75th percentile; *bottom of box*, 25th percentile). *Statistically significant difference. (Reprinted from Cassar K, Bachoo P, Ford I, et al: Markers of coagulation activation, endothelial stimulation and inflammation in patients with peripheral arterial disease. *Eur J Vasc Endovasc Surg* 29(2):171-176, 2005. Copyright 2005 by permission of the publisher.)

Results.—vWF and CRP levels were significantly higher in patients with intermittent claudication (1.9 U/ml, range 0.78–4.05; $p < 0.001$; 3.4 mg/l, range 0.15–24; $p > 0.001$, respectively) and critical ischaemia (2.36 U/ml; range 1.03–5.69; $p < 0.001$; 7.17 mg/ml, range 0.15–174; $p < 0.001$, respectively) compared to controls (1.28 U/ml, range 0.62–3.13; 1.04, range 0.15–7.59 mg/l). DD was also significantly higher in claudicants (48.6 μg/ml; range 2-N-1741; $p < 0.001$) and in patients with CLI (61.1 μg/ml, range 3.65–1963; $p < 0.001$) compared to controls (26.1 μg/ml, range 9.65–203.1). TAT levels were significantly higher in CLI (3.14 mg/l, range 2.09–58.11), compared to controls (2.36 mg/l, range 1.49–7.38; $p = 0.004$). Patients with CLI had significantly higher levels of CRP, vWF, and TAT than claudicants.

Conclusions.—Coagulation activation and endothelial stimulation are significantly increased in patients with peripheral arterial disease compared to healthy controls. Coagulation and endothelial activation increases with the severity of the arterial disease (Figs 1 and 3).

▶ Atherosclerosis is an inflammatory disease, and this descriptive article confirms a positive correlation between the severity of peripheral lower extremity ischemia and the elevation of inflammatory and procoagulant factors. None of these data are surprising. Although probably not statistically powered to do so, this article would have been significantly more useful if it had evaluated the effects of risk factor reduction (quitting smoking, adding appropriate medical therapy, or beginning a structured exercise program) on changes in these serum procoagulant and inflammatory factors over time.

P. K. Henke, MD

Endothelium-Intrinsic Requirement for *Hif-2α* During Vascular Development

Duan L-J, Zhang-Benoit Y, Fong G-H (Univ of Connecticut, Farmington)
Circulation 111:2227-2232, 2005   1–32

Background.—The development of the vascular system is a complex process that involves communications among multiple cell types. As such, it is important to understand whether a specific gene regulates vascular development directly from within the vascular system or indirectly from nonvascular cells. Hypoxia-inducible factor-2α (Hif-2α, or endothelial PAS protein-1 [EPAS-1]) is required for vascular development in mice, but it is not clear whether its requirement resides directly in endothelial cells.

Method and Results.—To address this issue, we expressed *Hif-2α* cDNA in the vascular endothelium of *Hif-2α$^{-/-}$*embryos by an embryonic stem (ES) cell–mediated transgenic approach and assessed whether endothelium-specific reexpression of *Hif-2α* could rescue vascular development. Here we report that although ES cell–derived *Hif-2α$^{-/-}$*embryos developed severe vascular defects by embryonic day (E) 11.5 and died in utero before E12.5, endothelium-specific expression of *Hif-2α* cDNA restored normal vascular development at all stages examined (up to E14.5) and allowed *Hif-2α$^{-/-}$*embryos to survive at a frequency comparable to that of *Hif-2α$^{+/-}$*embryos. Furthermore, we found that *Tie-2* expression was significantly reduced in *Hif-2α$^{-/-}$*mutants but was restored by *Hif-2α* cDNA expression.

Conclusions.—These data demonstrate an intrinsic requirement for *Hif-2α* by endothelial cells and imply that hypoxia may control endothelial functions directly via *Hif-2α*–regulated *Tie-2* expression.

▶ Hypoxia serves as the primary stimulator of embryonic vascular development via oxygen-sensitive mechanisms. By causing the expression of *Hif-2α* cDNA in the vascular endothelium (*Tie-2* promoter) of *Hif-2α*–deficient embryos, the researchers rescued vascular development. Therefore, *Hif-2α* is required in endothelial cells for vascular system development, and *Tie-2* may be a functionally relevant target for *Hif-2α*. Delineation of basic developmental mechanisms such as this via cell linage-specific re-expression in a null background may point to novel therapeutic strategies for vascular disease.

C. K. Ozaki, MD

Noninvasive Imaging of Angiogenesis With a ^{99m}Tc-Labeled Peptide Targeted at α$_v$β$_3$ Integrin After Murine Hindlimb Ischemia

Hua J, Dobrucki LW, Sadeghi MM, et al (Yale Univ, New Haven, Conn; Albert-Ludwigs Univ, Freiburg, Germany; GE Healthcare, Buckinghamshire, England)
Circulation 111:3255-3260, 2005   1–33

Background.—Noninvasive imaging strategies play a critical role in assessment of the efficacy of angiogenesis therapies. The α$_v$β$_3$ integrin is activated in angiogenic vessels and represents a potential target for noninvasive imaging of angiogenesis.

Method and Results.—We evaluated a ^{99m}Tc-labeled peptide (NC100692) targeted at α$_v$β$_3$ integrin for imaging in an established murine model of angiogenesis induced by hindlimb ischemia. Control mice (n=9) or mice with surgical right femoral artery occlusion (n=29) were injected with NC100692 (1.5±0.2 mCi IV) at different times after femoral occlusion (1, 3, 7, and 14 days) for in vivo pinhole planar gamma camera imaging. Tissue from hindlimb proximal and distal to occlusion was excised for gamma well counting and for immunostaining. On in vivo pinhole images, increased focal NC100692 activity was seen distal to the occlusion at days 3 and 7. This increase in relative NC100692 activity was confirmed by gamma well counting. Lectin staining confirmed increased angiogenesis in the ischemic hindlimb at these time points. A fluorescent analogue of NC100692 was used to confirm specificity and localization of the targeted tracer in cultured endothelial cells. In addition, endothelial cell specificity was confirmed on tissue sections with the use of dual immunofluorescent staining of endothelium and the fluorescent analogue targeted at the α$_v$β$_3$ integrin.

Conclusions.—A ^{99m}Tc-labeled peptide (NC100692) targeted at α$_v$β$_3$ integrin selectively localized to endothelial cells in regions of increased angiogenesis and could be used for noninvasive serial "hot spot" imaging of angiogenesis. This targeted radiotracer imaging approach is a major advance in tracking therapeutic myocardial angiogenesis and has an important clinical potential.

▶ This may be a major advance in the field of angiogenesis. The approach offers the capability to serially evaluate the angiogenic process in experimental animals without the need for euthanizing at distinct time points. In addition, it targets the angiogenic process itself rather than the more standard measures of the physiologic consequences of angiogenesis, such as an increase in tissue oxygenation. The favorable clearance kinetics of NC100692 may potentially allow noninvasive assessment of angiogenesis in patients undergoing various drug therapies for peripheral vascular disease.

G. L. Moneta, MD

Akt1/protein kinase Bα is critical for ischemic and VEGF-mediated angiogenesis
Ackah E, Yu J, Zoellner S, et al (Yale Univ, New Haven, Conn; Boston Univ; Univ of Pennsylvania, Philadelphia)
J Clin Invest 115:2119-2127, 2005   1–34

Akt, or protein kinase B, is a multifunctional serine-threonine protein kinase implicated in a diverse range of cellular functions including cell metabolism, survival, migration, and gene expression. However, the in vivo roles and effectors of individual Akt isoforms in signaling are not explicitly clear. Here we show that the genetic loss of Akt1, but not Akt2, in mice results in defective ischemia and VEGF-induced angiogenesis as well as severe peripheral vascular disease. Akt1 knockout (*Akt1 −/−*) mice also have reduced endothelial progenitor cell (EPC) mobilization in response to ischemia, and reintroduction of WT EPCs, but not EPCs isolated from *Akt1 −/−*mice, into WT mice improves limb blood flow after ischemia. Mechanistically, the loss of Akt1 reduces the basal phosphorylation of several Akt substrates, the migration of fibroblasts and ECs, and NO release. Reconstitution of *Akt1 −/−*ECs with Akt1 rescues the defects in substrate phosphorylation, cell migration, and NO release. Thus, the Akt1 isoform exerts an essential role in blood flow control, cellular migration, and NO synthesis during postnatal angiogenesis.

▶ The Akt signaling pathway has been implicated in multiple angiogenic mechanisms. However, mice lacking Akt1 develop relatively normally, which suggests redundancy with other pathways or a nonessential role for this pathway in embryonic angiogenesis. The authors examined several angiogenic/arteriogenic phenotypes in Akt1- or Akt2-deficient mice and found that Akt1 serves as a key regulator of postnatal angiogenesis. Thus, fundamental vascular biological signaling pathways not critical for development may exert profound effects postnatally in response to environmental perturbations such as ischemia.

C. K. Ozaki, MD

START Trial: A Pilot Study on STimulation of ARTeriogenesis Using Sub-cutaneous Application of Granulocyte-Macrophage Colony-Stimulating Factor as a New Treatment for Peripheral Vascular Disease
van Royen N, Schirmer SH, Atasever B, et al (Univ of Amsterdam; Univ of Freiburg, Germany; Max Planck Inst, Bad Nauheim, Germany; et al)
Circulation 112:1040-1046, 2005   1–35

Background.—Granulocyte-macrophage colony-stimulating factor (GM-CSF) was recently shown to increase collateral flow index in patients with coronary artery disease. Experimental models showed beneficial effects of GM-CSF on collateral artery growth in the peripheral circulation. Thus, in the present study, we evaluated the effects of GM-CSF in patients with peripheral artery disease.

Method and Results.—A double-blinded, randomized, placebo-controlled study was performed in 40 patients with moderate or severe intermittent claudication. Patients were treated with placebo or subcutaneously applied GM-CSF (10 µg/kg) for a period of 14 days (total of 7 injections). GM-CSF treatment led to a strong increase in total white blood cell count and C-reactive protein. Monocyte fraction initially increased but thereafter decreased significantly as compared with baseline. Both the placebo group and the treatment group showed a significant increase in walking distance at day 14 (placebo: 127 ± 67 versus 184 ± 87 meters, $P=0.03$, GM-CSF: 126 ± 66 versus 189 ± 141 meters, $P=0.04$) and at day 90. Change in walking time, the primary end point of the study, was not different between groups. No change in ankle-brachial index was found on GM-CSF treatment at day 14 or at day 90. Laser Doppler flowmetry measurements showed a significant decrease in microcirculatory flow reserve in the control group ($P=0.03$) and no change in the GM-CSF group.

Conclusions.—The present study does not support the use of GM-CSF for treatment of patients with moderate or severe intermittent claudication. Issues that need to be addressed are dosing, the selection of patients, and potential differences between GM-CSF effects in the coronary and the peripheral circulation.

▶ Animal studies support a positive role for GM-CSF in stimulating collateral artery recruitment (arteriogenesis). The results in this small, controlled GM-CSF trial involving patients with claudication were negative. This START trial again points out the importance of a placebo control arm in claudication studies, as illustrated by its ~50% increase in walking distance at 14 days for both groups. Medication side effect rates were high. The paradoxical aspect of this strategy is that arteriogenesis is driven largely by proinflammatory mechanisms. Treatment with agents like GM-CSF increase inflammatory marker levels (eg, C-reactive protein), which can potentially have negative long-term consequences. The results conflict with similar research in human coronary disease in which an increase in the coronary collateral flow index has been observed. There are biological differences between vascular beds and their responses to occlusive disease.

C. K. Ozaki, MD

Sympathetic innervation promotes vascular smooth muscle differentiation
Damon DH (Univ of Vermont, Burlington)
Am J Physiol Heart Circ Physiol 288:H2785-H2791, 2005   1–36

The sympathetic nervous system (SNS) is an important modulator of vascular smooth muscle (VSM) growth and function. Several lines of evidence suggest that the SNS also promotes VSM differentiation. The present study tests this hypothesis. Expression of smooth muscle myosin (SM2) and α-actin were assessed by Western analysis as indexes of VSM differentiation. SM2 expression (normalized to α-actin) in adult innervated rat femoral and tail arteries was $479 \pm 115\%$ of that in noninnervated carotid arteries. Expression of α-actin (normalized to GAPDH or total protein) in 30-day-innervated rat femoral arteries was greater than in corresponding noninnervated femoral arteries from guanethidine-sympathectomized rats. SM2 expression (normalized to α-actin) in neonatal femoral arteries grown in vitro for 7 days in the presence of sympathetic ganglia was greater than SM2 expression in corresponding arteries grown in the absence of sympathetic ganglia. In VSM-endothelial cell cultures grown in the presence of dissociated sympathetic neurons, α-actin (normalized to GAPDH) was $300 \pm 66\%$ of that in corresponding cultures grown in the absence of neurons. This effect was inhibited by an antibody that neutralized the activity of transforming growth factor-$\beta2$. All of these data indicate that sympathetic innervation increased VSM contractile protein expression and thereby suggest that the SNS promotes and/or maintains VSM differentiation.

▶ Vascular tone, modulated by the SNS, is often neglected in considerations of arterial response to injury. This basic laboratory investigation shows that smooth muscle cell denervation may be one mechanism whereby postinjury neointimal hyperplasia occurs. How this study may relate to the clinical situation is difficult to determine. For example, how often vascular denervation occurs with a peripheral bypass or whether periatherosclerotic inflammation causes this process has not been well studied in human beings.

P. K. Henke, MD

Sonoporation with Doxorubicin Enhances Suppression of Intimal Hyperplasia in a Vein Graft Model

Mizuno Y, Iwata H, Takagi H, et al (Gifu Univ, Japan)
J Surg Res 124:312-317, 2005
1–37

Background.—The purpose of the present study is to examine whether sonoporation with doxorubicin enhances suppression of intimal hyperplasia (IH) in a vein graft model.

Materials and Methods.—After the administration of 1.5 mg/kg doxorubicin intravenously, the right external jugular vein of six rabbits was exposed at 2 W/cm^2 and 1 MHz of ultrasound for 2 min (Sonoporation group). Tissue doxorubicin concentration was measured. In 48 rabbits, the right common carotid artery was ligated after performing a vein graft bypass. The animals were divided into the following four groups: the C0 group (surgical procedure only); the C0S (sonoporation without doxorubicin); the C1 (doxorubicin administration only); the C1S (sonoporation with doxorubicin). Twenty-four grafts were subjected to Elastic van Gieson staining for morphometric analysis 4 weeks after the operation; others were subjected to TdT-mediated X-dUTP nick end-labeling for detection of apoptotic cells and to staining with a monoclonal antibody against the proliferating cell nuclear antigen for assessment of cell proliferation 1 week after.

Results.—The tissue doxorubicin concentration was significantly higher in the Sonoporation group than in the Control group. Compared with the C0 group, IH was not suppressed in the C1 group but was significantly suppressed in the C1S group. Sonoporation with doxorubicin administration suppressed IH significantly (C1 group versus *C1S group: P* < 0.05). Cell apoptosis was induced and cell proliferation was suppressed significantly in the C1S group.

Conclusions.—Sonoporation with doxorubicin suppressed IH of the vein graft. Sonoporation may be effective in coronary or peripheral revascularization using vein grafts.

▶ Transcranial Doppler US has recently been shown clinically to improve thrombolysis in stroke patients treated with plasmin activators in the local artery tree. This experimental study of interposition vein grafts in rabbits shows that the systemic delivery of an antiproliferative agent can be enhanced by high-frequency US in the region of the vein graft. The systemic immunosuppressive effects were not discussed. Whether this methodology could work in deeper and/or diseased artery–graft anastomoses is not clear but certainly warrants further study.

P. K. Henke, MD

Nitric oxide modulates vascular inflammation and intimal hyperplasia in insulin resistance and the metabolic syndrome

Barbato JE, Zuckerbraun BS, Overhaus M, et al (Univ of Pittsburgh, Pa)
Am J Physiol Heart Circ Physiol 289:H228-H236, 2005   1–38

Type 2 diabetes mellitus (DM) and the metabolic syndrome, both characterized by insulin resistance, are associated with an accelerated form of atherosclerotic vascular disease and poor outcomes following vascular interventions. These vascular effects are thought to stem from a heightened inflammatory environment and reduced bioavailability of nitric oxide (NO). To better understand this process, we characterized the vascular injury response in the obese Zucker rat by examining the expression of adhesion molecules, the recruitment of inflammatory cells, and the development of intimal hyperplasia. We also evaluated the ability of exogenous NO to inhibit the sequela of vascular injury in the metabolic syndrome. Obese and lean Zucker rats underwent carotid artery balloon injury. ICAM-1 and P-selectin expression were increased following injury in the obese animals compared with the lean rats. The obese rats also responded with increased macrophage infiltration of the vascular wall as well as increased neointima formation compared with their lean counterparts (intima/media = 0.91 vs. 0.52, $P = 0.001$). After adenovirus-mediated inducible NO synthase (iNOS) gene transfer, ICAM-1, P-selectin, inflammatory cell influx, and oxidized low-density lipoprotein (LDL) receptor expression were all markedly reduced versus injury alone. iNOS gene transfer also significantly inhibited proliferative activity (54% and 73%; $P < 0.05$) and neointima formation (53% and 67%; $P < 0.05$) in lean and obese animals, respectively. The vascular injury response in the face of obesity and the metabolic syndrome is associated with increased adhesion molecule expression, inflammatory cell infiltration, oxidized LDL receptor expression, and proliferation. iNOS gene transfer is able to effectively inhibit this heightened injury response and reduce neointima formation in this proinflammatory environment.

▶ With the epidemic of type 2 diabetes and the metabolic syndrome, it is logical to focus on the vascular response to injury and the increased oxidative stress and inflammatory phenotype of the obese mammal with insulin resistance and hyperlipidemia. The authors nicely confirm the value of the Zucker rat model in reaching this goal. In addition to robustly characterizing obese rats' unique response to injury compared with that of lean control rats, these authors structured their experiments to probe mechanisms. The findings suggest the potential value of iNOS gene transfer therapy in the setting of insulin resistance and the metabolic syndrome.

C. K. Ozaki, MD

Sirolimus-Eluting Stents to Abolish Intimal Hyperplasia and Improve Flow in Porcine Arteriovenous Grafts: A 4-Week Follow-Up Study

Rotmans JI, Pattynama PMT, Verhagen HJM, et al (Univ Med Ctr, Utrecht, The Netherlands; Univ Med Ctr Rotterdam, The Netherlands; Academic Med Ctr, Amsterdam)
Circulation 111:1537-1542, 2005
1–39

Background.—The patency of arteriovenous (AV) expanded polytetrafluoroethylene (ePTFE) hemodialysis grafts is severely compromised by intimal hyperplasia (IH) at the venous anastomosis and in the venous outflow tract. We addressed the potential of primary placement of a sirolimus-eluting stent (SES) in a validated porcine model.

Method and Results.—In 25 pigs, ePTFE AV grafts were created bilaterally between the carotid artery and the jugular vein, whereupon a self-expandable nitinol stent (14 SESs and 11 bare-metal stents) was implanted over the venous anastomosis in 1 of the 2 grafts. After exclusion of technical failures and 1 unilateral occlusion, 16 pigs (9 SESs and 7 bare-metal stents) were included for further analysis. After 28 days, we measured graft flow and performed quantitative angiography. The pigs were then euthanized, and grafts with adjacent vessels were excised for histological analysis. Minimal luminal diameter was substantially larger in the SES group compared with unstented controls (5.9 ± 0.2 versus 3.8 ± 0.4 mm, respectively, $P=0.01$), which was accompanied by more prominent graft flow (SES, 1360 ± 89 mL/min versus unstented, 861 ± 83 mL/min, $P=0.05$). IH at the venous anastomosis was 77% less in the SES group compared with unstented controls (0.44 ± 0.05 versus 1.92 ± 0.5 mm^2, respectively, $P=0.01$), whereas IH increased markedly when bare-metal stents were used (5.7 ± 1.4 mm^2, $P=0.05$).

Conclusions.—SESs in the venous outflow of AV grafts significantly reduce IH and increase vessel diameter and graft flow compared with unstented grafts. These findings suggest that SESs have the potential to improve primary patency of AV grafts in hemodialysis patients.

▶ Oversizing of the stents may have contributed to the increased IH in the bare-metal stented group. The use of an SES stent appears to obviate the IH effects of the venous anastomotic stent and provide improved venous anastomotic diameters and flows over unstented venous anastomoses. Obviously, this is a porcine model with short, very high flow grafts. Nevertheless, data such as these certainly can, and likely will be, used to support a clinical trial in human beings.

G. L. Moneta, MD

Mitochondrial-dependent apoptosis in experimental rodent abdominal aortic aneurysms

Sinha I, Sinha-Hikim AP, Hannawa KK, et al (Univ of Michigan, Ann Arbor; Harbor-UCLA, Torrance, Calif)
Surgery 138:806-811, 2005   1–40

Objectives.—While extrinsic mechanisms of apoptosis in abdominal aortic aneurysms (AAAs) are recognized, this project hypothesizes that an intrinsic, mitochondrial-dependent mechanism of apoptosis also contributes to experimental AAA formation.

Methods.—Rat aortas were perfused with either saline or elastase (N = 5 per group) and harvested 7 days postperfusion. The aortas were placed in gluteraldehyde for subsequent transmission electron microscopy, Bouin's solution for TUNEL, or paraformaldehyde for immunohistochemical staining for caspase-9, caspase-3, and Bid.

Results.—Abdominal aortic diameters increased 168 ± 25% (mean ± SEM) after elastase perfusion. compared with 30 ± 5% after saline perfusion (*P* < .001). Apoptosis of aortic smooth muscle cells, macrophages, and neutrophils was evidenced by transmission electron microscopy and TUNEL in the elastase-perfused aneurysmal aortas. Quantitative analysis of the apoptotic cells revealed a significant (*P* < .01) increase in the number of total apoptotic cells in the elastase-perfused aortas (12 ± 3 cells per high-power field), compared with that of saline-infused controls (1.3 ± 0.2). Caspase-9,

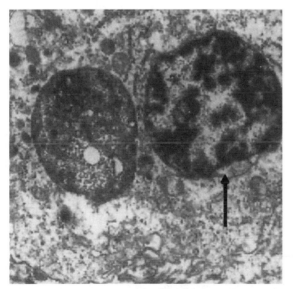

FIGURE 3. — Multiple apoptotic cell types are visualized in the elastase-perfused aortas by transmission electron microscopy. *Arrows* are pointing toward chromatin. **A**, An apoptotic macrophage shows chromatin fragmentation characteristic of apoptosis. (Reprinted by permission of the publisher from Sinha I, Sinha-Hikim AP, Hannawa KK, et al: Mitochondrial-dependent apoptosis in experimental rodent abdominal aortic aneurysms. *Surgery* 138.806-811, 2005. Copyright 2005 by Elsevier.)

the key initiator in the mitochondrial-dependent apoptotic pathway, stained positively in only elastase-perfused aortas. Bid staining was not detected in either the elastase-perfused aortas or the saline controls.

Conclusions.—Apoptosis is evident in multiple cell lines in elastase-perfused aneurysmal aortas, but rarely observed in control aortas. Caspase-9, the key initiator of intrinsic apoptosis, was documented only in elastase-perfused aortas. These results suggest that mitochondrial-dependent apoptosis is associated with abdominal aortic aneurysm formation (Fig 3).

▶ Although debate exists on the relevance of animal models of AAAs compared with human AAAs, this experimental study suggests that mitochondrial-associated apoptosis may play a role in AAA pathogenesis. However, whether this process is present early, is mechanistic, or is a manifestation of the late pathologic features of aneurysms is not answered in this study because only one later time was evaluated. Unfortunately, human studies will unlikely better clarify this, as the only aneurysmal tissue available for detailed histologic analysis is from late stages of AAA development. Apoptosis does play a role in vascular pathology. The important question is whether this process could be specifically manipulated to halt AAA growth.

P. K. Henke, MD

Neutrophil Depletion Inhibits Experimental Abdominal Aortic Aneurysm Formation

Eliason JL, Hannawa KK, Ailawadi G, et al (Univ of Michigan, Ann Arbor; Washington Univ, St Louis)
Circulation 112:232-240, 2005   1–41

Background.—Neutrophils may be an important source of matrix metalloproteinase-2 (MMP-2) and matrix metalloproteinase-9 (MMP-9), two matrix-degrading enzymes thought to be critical in the formation of an abdominal aortic aneurysm (AAA). The purpose of this investigation was to test the hypothesis that neutrophil depletion would limit experimental AAA formation by altering one or both of these enzymes.

Method and Results.—Control, rabbit serum–treated (RS; n=27) or anti-neutrophil-antibody–treated (anti-PMN; n=25) C57BL/6 mice underwent aortic elastase perfusion to induce experimental aneurysms. Anti-PMN–treated mice became neutropenic (mean, 349 cells/µL), experiencing an 84% decrease in the circulating absolute neutrophil count ($P<0.001$) before elastase perfusion. Fourteen days after elastase perfusion, control mice exhibited a mean aortic diameter (AD) increase of $104\pm14\%$ ($P<0.0001$), and 67% developed AAAs, whereas anti-PMN–treated mice exhibited a mean AD increase of $42\pm33\%$, with 8% developing AAAs. The control group also had increased tissue neutrophils (20.3 versus 8.6 cells per 5 high-powered fields [HPFs]; $P=0.02$) and macrophages (6.1 versus 2.1 cells per 5 HPFs, $P=0.005$) as compared with anti-PMN–treated mice. There were no differences in monocyte chemotactic protein-1 or macrophage inflammatory protein-1α chemokine levels between groups by enzyme-linked immunosorbent assay. Neutrophil collagenase (MMP-8) expression was detected only in the 14-day control mice, with increased MMP-8 protein levels by Western blotting ($P=0.017$), and MMP-8–positive neutrophils were seen almost exclusively in this group. Conversely, there were no statistical differences in MMP-2 or MMP-9 mRNA expression, protein levels, enzyme activity, or immunostaining patterns between groups. When C57BL/6 wild-type (n=15) and MMP-8–deficient mice (n=17) were subjected to elastase perfusion, however, ADs at 14 days were no different in size (134±7.9% versus 154±9.9%; $P=0.603$), which suggests that MMP-8 serves only as a marker for the presence of neutrophils and is not critical for AAA formation.

Conclusions.—Circulating neutrophils are an important initial component of experimental AAA formation. Neutrophil depletion inhibits AAA development through a non–MMP-2/9–mediated mechanism associated with attenuated inflammatory cell recruitment.

▶ Neutrophils are not thought to be a "smart leukocyte" like the monocyte. This leukocyte class has received less attention than monocytes in aneurysm pathogenesis. Histologic studies in human AAAs have suggested that the interface between the thrombus and arterial wall has a high concentration of neutrophils. This experimental study confirms the importance of the neutrophil in an elastase model of AAA genesis, although the exact mechanism is not discerned. However, it is unlikely that MMP-2, -8, and -9 play a significant role, at least at the later time points. It is more likely that another enzyme released by the neutrophil results in aneurysmal development in this model. Whether neutrophils are critical for AAA initiating events or appear at the end stage of the disease is not clear.

P. K. Henke, MD

Treatment With Simvastatin Suppresses the Development of Experimental Abdominal Aortic Aneurysms in Normal and Hypercholesterolemic Mice

Steinmetz EF, Buckley C, Shames ML, et al (Washington Univ, St Louis)
Ann Surg 241:92-101, 2005   1–42

Objective.—To determine if treatment with hydroxymethylglutaryl-coenzyme A reductase inhibitors (statins) can influence the development of experimental abdominal aortic aneurysms (AAAs).

Summary Background Data.—AAAs are associated with atherosclerosis, chronic inflammation, and matrix metalloproteinase (MMP)-mediated connective tissue destruction. Because statins exert antiinflammatory activities independent of their lipid-lowering effects, these agents may help suppress aneurysmal degeneration.

Methods.—C57Bl/6 wild-type and hypercholesterolemic apoE-deficient mice underwent transient perfusion of the aorta with elastase followed by subcutaneous treatment with either 2 mg/kg simvastatin per day or vehicle.

Aortic diameter (AD) was measured before and 14 days after elastase perfusion. The extent of aortic dilatation (ΔAD) was determined with AAAs defined as ΔAD >100%.

Results.—Wild-type mice treated with simvastatin exhibited a 21% reduction in ΔAD and a 33% reduction in AAAs compared with vehicle-treated controls. Suppression of AAAs in simvastatin-treated mice was associated with preservation of medial elastin and vascular smooth muscle cells, as well as a relative reduction in aortic wall expression of MMP-9 and a relative increase in expression of TIMP-1. In hypercholesterolemic apoE-deficient mice, treatment with simvastatin was associated with a 26% reduction in ΔAD and a 30% reduction in AAAs. Treatment with simvastatin had no effect on serum cholesterol levels in either normal or hypercholesterolemic mice.

Conclusions.—Treatment with simvastatin suppresses the development of experimental AAAs in both normal and hypercholesterolemic mice. The mechanisms of this effect are independent of lipid-lowering and include preservation of medial elastin and smooth muscle cells, as well as altered aortic wall expression of MMPs and their inhibitors.

▶ These authors have previously documented suppression of elastin-induced aneurysm formation using the MMP inhibitor doxycycline. The current results may ultimately translate into a clinical recommendation for statin treatment for patients with small AAAs to lower the rates at which aneurysm diameters increase. However, I am not holding my breath.

G. L. Moneta, MD

Systemic Dilation Diathesis in Patients with Abdominal Aortic Aneurysms: A Role for Matrix Metalloproteinase-9?
van Laake LW, Vainas T, Dammers R, et al (Univ of Maastricht, The Netherlands; Cardiovascular Research Inst Maastricht, The Netherlands)
Eur J Vasc Endovasc Surg 29:371-377, 2005   1–43

Introduction.—Accumulating evidence suggests that patients with abdominal aortic aneurysm (AAA) suffer from a systemic dilating condition affecting all arteries. Matrix metalloproteinases (MMPs) and their natural inhibitors, the tissue inhibitors of metalloproteinases (TIMPs), appear to be involved in aneurysm formation, as evidenced by increased aortic tissue MMP activity and plasma MMP levels in patients with AAA. Hypothesizing that an imbalance in plasma MMP/TIMP level might be associated with a systemic dilation diathesis, we studied mechanical vessel wall properties of non-affected arteries of patients with either AAA or aorto-iliac obstructive lesions in association with plasma MMP-9 and TIMP-1 levels.

Methods.—Twenty-two patients with AAA and 12 with aorto-iliac occlusive disease (AOD) were included. Diastolic diameter (d) and distension (Δd) were measured at the level of the common carotid artery (CCA) and suprarenal aorta (SA) using ultrasonography. Distensibility (DC) and compliance

(CC) were calculated from d, Δd and brachial pulse pressure. Plasma MMP-9 and TIMP-1 were determined with specific immunoassays.

Results.—The average (±SD) age was 72.3±5.6 and 65.0±8.2 years for the AAA and AOD patients, respectively, ($P=0.005$). CCA diameter was 9.1±1.3 mm in AAA patients and 7.8±1.4 mm in AOD patients, $P=0.009$. This difference persisted after correction for age. Plasma MMP-9 and TIMP-1 did not differ significantly between AAA and AOD patients. In the total 34 patients, the MMP-9/TIMP-1 ratio was correlated inversely with distensibility ($r=-0.74$, $P=0.002$) and to compliance ($r=-0.58$, $P=0.024$) of the suprarenal aorta.

Conclusions.—The CCA diameter was larger in AAA patients compared to AOD patients. MMP-9/TIMP-1 ratio was associated with decreased distensibility and compliance of the suprarenal aorta. These data support the idea that AAA patients exhibit a systemic dilation diathesis, which might be attributable to MMP/TIMP imbalances.

▶ Consistent with the current working hypothesis of AAA progression, this study correlates two measures of arterial biomechanics with the MMP-9 and TIMP-1 ratio. However, no differences were found in absolute levels of these mediators in those patients with AOD or AAA. Further, no correlation was seen between the serum level of MMP-9 or TIMP-1 and typical risk factors for AAA size. The only positive finding was decreased arterial DC and the MMP-9/TIMP-1 ratio. This is weak epidemiological evidence that MMPs may play a role in AAAs. A much better study would be a longitudinal evaluation in patients at high risk of developing AAAs or following the growth of small AAAs and serially measuring these variables.

P. K. Henke, MD

MMP-12 has a role in abdominal aortic aneurysms in mice

Longo GM, Buda SJ, Fiotta N, et al (Univ of Nebraska, Omaha; Brigham and Women's Hosp, Boston)
Surgery 137:457-462, 2005   1–44

Background.—Matrix metalloproteinase (MMP)-12 levels are increased in the abdominal aortic aneurysm (AAA), implicating this protease in AAA pathogenesis. The purpose of this study was to assess the role of MMP-12 in aneurysm formation.

Methods.—A murine aneurysm model was generated by periaortic application of 0.25 mol/L calcium chloride ($CaCl_2$) for 15 minutes. Aortic diameters were measured and compared before and 10 weeks after aneurysm induction. Aortic diameter changes for wild type (WT) and MMP-12 knockout (MMP-12$^{-/-}$) mice were determined. MMP-12 production in mouse aorta was analyzed by casein zymography. MMP-2 and MMP-9 expressions were examined by gelatin zymography. Immunohistochemical study was used to measure macrophage infiltration into the aorta.

Results.—There is an increase of 63 ± 5% (mean ± SEM) in aortic diameters of WT mice after $CaCl_2$ inductions, while MMP-12$^{-/-}$ mice increased only 26 ± 14%. Connective tissue staining of aortic sections from WT mice showed disruption and fragmentation of medial elastic fibers, while MMP-12$^{-/-}$ mice showed only focal elastic lamellae breakdown. MMP-12 levels in WT mice were significantly increased after $CaCl_2$ treatment, whereas no MMP-12 was detected in MMP-12$^{-/-}$ mice. There was no difference in the MMP-2 and MMP-9 productions between WT and MMP-12$^{-/-}$ mice. Immunohistochemical analysis demonstrated that infiltrating macrophages in the aorta of MMP-12$^{-/-}$ mice were significantly less than WT controls.

Conclusions.—MMP-12 deficiency attenuates aneurysm growth, possibly by decreasing macrophage recruitment.

▶ This study supports the hypothesis that MMP-12 plays some role in aneurysm pathogenesis. The major source of MMP-12 in vivo is the macrophage. The macrophage may, thus, play an important role in aneurysm formation. Macrophages can convert pro-MMP-12 to an active form and trigger lysis of the elastic component of the aortic wall, which results in medial destruction and aneurysm formation.

G. L. Moneta, MD

Enhanced Abdominal Aortic Aneurysm in TIMP-1-Deficient Mice

Eskandari MK, Vijungco JD, Flores A, et al (Northwestern Univ, Chicago)
J Surg Res 123:289-293, 2005   1–45

Background.—Matrix metalloproteinases (MMPs) are known elastolytic mediators of abdominal aortic aneurysm (AAA) degeneration, and their activity is tightly regulated by the presence of tissue inhibitors of MMPs (TIMPs). Imbalances in this system may be instrumental in compromising arterial wall integrity. The aim of this study was to show that, in an elastase-induced murine model of aneurysm formation, TIMP-1 has a protective effect.

Materials and Methods.—Twenty-four wild-type (TIMP-1$^{+/+}$) and 22 knockout (TIMP-1$^{-/-}$) mice underwent laparotomy and isolation of the infrarenal aorta. A polyethylene catheter was inserted into the aorta and dilute pancreatic elastase (0.39 Units/ml) was infused over 5 min using a perfusion pump. Pre- and postinfusion maximal aortic diameters were obtained in triplicate for each animal using NIH Image. Final aortic measurements were obtained 14 days later, prior to perfusion fixation with 10% buffered Formalin. Aortic specimens were sectioned and stained. Statistical analysis was performed using the Student's *t* test.

Results.—TIMP-1$^{-/-}$ mice demonstrated a significant postinfusion diameter increase compared to wild-types after elastase, which was not seen after saline infusion. At sacrifice, TIMP-1$^{-/-}$ mice, following both saline and elastase infusion, showed a significant increase in maximal aortic diameter relative to postinfusion measurements compared to TIMP-1$^{+/+}$ mice.

Conclusions.—TIMP-1$^{-/-}$ mice develop larger aneurysms than TIMP-1$^{+/+}$ mice. This study illustrates the protective effects of TIMP-1 in an experimental AAA model and may provide a means for pharmacologically controlling aneurysm growth.

▶ While the role of MMPs in AAA pathogenesis has been confirmed, the impact of the endogenous TIMPs remains less established. Taking advantage of TIMP-1 deficient mice, the authors reveal a protective role for TIMP-1 on the aneurysm-prone artery wall. Understanding TIMP biology in parallel with MMP dynamics will enhance understanding of the imbalance of local proteolytic activity in aneurysm development.

C. K. Ozaki, MD

Association of Osteoprotegerin With Human Abdominal Aortic Aneurysm Progression

Moran CS, McCann M, Karan M, et al (James Cook Univ, Townsville, Australia; Univ of Western Australia, Fremantle)
Circulation 111:3119-3125, 2005   1–46

Background.—Abdominal aortic aneurysm (AAA) is characterized by destruction of the arterial media associated with loss of vascular smooth muscle cells, infiltration of mononuclear cells, and high concentration of metalloproteinases (MMPs) and cytokines. Osteoprotegerin (OPG) has recently been identified in atherosclerosis. The presence and functional importance of OPG in human AAA was investigated.

Method and Results.—In 146 men with small AAA followed up by ultrasound for 3 years, serum OPG was weakly correlated with aneurysm growth rate. Western analysis showed 3-, 8-, and 12-fold-greater OPG concentrations in human AAA biopsies compared with biopsies of atherosclerotic narrowed aorta (1.4 ± 0.1 versus 0.5 ± 0.1 ng/mg tissue; $P=0.002$), postmortem nondiseased abdominal aorta (1.4 ± 0.1 versus 0.2 ± 0.1 ng/mg tissue; $P<0.001$), and nondiseased thoracic aorta (1.4 ± 0.1 versus 0.1 ± 0.06 ng/mg tissue; $P<0.001$). Healthy human aortic vascular smooth muscle cells incubated with recombinant human (rh)OPG (0 to 20 ng rhOPG/10^5) cells per 1 mL per 24 hours) developed an aneurysmal phenotype defined by impaired cell proliferation ($P<0.001$), increased apoptosis ($P<0.01$), and increased MMP-9 (92 kDa) expression ($P<0.001$). Incubation of monocytic THP-1 cells with 1 ng rhOPG/10^5 cells per 1 mL per 24 hours induced a 2-fold increase in MMP-9 expression ($P<0.001$), a 1.5-fold increase in MMP-2 activity ($P=0.005$), and a 2-fold stimulation of IL-6 production in these cells ($P=0.02$). Finally, secretion of OPG from human AAA explant was abrogated by treatment with the angiotensin II blocker irbesartan, with the reduction in secreted levels averaging 63.0 ± 0.9 ng/mg tissue per 48-hour period.

Conclusions.—These findings support a role for OPG in the growth of human AAA and suggest a potential benefit for angiotensin II blockade in slowing aneurysm expansion.

▶ OPG has been implicated in human atherosclerosis, and now evidence is provided that it also drives aortic aneurysm progression. The authors give in vitro results that support OPG having a role in aneurysm genesis: it appears to lead to smooth muscle cell and monocyte phenotypes that are thought to participate in pathobiological aneurysm features. Angiotensin II upregulates OPG. In the current article, angiotensin II blockade attenuated AAA tissue OPG secretion. Distinctive OPG signaling pathways that result in an atherosclerotic versus an aneurysmal aorta are not defined, which makes it unclear how OPG could participate in both processes. We have seen medical therapies for occlusive atherosclerosis emerge over the last few decades. One can envision a similar emergence of medical treatment for patients with aortic aneurysmal disease.

C. K. Ozaki, MD

Overexpression of Transforming Growth Factor-β1 Stabilizes Already-Formed Aortic Aneurysms: A First Approach to Induction of Functional Healing by Endovascular Gene Therapy

Dai J, Losy F, Guinault A-M, et al (Université Paris XII; Assistance Publique des Hôpitaux de Paris; Hôpital H Mondor, Créteil, France; et al)
Circulation 112:1008-1015, 2005   1–47

Background.—The cell response to transforming growth factor-β1 (TGF-β1), a multipotent cytokine with healing potential, varies according to tissue context. We have evaluated the ability of TGF-β1 overexpression by endovascular gene therapy to stabilize abdominal aortic aneurysms (AAAs) already injured by inflammation and proteolysis.

Method and Results.—Active TGF-β1 overexpression was obtained in already-developed experimental AAAs in rats after endovascular delivery of an adenoviral construct encoding for a mutated form of active simian TGF-β1 and in an explant model using human atherosclerotic AAA fragments incubated with recombinant active TGF-β1. Transient exogenous TGF-β1 overexpression by endovascular gene delivery was followed by induction of endogenous rat TGF-β1. Overexpression of active TGF-β1 in experimental AAAs was associated with diameter stabilization, preservation of medial elastin, decreased infiltration of monocyte-macrophages and T lymphocytes, and a decrease in matrix metalloproteinase-2 and -9, which was also observed in the explant model, in both thrombus and wall. In parallel with downregulation of the destructive process, active TGF-β1 overexpression triggered endoluminal reconstruction, replacing the thrombus by a vascular smooth muscle cell–, collagen-, and elastin-rich intima.

Conclusions.—Local TGF-β1 self-induction after transient exogenous overexpression reprograms dilated aortas altered by inflammation and proteolysis and restores their ability to withstand arterial pressure without further dilation. This first demonstration of stabilization of expanding AAAs by delivery of a single multipotent self-promoting gene supports the view that endovascular gene therapy should be considered for treatment of aneurysms.

▶ TGF-β1 stands as a central mediator of wound healing processes. The authors utilize genetic approaches to support that TGF-β1 can stabilize established AAAs via specific cellular and biochemical mechanisms. With the wide range of clinically positive and negative effects of TGF-β1 overexpression and the uncertainties of contemporary endovascularly delivered adenoviral gene therapy, attention to side effects will be necessary. Beyond extension of this direct gene therapy approach, this work should stimulate investigations into why human beings fail to upregulate endogenous TGF-β1 activity to counterbalance the destructive local environment of the expanding AAA.

C. K. Ozaki, MD

AIDS-related vasculopathy: evidence for oxidative and inflammatory pathways in murine and human AIDS
Baliga RS, Chaves AA, Jing L, et al (Ohio State Univ, Columbus)
Am J Physiol Heart Circ Physiol 289:I11373-H1380, 2005   1–48

Increased life expectancy of human immunodeficiency virus (HIV)-positive patients has led to evidence of complications apparently not directly related to immunodeficiency or opportunistic infection, including increased cardiovascular risk. We tested the hypothesis that vascular dysfunction occurs in the murine acquired immune deficiency syndrome (AIDS) model and evaluated potential mechanisms in murine AIDS tissues and relevant human HIV/AIDS vascular tissues. We also investigated endothelial activation and/or endothelial protein nitration and their association with time-dependent vascular dysfunction. At 1 and 5 wk of murine AIDS, statistically significant decreases in KCl contractility and time-dependent contractile deficits in response to phenylephrine were observed. The maximal response (E_{max}) was reduced by ~40% at 10 wk, and EC_{50} values were significantly changed: 102 ± 7.3 ng for control vs. 190 ± 37 and 130 ± 22 ng at 5 and 10 wk, respectively ($P < 0.05$). Endothelium-dependent relaxation to ACh was decreased (EC_{50} = 120 ± 27 and 343 + 94 nM for control and at 10 wk, respectively), whereas the response to an exogenous nitric oxide donor, sodium nitroprusside, remained unchanged, suggesting a specific endothelial dysfunction. Histochemical investigations of the same vascular tissues as well as corresponding coronary endothelium showed an increase in protein 3-nitrotyrosine, intercellular adhesion molecule, and nitric oxide synthase isoforms 2 and 3. These findings were corroborated in concurrent experiments in a cohort of well-cataloged human cardiac microvascular tissues. We have demonstrated, for the first time, a specific functional vasculopathy with endothelial involvement in a murine model of AIDS that was also associated with and correlated to increased oxidative stress and specific endothelial activation. This finding was echoed in a relevant population of human HIV/AIDS patients. Research into sources and intracellular targets of oxidants in this disease could provide important mechanistic insights and may reveal new therapeutic opportunities for this increasingly important cardiovascular disease state.

▶ Successful medical therapies for HIV infection have brought vascular complications to the forefront for these patients. The authors utilized a murine AIDS model to qualify and dissect the molecular mechanisms of this vasculopathy. They found general alterations in reactive nitrogen species appear to contribute to vascular dysfunction. Some of the observations suggest that the host inflammatory–oxidative response to the virus, rather than the specific pathogen, may drive cardiovascular abnormalities in this model. They also found gross overall homology of the vascular changes they observed in the murine model with coronary artery endothelium from HIV/AIDS human autopsy samples. The murine model may, thus, be useful in preclinical therapeutic trials directed toward developing treatment for AIDS-related vasculopathy.

C. K. Ozaki, MD

Elevation of Endothelial Microparticles, Platelets, and Leukocyte Activation in Patients With Venous Thromboembolism

Chirinos JA, Heresi GA, Velasquez H, et al (Univ of Miami, Fla)

J Am Coll Cardiol 45:1467-1471, 2005   1–49

Objectives.—The purpose of this research was to determine the levels of platelet, leukocyte, and endothelial activation and markers of cellular interactions in patients with venous thromboembolism (VTE).

Background.—The details of interactions between endothelium, platelets, and leukocytes in VTE are not well understood.

Methods.—We studied 25 patients with VTE and compared 25 healthy controls. We used flow cytometry to measure: 1) endothelial microparticles (EMP) identified by CD31+/CD42b− (EMP_{31}) or E-selectin (EMP_{62E}); 2) platelet microparticles (CD31+/CD42b+); 3) surface expression of P-selectin in platelets and CD11b in leukocytes; 4) EMP-monocyte conjugates (percentage of monocytes positive for E-selectin); and 5) platelet-leukocyte conjugates (PLC) expressed as percentage of leukocytes positive for CD41.

Results.—Patients with VTE had marked elevations of EMP_{31} (2,193 vs. 383 counts/µl; $p = 0.003$), EMP_{62E} (368 vs. 223 counts/µl; $p = 0.001$), and EMP-monocyte conjugates (3.3% vs. 2.5%; $p = 0.002$), as well as increased activation of platelets (35.2 vs. 5.0 fluorescence intensity units for P-selectin; $p < 0.0001$) and leukocytes (13.9 vs. 7.7 U for CD11b; $p = 0.004$). Also elevated in VTE were PLC (61.7% vs. 39.6%; $p = 0.01$). Expression of CD11b in leukocytes strongly correlated with PLC ($r = 0.74$; $p < 0.0001$).

Conclusions.—Marked activation of endothelium, platelets, and leuko-cytes occurs in VTE, and VTE, or the accompanying inflammatory process, involves the release of EMP and formation of EMP-monocyte conjugates and PLC. These findings support prior studies suggesting that release of EMP and their binding to monocytes are key events in thrombogenesis. Our findings also support the concept that the formation of PLC regulates leuko-cyte activation and participates in linking thrombosis with inflammation.

▶ The complexity and dynamic state of VTE are now better known, and basic and clinical studies are forthcoming. This article highlights a specific endothelial-platelet mechanism of microparticles associated with the patho-genesis of VTE. It would be very useful if these measured laboratory markers could be adapted to clinical practice to predict the preclinical occurrence of deep vein thrombosis. However, all patients in this study had evidence of VTE, and the timing of the blood draw for these laboratory parameters and the onset of clinical symptoms was not presented in this study. Overall, more and more laboratory parameters will likely be available to predict those at high risk of VTE outside standard risk factor analysis, with the idea that more aggressive pro-phylactic therapy would be delivered.

P. K. Henke, MD

Identification of Differentially Expressed Genes in Primary Varicose Veins
Kim D-I, Eo H-S, Joh J-H (Sungkyunkwan Univ, Seoul, Korea; Samsung Bio-medical Research Inst, Seoul, Korea)
J Surg Res 123:222-226, 2005   1–50

Background.—A number of changes in protein expression have been de-scribed in primary varicose veins, but the altered gene expressions in this dis-ease are unknown. The aim of this study was to identify differentially ex-pressed genes in primary varicose veins.

Materials and Methods.—Total RNAs were isolated from two groups of greater saphenous veins (four primary varicose veins and three normal) and then were reverse transcribed into cDNAs. We used the differential display reverse transcription–polymerase chain reaction technique to screen the dif-ferences in the mRNA expression profiles of the groups.

Results.—We found that three cDNAs showed differences in expression patterns between normal and diseased saphenous veins. The cDNAs are prominently expressed only in patients with varicose veins. We identified that the cDNAs had significant similarities to the L1M4 repeat sequence of clone RP11-57L9, clone RP11-299H13, and Alu repetitive sequence of hu-man tropomyosin 4 mRNA.

Conclusions.—Our results suggest that the screened cDNA clones are use-ful disease markers in the genetic diagnosis of primary varicose vein and that the L1 and Alu elements possibly participated in the development of primary varicose veins through their expression patterns in genes encoded with structural proteins, such as collagen, elastin, and tropomyosin. Further studies are required to elucidate the potential relationship between repeat sequences and primary varicose veins.

▶ Varicose veins tend to run in families. This article, although with small patient numbers, shows that 3 genetic differences exist between control subjects and those with mild varicose veins. This study is controlled for CEAP class but not ongoing therapies. It is doubtful, given the relatively benign nature of venous varicosities, whether prospective genetic analysis in the clinical setting would be cost-effective or would alter therapy.

P. K. Henke, MD

2 Vascular Laboratory and Imaging

Diagnostic Performance of Duplex Ultrasound in Patients Suspected of Carotid Artery Disease: The Ipsilateral Versus Contralateral Artery
Heijenbrok-Kal MH, Nederkoorn PJ, Buskens E, et al (Erasmus MC-Univ Med Ctr, Rotterdam, the Netherlands; Academic Med Ctr Amsterdam; Harvard School of Public Health, Boston)
Stroke 36:2105-2109, 2005   2–1

Background and Purpose.—To evaluate duplex ultrasonographic thresholds for the determination of 70% to 99% stenosis of the ipsilateral and contralateral internal carotid artery in patients with symptoms of amaurosis fugax, transient ischemic attack (TIA), or minor stroke based on 2 criteria: maximizing accuracy and optimizing cost-effectiveness and to compare these with current recommendations.

Methods.—From January 1997 to January 2000, a prospective multicenter study was conducted including 350 consecutive patients with symptoms of amaurosis fugax, TIA, or minor stroke who underwent bilateral duplex ultrasonography and digital subtraction angiography. A linear regression analysis was performed to estimate the degree of angiographic stenosis as a function of the peak systolic velocity (PSV). PSV thresholds were calculated for the ipsilateral and contralateral carotid arteries based on maximizing accuracy and optimizing cost-effectiveness.

Results.—The PSV measurements significantly overestimated the angiographic stenosis in the contralateral artery (9.5%; 95% CI, 6.3% to 12.7%) compared with the ipsilateral carotid artery. The recommended PSV threshold for the diagnosis of 70% to 99% stenosis is 230 cm/s. Maximizing accuracy, the optimal PSV threshold for the ipsilateral artery was 280 cm/s, and for the contralateral artery, 370 cm/s for diagnosing a 70% to 99% stenosis. Optimizing cost effectiveness, the optimal PSV threshold was 220 cm/s for ipsilateral and 290 cm/s for contralateral carotid arteries.

Conclusions.—PSV measurements overestimate the degree of angiographic stenosis in the contralateral carotid artery in patients with symptoms of amaurosis fugax, TIA, or minor stroke. Separate PSV thresholds should be used for the ipsilateral and contralateral carotid artery. PSV thresholds that optimize cost-effectiveness differ from the recommended thresholds and from thresholds that maximize accuracy.

▶ In 2002, the Society for Radiologists and Ultrasound (SRU) convened a consensus conference and suggested a PSV of 230 cm/s as the criterion for detecting a 70% to 99% internal carotid artery (ICA) stenosis. There has, however, been a buzz that this criterion, while highly sensitive, had a poor positive predictive value. In our laboratory, a PSV of 230 cm/s would have a positive predictive value for 70% angiographic ICA stenosis of only 69%. This study confirms some of that "buzz." I think there will be more studies appearing suggesting the SRU PSV criterion for 70% ICA stenosis is too low. This would especially be the case if this criterion is used to select asymptomatic patients for a prophylactic carotid intervention.

G. L. Moneta, MD

Accuracy of Color Duplex Ultrasound Diagnosis of Spontaneous Carotid Dissection Causing Ischemia
Benninger DH, Georgiadis D, Gandjour J, et al (Univ Hosp of Zürich, Switzerland)
Stroke 37:377-381, 2006   2–2

Background and Purpose.—Spontaneous dissection of the cervical internal carotid artery (sICAD) is mainly assessed with MRI and magnetic resonance angiography (MRA), which are not always at hand. In contrast, color duplex sonography (CDS) is readily available. We undertook this prospective study to examine the accuracy of CDS to diagnose sICAD in patients with first carotid territory ischemia.

Methods.—Consecutive patients with first carotid territory stroke or transient ischemic attack or retinal ischemia underwent clinical and laboratory examinations, ECG, CDS of the cerebral arteries, cranial computed tomography in case of stroke or transient ischemic attack, and echocardiography and 24-hour ECG in selected cases. Patients were included, if they were <65 years of age, CDS showed a probable sICAD (cervical internal carotid artery stenosed or occluded), or had no determined etiology of ischemia. All of the included patients underwent cervical MRI and MRA±cerebral catheter angiography. The sonographer was blinded to the results of MRI and angiography studies.

Results.—We included 177 of 1652 screened patients. Excluded patients (n=1475) were ≥65 years old (n=818), had another determined cause of ischemia (n=1475), and had intracranial hemorrhage (n=58). CDS diagnosed sICAD in 77 of 177 patients, and the etiology of ischemia was undetermined in the remaining 100 patients. Cervical MRI and angiography showed 74 sICAD; there were 6 falsely positive and 3 falsely negative CDS findings. Thus, sensitivity, specificity, and positive and negative predictive values for CDS diagnosis of patients with sICAD causing carotid territory ischemia was 96%, 94%, 92%, and 97%, respectively.

Conclusions.—Color duplex ultrasound allows the reliable exclusion of sICAD in patients with carotid territory ischemia, whereas diagnosis of CDS of sICAD must be confirmed with cervical MRI and MRA.

▶ The very high negative predictive value for excluding sICAD with CDS, essentially, allows withholding of treatment for sICAD in patients where that diagnosis is suspected but in whom the duplex US shows no evidence of dissection. Positive predictive value is also excellent, but because such patients will be treated with anticoagulants or perhaps other interventions, patients in whom sICAD is diagnosed by CDS should have a confirmatory study before initiating treatment.

G. L. Moneta, MD

Duplex Ultrasound Remains a Reliable Test Even After Carotid Stenting
Peterson BG, Longo GM, Kibbe MR, et al (Northwestern Univ, Chicago)
Ann Vasc Surg 19:793-797, 2005   2–3

Transluminal arterial stenting reduces vessel compliance and may alter accurate interpretation of flow velocities. We reviewed duplex ultrasonography (DUS) following carotid stenting to identify criteria indicative of severe recurrent stenosis. This is a single-center retrospective review of 158 carotid stenoses treated with carotid angioplasty and stenting (CAS) from April 2001 to December 2004. DUS was obtained preoperatively, postoperatively, and at 3-month intervals thereafter. Peak systolic velocity (PSV) and end diastolic velocity (EDV) were analyzed. Mean follow-up was 12 months (range 1-40). Mean age was 71 ± 9 years (range 51-91; 74% men, 26% women). Three patients (1.9%) developed restenosis and one (0.6%) developed an asymptomatic occlusion during follow-up. Average preoperative PSV was 373 ± 123 cm/sec (mean ± SD) and EDV was 148 ± 63 cm/sec. Immediate postoperative PSV and EDV decreased by an average of 70% (average 118 ± 45 cm/sec) and 72% (average 32 ± 15 cm/sec), respectively. In patients free from restenosis or occlusion, these reductions (range 65-80%) were maintained throughout follow-up and remained within 1-25% of immediate postoperative values. In patients suffering restenosis or occlusion, follow-up PSV and EDV increased 34% and 28%, respectively, compared to preoperative values. PSV and EDV increased by an average of 287% and 500%, respectively, compared to immediate postoperative values. Using criteria of PSV >170 cm/sec and a 50% increase of PSV over immediate postoperative values, restenosis or occlusion was detected with 100% sensitivity and specificity in our patients. Additionally, EDV >120 cm/sec and a 50% increase in EDV over immediate postoperative values detected restenosis and occlusion with 100% sensitivity and specificity. Presumed restenosis and occlusion detected by DUS were confirmed in all cases with angiography. Restenosis or occlusion after CAS at our institution can reliably be detected by carotid duplex using cut-off values of 170 cm/sec PSV, 120 cm/sec EDV, and >50% increase over immediate postoperative values. While these criteria are applied to patients undergoing CAS at our institution, they serve only as suggested guidelines for patient populations at other centers and must be customized to each Intersocietal Commission for the Accreditation of Vascular Laboratories-accredited vascular laboratory.

▶ Several papers have suggested slightly different criteria to detect stenosis in stented versus nonstented carotid arteries. This article shows that recommended velocity thresholds to detect stenosis in stented arteries should be higher than in native arteries. A slightly new twist is comparison of late velocities to immediate poststent placement velocities. This comparison seems to work in this analysis, but I wonder whether criteria for stenosis in stented carotid arteries will need to be indexed to disease in the opposite internal carotid artery.

G. L. Moneta, MD

Sensitivity and specificity of color duplex ultrasound measurement in the estimation of internal carotid artery stenosis: A systematic review and meta-analysis

Jahromi AS, Ciná CS, Liu Y, et al (McMaster Univ, Hamilton, Ont, Canada; Univ of Toronto)

J Vasc Surg 41:962-972, 2005   2–4

Background.—Duplex ultrasound is widely used for the diagnosis of internal carotid artery stenosis. Standard duplex ultrasound criteria for the grading of internal carotid artery stenosis do not exist; thus, we conducted a systematic review and meta-analysis of the relation between the degree of internal carotid artery stenosis by duplex ultrasound criteria and degree of stenosis by angiography.

Methods.—Data were gathered from Medline from January 1966 to January 2003, the Cochrane Central Register of Controlled Trials and Database of Systematic Reviews, Database of Abstracts of Reviews of Effects, ACP Journal Club, UpToDate, reference lists, and authors' files. Inclusion criteria were the comparison of color duplex ultrasound results with angiography by the North American Symptomatic Carotid Endarterectomy Trial method; peer-reviewed publications, and ≥10 adults.

Results.—Variables extracted included internal carotid artery peak systolic velocity, internal carotid artery end diastolic velocity, internal carotid artery/common carotid artery peak systolic velocity ratio, sensitivity and specificity of duplex ultrasound scanning for internal carotid artery stenosis by angiography. The Standards for Reporting of Diagnostic Accuracy (STARD) criteria were used to assess study quality. Sensitivity and specificity for duplex ultrasound criteria were combined as weighted means by using a random effects model. The threshold of peak systolic velocity ≥130 cm/s is associated with sensitivity of 98% (95% confidence intervals [CI], 97% to 100%) and specificity of 88% (95% CI, 76% to 100%) in the identification of angiographic stenosis of ≥50%. For the diagnosis of angiographic stenosis of ≥70%, a peak systolic velocity ≥200 cm/s has a sensitivity of 90% (95% CI, 84% to 94%) and a specificity of 94% (95% CI, 88% to 97%). For each duplex ultrasound threshold, measurement properties vary widely between laboratories, and the magnitude of the variation is clinically important. The heterogeneity observed in the measurement properties of duplex ultrasound may be caused by differences in patients, study design, equipment, techniques or training.

Conclusions.—Clinicians need to be aware of the limitations of duplex ultrasound scanning when making management decisions.

► This article is roughly modeled along the lines of a Cochrane Library Review. The mathematics and statistics are sophisticated but, unfortunately, the result is not very useful. Meta-analysis works best when data are uniformly acquired. This is not the case with duplex US where data are always technician dependent, machine dependent, and will vary with the composition of the study population. This study confirms the fact that duplex criteria are variable and will be subject to local variation. I think we already knew that.

G. L. Moneta, MD

Human factors as a source of error in peak Doppler velocity measurement
Lui EYL, Steinman AH, Cobbold RSC, et al (Univ of Toronto)
J Vasc Surg 42:972-979, 2005   2–5

Objective.—The study was conducted to assess the error and variability that results from human factors in Doppler peak velocity measurement. The positioning of the Doppler sample volume in the vessel, adjustment of the Doppler gain and angle, and choice of waveform display size were investigated. We hypothesized that even experienced vascular technologists in a laboratory accredited by the Intersocietal Commission for Accreditation of Vascular Laboratories make significant errors and have significant variability in the subjective adjustments made during measurements.

Methods.—Problems of patient variability were avoided by having the four technologists measure peak velocities from an in vitro pulsatile flow model with unstenosed and 61% stenosed tubes. To evaluate inaccurate angle and sample volume positioning, a probe holder was used in some of the experiments to fix the Doppler angle at 60°. The effect of Doppler gain was studied at three settings—low, ideal, and saturated gains—that were standardized from the ideal level chosen by consensus amongst the technologists. Two waveform display sizes were also investigated. Peak velocity measurement was assessed by comparison with true peak velocities. For each variable studied, average peak velocities were calculated from the 10 measurements made by each technologist and used to find the percent error from the true value, and the coefficient of variation was used to measure the variability.

Results.—Doppler angle, sample volume placement, and the Doppler gain were the most significant sources of error and variability. Inaccurate angle and placement increased the variability in measurements from 1% to 2% (range) to 4% to 6% for the straight tube and from 1% to 2% to 3% to 9% for the 61% stenosis. The peak velocity error was increased from 9% to 13% to 7% to 28% for the stenosis. Both measurement error and variability were strongly dependent on the Doppler gain level. At low gain, the error was approximately 10% less than the true value and at saturated gain, 20% greater. The display size only affected measurements from the stenosed tube, increasing the error from 9% to 13% to 15% to 24%.

Conclusions.—Major factors affecting Doppler peak velocity measurement error and variability were identified. Inaccurate angle and sample volume placement increased the variability. The presence of a stenosis was found to increase the measurement errors. The error was found to depend on the Doppler gain setting, with greater variability at low and saturated gains and on the display size with a stenosis.

Clinical Relevance.—Doppler ultrasound peak velocity measurements are widely used for the diagnostic assessment of the severity of arterial stenoses. However, it is known that these measurements are often in error. We have identified subjective human factors introduced by the technologist and assessed their contribution to peak velocity measurement error and variability. It is to be hoped that by understanding this, improvements in the machine design and measurement methods can be made that will result in improved measurement accuracy and reproducibility.

▶ Carotid duplex studies are known to be technologist dependent. There are, however, many steps used by the technologists from machine settings to patient positioning and manipulating of the scan head that, to varying degrees, may lead to potential error and variability in the examination. This article describes a laboratory model for studying technologist-induced variations in duplex scanning. One needs to be well rested to read it. Nevertheless, it may help standardize carotid testing by identifying specific technologist-related variables that can be targeted for standardization.

G. L. Moneta, MD

3D Ultrasound Measurement of Change in Carotid Plaque Volume: A Tool for Rapid Evaluation of New Therapies
Ainsworth CD, Blake CC, Tamayo A, et al (Robarts Research Inst, London, Ont, Canada)
Stroke 35:1904-1909, 2005   2–6

Background and Purpose.—New therapies are being developed that are antiatherosclerotic but that lack intermediate end points, such as changes in plasma lipids, which can be measured to test efficacy. To study such treatments, it will be necessary to directly measure changes in atherosclerosis. The study was designed to determine sample sizes needed to detect effects of treatment using 3D ultrasound (US) measurement of carotid plaque.

Methods.—In 38 patients with carotid stenosis >60%, age±SD 69.42±7.87 years, 15 female, randomly assigned in a double-blind fashion to 80 mg atorvastatin daily (n=17) versus placebo (n=21), we measured 3D plaque volume at baseline and after 3 months by disc segmentation of voxels representing carotid artery plaque, after 3D reconstruction of parallel transverse duplex US scans into volumetric 3D data sets.

Results.—There were no significant differences in baseline risk factors. The rate of progression was 16.81±74.10 mm³ in patients taking placebo versus regression of −90.25±85.12 mm³ in patients taking atorvastatin (*P*<0.0001).

Conclusions.—3D plaque volume measurement can show large effects of therapy on atherosclerosis in 3 months in sample sizes of approximately 20 patients per group. Sample sizes of 22 per group would be sufficient to show an effect size of 25% that of atorvastatin in 6 months. This technology promises to be very useful in evaluation of new therapies.

▶ This technology looks promising for testing drug therapy for atherosclerosis. It appears better than measurement of intimal medial thickness (IMT). IMT measurements require longer follow-ups and greater sample sizes. Plaques tend to grow longitudinally and circumferentially more rapidly than they do in thickness. Therefore, 3-D US, which can assess these more rapid patterns of growth and regression, would appear better than IMT for monitoring potential drug effects on atherosclerosis.

G. L. Moneta, MD

Asymptomatic Embolization Detected by Doppler Ultrasound Predicts Stroke Risk in Symptomatic Carotid Artery Stenosis

Markus, HS, MacKinnon A (St George's Hosp Med School, London)
Stroke 36:971-975, 2005   2–7

Background and Purpose.—Asymptomatic cerebral emboli can be detected using transcranial Doppler ultrasound (TCD). These embolic signals have potential as a marker of stroke risk and as a surrogate marker to evaluate antiplatelet agents. Small studies have demonstrated that they predict the combined endpoint of stroke and transient ischemic attack (TIA), but no studies have shown that they predict the more important endpoint of stroke alone.

Methods.—TCD was used to record for 1 hour from the ipsilateral middle cerebral artery in 200 patients with >50% symptomatic carotid stenosis. The Doppler audio signal was recorded for later analysis blinded to clinical details. Subjects were followed-up prospectively until surgical intervention, stroke, or study end at 90 days.

Results.—Embolic signals (ES) were detected in 89 (44.5%). During follow-up, 31 subjects experienced recurrent ipsilateral ischemic events: 7 strokes and 24 TIAs. The presence of ES predicted stroke alone (*P*=0.001) and the combined endpoint of stroke and TIA (*P*=0.00001). This remained significant, with an odds ratio of 4.67 (*95% CI, 1.99 to 11.01; P<0.0001*) after Cox regression to control for age, sex, smoking, hypertension, time from last symptoms, and degree of stenosis. The absence of ES identified a group at low risk for stroke alone and stroke and TIA during follow-up: 0% and 7.5%, respectively, versus 3.5% and 15.5% in all 200 subjects.

Conclusions.—Asymptomatic embolization in carotid stenosis predicts short-term ipsilateral stroke risk. This supports use of the technique to identify patients at high-risk for recurrent stroke for therapeutic interventions and as a surrogate marker to evaluate antithrombotic medication.

▶ Obviously, if one identifies a patient with symptomatic internal carotid artery (ICA) stenosis more than 50%, and that patient is a reasonable risk, the carotid stenosis should be treated. This article suggests that patients in whom treatment may need to be delayed, or patients who are marginal candidates for intervention, might be studied with TCD to further stratify their risk for a neurologic event. The need for this ought to occur in a relatively small number of patients with symptomatic ICA stenosis. Any effort to better target who should have a carotid intervention is a step in the right direction.

G. L. Moneta, MD

The Significance of Incidental Thyroid Abnormalities Identified During Carotid Duplex Ultrasonography

Steele SR, Martin MJ, Mullenix PS, et al (Madigan Army Med Ctr, Fort Lewis, Wash)

Arch Surg 140:981-985, 2005   2–8

Hypothesis.—Incidental thyroid masses identified during carotid duplex ultrasonography may represent clinically significant lesions.

Design and Setting.—Retrospective review of a prospective database in a tertiary care referral center.

Patients.—A total of 2004 consecutive patients from January, 2000, through January, 2002, undergoing carotid duplex ultrasonography.

Interventions.—After bilateral carotid duplex ultrasonography, selected patients additionally underwent 1 or more of the following: dedicated thyroid ultrasound, fine-needle aspiration biopsy, and/or partial or total thyroidectomy.

Main Outcome Measures.—The prevalence and type of thyroid abnormalities, correlation with a dedicated thyroid ultrasound, and results of histopathologic diagnosis.

Results.—One or more thyroid abnormalities were identified in 188 duplexes (9.4%) involving 168 patients. Abnormalities were unilateral in 84 patients (50.6%) and bilateral in 81 patients (49.4%). Seventy-seven abnormalities (47%) were cystic, 72 (43%) were solid, and 16 (10%) were of mixed consistency. Sixty-six of the patients (40%) went on to have formal thyroid ultrasounds. Forty-five patients (70.3%) had masses greater than 1 cm on ultrasound. Based on ultrasound findings, 29 of 66 (44%) underwent fine-needle aspiration biopsy, with 13 of 66 (19.7%) eventually undergoing surgery. Surgical pathology included 5 patients with cancer (3 with papillary cancer, 2 with follicular cancer), 4 patients with a follicular adenoma, and 2 with lymphocytic thyroiditis). Two additional patients were discovered to have parathyroid adenomas following further workup and surgery. Thyroid abnormalities identified during carotid duplex ultrasonography correlated with formal ultrasound in 64 of 66 (97%) patients. Measurement of the thyroid mass by carotid duplex strongly correlated with measurement by formal thyroid ultrasound (r = 0.95, P<.001). Two patients with unilateral masses noted on carotid duplex had a normal thyroid formal ultrasound.

Conclusions.—Incidental thyroid abnormalities identified during carotid duplex ultrasound are common and contain clinically significant pathology. A multidisciplinary clinical pathway may facilitate the appropriate evaluation of these abnormalities.

▶ Some of those thyroid masses seen on carotid duplex studies turn out to be important. Physicians interpreting vascular laboratory studies should mention the presence of the mass in their report, and, perhaps, suggest a formal thyroid US to a referring physician. In this study population, on the basis of the numbers of people who did not get follow up, there were certainly some thyroid cancers missed that could have been diagnosed.

G. L. Moneta, MD

Vertebrobasilar Ischemia and Structural Abnormalities of the Vertebral Arteries in Active Temporal Arteritis and Polymyalgia Rheumatica—An Ultrasonographic Case-Control Study

Pfadenhauer K, Esser M, Berger K (Klinikum Augsburg, Germany; Univ of Muenster, Germany)
J Rheumatol 32:2356-2360, 2005   2–9

Objective.—Temporal arteritis (TA) affects large arteries, including the vertebral arteries in up to 15% of cases. High resolution ultrasonography (US) is widely used for noninvasive imaging of the extracranial vertebral arteries. We assessed the prevalence of vertebrobasilar ischemia and structural abnormalities of the extracranial vertebral arteries by US in patients with TA and polymyalgia rheumatica (PMR) and in healthy controls.

Methods.—This prospective study included clinical and US data from 93 patients with TA and 34 with PMR. A comparison was made with US findings in a population based, age matched group of 203 elderly subjects.

Results.—Vertebrobasilar ischemia in 4 patients with TA was less frequent (4.3%) than neuroophthalmological complications (27.9%). In all 4 patients vertebrobasilar ischemia was associated with proximal vertebral artery occlusive disease. The rate of stenosis (>50%) and occlusions of the vertebral arteries was significantly higher in the TA patients (12.9%) than in the PMR patients (2.9%) and controls (3%). Concentric hypoechogenic mural thickening of the proximal segments V0/V1 of the vertebral artery was found in only one PMR patient and 2 TA patients.

Conclusion.—Vertebrobasilar ischemia is an uncommon complication of TA. Color duplex sonography can help to detect temporal arteritis of the vertebral arteries. Hypoechogenic mural thickening in TA can be indistinguishable from wall hematoma caused by vertebral artery dissection and atherothrombotic occlusive disease.

▶ The point of this study is to evaluate the vertebral arteries for wall thickening in patients with possible TA. Some abnormalities will be found. The percent of patients with TA and vertebral abnormalities is, however, probably too low to be of any use in making the initial diagnosis of TA.

G. L. Moneta, MD

Characterization of Human Atherosclerotic Plaques by Intravascular Magnetic Resonance Imaging
Larose E, Yeghiazarians Y, Libby P, et al (Harvard Med School, Boston; VA Boston Healthcare System, West Roxbury, Mass)
Circulation 112:2324-2331, 2005   2–10

Background.—Development and validation of novel imaging modalities to assess the composition of human atherosclerotic plaques will improve the understanding of atheroma evolution and could facilitate evaluation of therapeutic strategies for plaque modification. Surface MRI can characterize tissue content of carotid but not deeper arteries. This study evaluated the usefulness of intravascular MRI (IVMRI) to discern the composition of human iliac arteries in vivo.

Method and Results.—Initial studies validated IVMRI against histopathology of human atherosclerotic arteries ex vivo. A 0.030-inch-diameter IVMRI detector coil was advanced into isolated human aortoiliac arteries and coupled to a 1.5-T scanner. Information from combined T1-, moderate T2-, and proton-density-weighted images differentiated lipid, fibrous, and calcified components with favorable sensitivity and specificity and allowed accurate quantification of plaque size. The validated approach was then applied to image iliac arteries of 25 human subjects in vivo, and results were compared with those of intravascular ultrasound (IVUS). IVMRI readily visualized inner and outer plaque boundaries in all arteries, even those with extensive calcification that precluded IVUS interpretation. It also revealed the expected heterogeneity of atherosclerotic plaque content that was noted during ex vivo validation. Again, IVUS did not disclose this heterogeneity. The level of interobserver and intraobserver agreement in the interpretation of plaque composition was high for IVMRI but poor for IVUS.

Conclusions.—IVMRI can reliably identify plaque composition and size in arteries deep within the body. Identification of plaque components by IVMRI in vivo has important implications for the understanding and modification of human atherosclerosis.

▶ This is very interesting technology. It is becoming obvious that, as time goes by, MRI technology is improving and is going to be very competitive with US. MRI can provide much of the same information as US and what appears to be better plaque characterization. The particular technology used in this study is not going to be widely available for some time. However, stay tuned.

G. L. Moneta, MD

Value of the duplex waveform at the common femoral artery for diagnosing obstructive aortoiliac disease

Spronk S, den Hoed PT, de Jonge LCW, et al (Ikazia Hosp, Rotterdam, Netherlands; Erasmus Med Ctr, Rotterdam, Netherlands)
J Vasc Surg 42:236-242, 2005   2–11

Purpose.—To evaluate the accuracy, predictive value, and observer agreement of the duplex ultrasound waveform at the common femoral artery as a marker of significant aortoiliac disease in a large group of consecutive patients who underwent a diagnostic workup for peripheral arterial disease in a vascular unit.

Methods.—In 191 consecutive patients (381 aortoiliac segments), we classified the duplex ultrasound waveform at the common femoral artery as triphasic, biphasic, sharp monophasic, or poor monophasic. The waveforms were then compared with the findings of magnetic resonance angiography of the aortoiliac segment and peripheral runoff vessels. We calculated the diagnostic accuracy of the duplex waveform for detecting >50% obstructive disease of the aortoiliac segment and determined the observer agreement for classifying the duplex waveforms done by two independent observers.

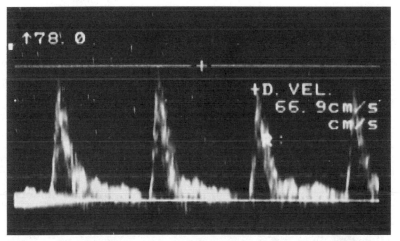

FIGURE 3.—Sharp monophasic consists of a sharp systolic rise, the lack of a reverse diastolic element, and a fast diastolic fall. (Reprinted by permission of the publisher from Spronk S, den Hoed PT, de Jonge LCW, et al: Value of the duplex waveform at the common femoral artery for diagnosing obstructive aortoiliac disease. *J Vasc Surg* 42:236-242, 2005. Copyright 2005 by Elsevier.)

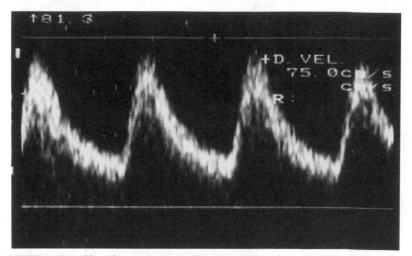

FIGURE 4.—Poor (blunted) monophasic waveform shows the loss of ?sharpness? in systole, the lack of a reverse diastolic element, and a slow diastolic fall. (Reprinted by permission of the publisher from Spronk S, den Hoed PT, de Jonge LCW, et al: Value of the duplex waveform at the common femoral artery for diagnosing obstructive aortoiliac disease. *J Vasc Surg* 42:236-242, 2005. Copyright 2005 by Elsevier.)

Results.—Magnetic resonance angiography showed obstruction in 152 (39.9%) of 381 aortoiliac segments in 191 patients. The presence of a poor monophasic waveform, encountered in 91 (24.3%) of 375 segments, was a reliable sign of significant aortoiliac disease, with a positive predictive value of 92%. Other waveforms were nondiagnostic for aortoiliac obstructive disease. The sharp monophasic waveform reliably predicted occlusive disease of the superficial femoral artery that was seen in 17 of 23 instances. There was good observer agreement for classifying duplex waveforms ($\kappa_w = 0.85$; 95% confidence interval, 0.80 to 0.89).

Conclusion.—The poor monophasic duplex waveform at the common femoral artery is in itself an accurate marker of aortoiliac obstructive disease. Other waveforms are nondiagnostic for aortoiliac disease (Figs 3 and 4).

▶ I am sure a monophasic femoral artery waveform indicates proximal occlusive disease. However, it gives no information regarding extent or location of that disease. If one wants only to document disease, a common femoral waveform can do that if it is very abnormal; otherwise, it does not help much. If one really wants to know what is going on with the iliac arteries, an MRA or duplex scan provides much more information. This is 2007; there is no need to guess.

G. L. Moneta, MD

Comparison Between Duplex Scanning and Angiographic Findings in the Evaluation of Functional Iliac Obstruction in Top Endurance Athletes
Alimi YS, Accrocca F, Barthèlemy P, et al (Univ Hôpital Nord, Marseilles, France)
Eur J Vasc Endovasc Surg 28:513-519, 2004   2–12

Objective.—Review of a 10 year-experience, to evaluate the efficacy of pre-operative investigations in the detection of external iliac artery (EIA) endofibrosis in top endurance athletes.

Design.—Retrospective study.

Materials.—From September 1995 to March 2004, 13 highly-trained athletes (all men, mean age 32.3 years) underwent surgery for disease involving 14 lower limbs (11 left, one right, one bilateral).

Methods.—We compared ultrasound scan (US) and digital subtraction angiography (DSA) data, at rest and at hip flexion with intra-operative findings for all 14 lower limbs. We analyzed the presence of stenosis in the external and common iliac arteries, the presence of psoas muscle arteries and the presence of excessive EIA length.

Results.—In the affected limbs, before treatment, the mean ankle brachial index (ABI) at rest was 0.98 compared with 0.56 after exercise, $p=0.0001$. The sensitivities of the US vs DSA examination in the detection of external and common iliac artery stenosis were, respectively, 84.6 and 53.8% vs 53.8 and 12.5%. The muscle psoas artery was detected by DSA with a sensitivity of 57.1 and 100% specificity. For the detection of excessive EIA length, the sensitivity of US was 85.7% with 57.1% specificity.

Conclusions.—A fall of ABI after exercise proves the presence of a significant stenosis in symptomatic athletes. Color coded duplex ultrasonography is recommended for non-invasive imaging of suspected endofibrotic stenosis in young athletes, since it detects reliably both stenosis and elongation of iliacal arteries (Fig 2).

▶ Endofibrosis is a rare problem primarily, but not exclusively, affecting professional cyclists. It is characterized by stenosis and elongation and sometimes kinking of the iliac arteries. The diagnosis is suggested by a fall in ankle brachial index after heavy exercise and a normal resting physical examination. The data show duplex US works reasonably well to detect EIA involvement with endofibrosis but not particularly well for assessing common iliac involvement. A combination of imaging modalities is recommended for preoperative planning as neither angiographic imaging or duplex US alone appears sufficient.

G. L. Moneta, MD

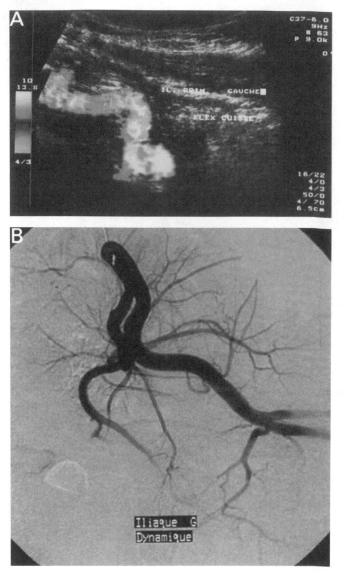

FIGURE 2.—Excessive length of internal iliac artery shown in the same patient by ultrasound scan at hip flexion (A) and by digital subtraction angiography at hip flexion (B). (Reprinted from Alimi YS, Accrocca F, Barthèlemy P, et al: Comparison between duplex scanning and angiographic findings in the evaluation of functional iliac obstruction in top endurance athletes. *Eur J Endovasc Surg* 28:513-519, 2004. Copyright 2004, by permission of the publisher W B Saunders Company Limited London.)

Peripheral Arterial Disease: Comparison of Color Duplex US and Contrast-enhanced MR Angiography for Diagnosis
Leiner T, Kessels AGH, Nelemans PJ, et al (Maastricht Univ, the Netherlands)
Radiology 235:699-708, 2005   2–13

Purpose.—To prospectively compare the diagnostic accuracies of color duplex ultrasonography (US) and contrast material-enhanced magnetic resonance (MR) angiography and to assess interobserver agreement regarding contrast-enhanced MR angiographic findings in patients suspected of having peripheral arterial disease (PAD).

Materials and Methods.—The institutional review board approved the study, and all patients provided signed informed consent. Two hundred ninety-five patients referred for diagnostic and preinterventional work-up of PAD with duplex US also underwent gadolinium-enhanced MR angiography. Data sets were reviewed for presence or absence of 50% or greater luminal reduction, which indicated hemodynamically significant stenosis, and to determine interobserver agreement. At duplex US, a peak systolic velocity ratio of 2.5 or greater indicated significant stenosis. Primary outcome measures were differences between duplex US and contrast-enhanced MR angiography in sensitivity and specificity for detection of significant stenosis, as assessed with the McNemar test, and interobserver agreement between the two contrast-enhanced MR angiogram readings, expressed as quadratic weighted κ values. Intraarterial digital subtraction angiography (DSA) was the reference standard.

Results.—Two hundred forty-nine patients had at least one hemodynamically significant stenotic lesion at contrast-enhanced MR angiography, duplex US, or both examinations. One hundred fifty-two patients underwent intraarterial DSA. The quadratic weighted κ for agreement regarding the presence of 50% or greater stenosis at contrast-enhanced MR angiography was 0.89 (95% confidence interval [CI]: 0.87, 0.91). Sensitivity of duplex US was 76% (95% CI: 69%, 82%); specificity, 93% (95% CI: 91%, 95%); and accuracy, 89%. Sensitivity and specificity of contrast-enhanced MR angiography were 84% (95% CI: 78%, 89%) and 97% (95% CI: 95%, 98%), respectively; accuracy was 94%. Sensitivity ($P - .002$) and specificity ($P = .03$) of contrast-enhanced MR angiography were significantly higher.

Conclusion.—Results of this prospective comparison between contrast-enhanced MR angiography and duplex US provide evidence that contrast-enhanced MR angiography is more sensitive and specific for diagnosis and preinterventional work-up of PAD.

► Both this abstract (Abstract 2–13) and the next abstract (Abstract 2 14) suggest duplex US and MRA should not be considered exclusive but rather complementary tests in the evaluation of PAD. For assessing the superficial femoral artery, duplex US is excellent, whereas MRA is probably better for iliac arteries in many patients, especially obese individuals. It is incumbent upon surgeons performing peripheral artery interventions to be familiar with the strengths and limitations of all imaging modalities and to choose the least toxic, most cost-effective method for each individual patient.

G. L. Moneta, MD

Gadolinium-enhanced Magnetic Resonance Angiography, Colour Duplex and Digital Subtraction Angiography of the Lower Limb Arteries from the Aorta to the Tibio-peroneal Trunk in Patients with Intermittent Claudication

Gjønnæss E, Morken B, Sandbæk G, et al (Aker Univ, Oslo, Norway; Ullevål Univ, Oslo, Norway)

Eur J Vasc Endovasc Surg 31:53-58, 2006   2–14

Objectives.—To evaluate the sensitivity, specificity, positive and negative predictive value of contrast-enhanced (gadolinium) magnetic resonance imaging (CE-MRA) and colour duplex ultrasound (CDU) of lower limb arteries.

Design.—Prospective, single centre study.

Material and Methods.—A consecutive series of 58 patients with intermittent claudication (IC) were examined with CE-MRA and CDU from the infrarenal aorta to the tibio-peroneal trunk with digital subtraction angiography (DSA) as reference. The arterial tree was divided into 15 segments, pooled into three regions; suprainguinal, thigh and knee. Sensitivity, specificity, positive and negative predictive values for significant obstructions were calculated. Cohen Kappa statistics was used to establish agreement between the three methods.

Results.—The sensitivity (specificity in parentheses) for significant obstructions in the suprainguinal region were 96% (94%) for CE-MRA and 91% (96%) for CDU, in the thigh region 92% (95%) for CE-MRA and 76% (99%) for CDU, and in the knee region 93% (96%) for CE-MRA and 33% (98%) for CDU. CDU failed to visualize 10% of suprainguinal, 2% of thigh and 13% of knee-region arterial segments.

Conclusions.—Both CE-MRA and CDU are good alternatives to DSA in the suprainguinal- and thigh-region. In the knee region only CE-MRA can be relied upon as an alternative to DSA. Imaging by CDU is not suited to situations were evaluation of runoff vessels is important.

▶ Basically, the same comments apply to this and to the previous abstract (Abstract 2–13). An interesting bit of information in this study is that both duplex US and MRA tend to overestimate the length of peripheral arterial occlusions. This may be of some importance if duplex US and/or MRA are used to screen patients for selection for a possible catheter-based intervention.

G. L. Moneta, M.D.

The limitations of magnetic resonance angiography in the diagnosis of renal artery stenosis: Comparative analysis with conventional arteriography

Patel ST, Mills JL Sr, Tynan-Cuisinier G, et al (Univ of Arizona, Tucson)
J Vasc Surg 41:462-468, 2005   2–15

Purpose.—Gadolinium-enhanced magnetic resonance angiography (MRA) is commonly used as a screening modality for the detection of renal artery stenosis. However, evidence supporting its utility in clinical practice is lacking; few rigorous studies have compared MRA with contrast arteriography (CA). After making anecdotal clinical observations that MRA sometimes overestimated the degree of renal artery stenosis, we decided to determine the interobserver variability, sensitivity, specificity, and diagnostic accuracy of MRA compared with CA.

Methods.—From September 1999 to April 2003, we evaluated 68 renal arteries in 34 patients with clinically suspected renal artery stenosis using both MRA and CA. All studies were independently reviewed by four blinded observers. Renal arteries were categorized by MRA as normal, <50%, and >50% stenosis/occlusion. The sensitivity, specificity, and accuracy of MRA detection of renal artery stenosis were compared to CA as the gold standard. Interobserver variability (κ) was also calculated.

Results.—MRA demonstrated 87% sensitivity, 69% specificity, 85% accuracy, 95% negative predictive value, and 51% positive predictive value for the diagnosis of renal artery stenosis. Interobserver agreement was moderate for MRA ($\kappa = 0.53$) and good for CA ($\kappa = 0.76$). In 21 arteries (31%), MRA was falsely positive.

Conclusions.—In patients with a high clinical suspicion of renal artery stenosis, MRA is 87% sensitive in the detection of 50% stenosis. However, MRA is relatively nonspecific compared with CA and results in significant overestimation of renal artery stenosis in nearly one third of patients. To re-

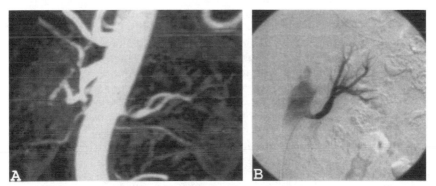

FIGURE 2.—A, Magnetic resonance angiography indicates high-grade stenosis of the left renal artery. B, Selective contrast arteriography indicates a normal left renal artery. (Reprinted by permission of the publisher from Patel ST, Mills JL Sr, Tynan-Cuisinier G, et al: The limitations of magnetic resonance angiography in the diagnosis of renal artery stenosis: Comparative analysis with conventional arteriography. *J Vasc Surg* 41:462-468, 2005. Copyright 2005 by Elsevier.)

duce unnecessary CA, clinicians should consider supplemental studies (Fig 2).

▶ The Achilles heel of MRA in virtually every location is its tendency to over-estimate stenosis. The author's conclusion to obtain additional noninvasive imaging before CA after an MRA identified renal artery stenosis makes sense. What probably makes most sense is to screen patients for renal artery steno-sis with a duplex US scan and, if positive, to go to CA and skip the MRA study altogether.

G. L. Moneta, MD

Hemodynamic changes associated with bypass stenosis regression
Taggert JB, Kupinski AM, Darling RC III, et al (Inst for Vascular Health and Dis-ease, Albany, NY)
J Vasc Surg 41:1013-1017, 2005   2–16

Background.—The long-term patency of vein bypasses in the lower ex-tremities can be improved by detection and correction of stenotic lesions. Five-year patency rates of 80% have been reported when stenotic lesions were corrected before graft thrombosis, compared with 40% when correc-tion of the lesion occurred after thrombosis. Duplex US scanning has been used to detect velocity increases, which are indicative of a bypass stenosis. However, subsequent examinations have, in some cases, shown regression of some stenotic lesions. In the present study, the hemodynamic changes that coincided with stenosis regression were examined in patients with elevated lower extremity vein bypass velocities discovered during surveillance.

Methods.—A retrospective review was conducted of patients with infra-inguinal autogenous vein bypass grafts who were in active follow-up in a pri-mary vascular laboratory. Duplex US scans were used to record the peak sys-tolic velocity (PSV) and volume flow from proximal and distal segments of the bypass grafts. The presence of valve remnants or other image defects was also noted. The PSV ratio (Vr) was calculated as the PSV at a stenosis divided by the PSV proximal to the lesion. A stenosis was defined as a Vr of 2.0 or greater.

Results.—The initial US scan identified a stenosis in 68 of 565 bypasses. The stenosis was repaired in 27 bypasses with a PSV of 335 ± 61 cm/s and a Vr of 4.0 ± 1.6. US image abnormalities were noted in 4 bypasses (67%) with persistent stenoses, 14 (52%) with repaired stenoses, and 10 (29%) with re-solved stenoses.

Conclusions.—The clinical course is unpredictable for patients with mod-erate PSV elevations identified during lower extremity vein bypass surveil-lance. Data in this study showed a much greater percentage of moderate ve-locity abnormalities undergoing regression. However, these increases in velocity may result from the action of the bypass conduit as a flow-limiting lesion until the hyperemia subsides. In this setting, the PSV is decreased with the reduction in blood flow, which gives the appearance of stenosis regression.

▶ The message here is that moderate elevations in PSV and Vr in vein grafts that are detected early in the postoperative period can be safely followed with serial duplex scans. Often the velocities will decrease. The data do not apply to lesions discovered later in the life of a bypass graft. The authors' idea that later decreases in PSV are secondary to a reduction of hyperemic flow through a moderate stenosis may be true but is no more than speculation.

G. L. Moneta, MD

Is Duplex Surveillance of Value After Leg Vein Bypass Grafting? Principal Results of the Vein Graft Surveillance Randomised Trial (VGST)
Davies AH, for the VGST Participants (Imperial College London; et al)
Circulation 112:1985-1991, 2005   2–17

Background.—The purpose of this study was to assess the benefits of duplex compared with clinical vein graft surveillance in terms of amputation rates, quality of life, and healthcare costs in patients after femoropopliteal and femorocrural vein bypass grafts.

Methods and Results.—This was a multicenter, prospective, randomized, controlled trial. A total of 594 patients with a patent vein graft at 30 days after surgery were randomized to either a clinical or duplex follow-up program at 6 weeks, then 3, 6, 9, 12, and 18 months postoperatively. The clinical and duplex surveillance groups had similar amputation rates (7% for each group) and vascular mortality rates (3% versus 4%) over 18 months. More patients in the clinical group had vein graft stenosis at 18 months (19% versus 12%, $P=0.04$), but primary patency, primary assisted patency, and secondary patency rates, respectively, were similar in the clinical group (69%, 76%, and 80%) and the duplex group (67%, 76%, and 79%). There were no apparent differences in health-related quality of life, but the average health service costs incurred by the duplex surveillance program were greater by £495 pound (95% CI £83 to £807) per patient.

Conclusions.—Intensive surveillance with duplex scanning did not show any additional benefit in terms of limb salvage rates for patients undergoing vein bypass graft operations, but it did incur additional costs.

▶ Vein graft stenoses develop more frequently in long grafts (ie, distal targets), grafts placed for limb salvage, disadvantaged grafts (composite grafts, arm vein grafts), and perhaps in patients undergoing repeat procedures. In this article, most of the patients probably had primary operations as evidenced by the high level of use of the ipsilateral greater saphenous vein, two thirds of the anastomoses were to the popliteal artery, and amputation rates appear to have been analyzed using both patients with claudication and patients with limb salvage indications for surgery, a bit of a "no-no." In short, if there was ever a group of patients who were unlikely to benefit from duplex US surveillance, this would be the group. This article should not lead one to abandon vascular laboratory duplex US surveillance for vein grafts at increased risk for stenosis. However, the data suggest that when a vein graft is placed to a popliteal artery using ipsilateral saphenous vein, duplex surveillance may not be of much benefit in reducing amputations over the short run.

G. L. Moneta, MD

Reproducibility of Duplex Ultrasonography and Air Plethysmography Used for the Evaluation of Chronic Venous Insufficiency
Asbeutah AM, Riha AZ, Cameron JD, et al (Monash Univ and Southern Health, Melbourne, Victoria, Australia; The Wesley Vascular Centre, Brisbane, Queensland, Australia)
J Ultrasound Med 24:475-482, 2005   2–18

Objective.—The purpose of this study was to determine the reproducibility of measurements on duplex ultrasonography (DU) and air plethysmography (APG) in subjects with post-thrombotic syndrome.

Methods.—Duplex ultrasonography and APG were used to measure indices of lower limb venous reflux in 15 limbs with a history of deep vein thrombosis and evidence of venous insufficiency as diagnosed by ultrasonography. Three limbs were in class 0; 4 were in classes 1 to 3; and 8 were in classes 4 to 6, according to clinical, etiologic, anatomic, and pathophysiologic clinical classification. Duplex ultrasonography was performed 3 times on the same day, and venous diameter, area, peak reflux velocity, reflux flow volume, and reflux duration measurements were obtained. Air plethysmography was performed on 2 days, 7 to 10 days apart, with 1 measurement on the first day and 2 measurements on the second day. Values obtained from APG included outflow fraction, venous filling index, ejection fraction, and residual volume fraction. The measurements were performed by a vascular technologist blinded to the previous test results. One-way analysis of variance, the Student paired *t* test, and Bland-Altman plots were used to examine the statistical differences of the DU and APG parameters for all measurements.

Results.—The mean coefficient of variation for within-subject measurements of all DU and APG parameters measured was less than 10%. Bland-Altman plots showed that there were no apparent trends with increasing values over a wide range for any of the DU parameters, nor were there any for the APG parameters.

Conclusions.—Under ideal conditions, when measured by a highly trained technologist, both DU and APG showed satisfactory reproducibility.

▶ Many of us involved in venous testing have the anecdotal impression that APG findings are not very reproducible. In that regard, this study is encouraging in that the APG seemed to be reproducible, at least within the context of this study design. However, only one vascular technologist performed the examinations. Therefore, the question of interobserver variability was not addressed. In addition, patients were studied relatively close in time, and the effects of diurnal variation were not studied. Overall, the question of the reproducibility of APG results still remains.

G. L. Moneta, MD

Interobserver agreement on ultrasound measurements of residual vein diameter, thrombus echogenicity and Doppler venous flow in patients with previous venous thrombosis
Linkins L-A, Stretton R, Probyn L, et al (McMaster Univ, Hamilton, Ont, Canada; Univ of Aberdeen, England)
Thromb Res 117:241-247, 2006   2–19

Introduction.—In patients with new symptoms in a leg previously affected by deep vein thrombosis (DVT), the presence of thrombus on ultrasound cannot be assumed to be due to recurrent thrombosis. Several parameters have been suggested to differentiate between acute and chronic thrombus on ultrasound, including measurement of residual vein diameter during compression, thrombus echogenicity and Doppler assessment of venous flow, but studies on the reproducibility of these measurements are sparse.

Objective.—To determine interobserver agreement on measurement of residual vein diameter, thrombus echogenicity and Doppler venous flow in patients with residual thrombus in the veins of the lower limb.

Materials and Methods.—Patients with previous proximal DVT who had a high likelihood of residual thrombosis, but without symptoms of recurrent DVT, had ultrasound examinations independently performed by two examiners on the same day. Interobserver agreement on measurement of residual vein diameter, thrombus echogenicity and Doppler venous flow was evaluated.

Results.—We determined that interobserver agreement on these measurements was moderate. The mean difference between paired measurements of residual vein diameter was 2.2 mm (95th centile, 8.0 mm). When both examiners agreed residual thrombus was present, 54% of the variance of the measurement of residual vein diameter was accounted for by the paired measurements. The weighted kappa coefficient for thrombus echogenicity was 0.01 and for Doppler venous flow was 0.51.

Conclusions.—The error associated with ultrasound measurements of residual vein diameter, thrombus echogenicity and flow appears to be considerable.

▶ There are no standard US variables to differentiate an acute on chronic venous thrombus from a chronic venous thrombus alone. To address this question, there must be US variables that change over time and can be quantified. This study attempted to evaluate interobserver reproducibility of several potential US variables to distinguish acute from acute on chronic thrombus. The overall results were disappointing. At this point, when serial US tests are similar, some other measure of thrombus activity must be used. Perhaps D-dimer, or even signal intensity on MRV studies, may be used as a measure of inflammation associated with an acute thrombotic process superimposed on an older chronic thrombus.

G. L. Moneta, MD

Noncontrast three-dimensional magnetic resonance imaging vs lymphoscintigraphy in the evaluation of lymph circulation disorders: A comparative study

Liu N, Wang C, Sun M (Shanghai Second Med Univ, China; Shanghai Chang Zheng Hosp, China)
J Vasc Surg 41:69-75, 2005

2–20

Background.—Visualization of the lymphatic vessels is a challenge in patients with disorders of the lymphatic circulation. In an effort to improve the diagnostic scope of lymphatic imaging, we compared traditional lympho-

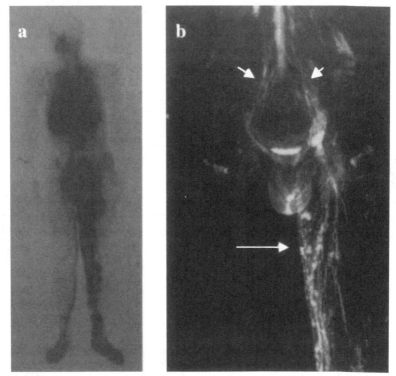

FIGURE 2.—A 34-year-old man with lymphatic hyperplasia of the left leg. a, Lymphoscintigraphy shows an intensive radioactive signal along the medial part of the left lower extremity and in the pelvis, groin, and scrotum. b, Three-dimensional magnetic resonance imaging depicts enlarged lymphatics in the thigh (*arrow*). The estimated diameter of the lymphatics is 2 to 5 mm. Clusters of dilated inguinal, iliac, scrotum, and lumbar trunks (*arrowhead*) are also visualized. (Reprinted by permission of the publisher from Liu N, Wang C, Sun M: Noncontrast three-dimensional magnetic resonance imaging vs lymphoscintigraphy in the evaluation of lymph circulation disorders: A comparative study. *J Vasc Surg* 41:69-75, 2005. Copyright 2005 by Elsevier.)

scintigraphy (LSG) with three-dimensional magnetic resonance imaging (3D MRI).

Methods.—From October 1, 2002, to May 30, 2004, 39 patients (27 males and 12 females) with lower extremity lymphedema and/or skin lymphorrhea in the abdominal wall or the external genitalia underwent LSG and 3D MRI. Patients' ages ranged from 3 to 71 years. Assessment of the imaging studies included the degree and quality of visualization of the malformations of the lymphatic collectors, lymphatic trunks, lymph nodes, and tissue edema.

Results.—In patients with lymphedema, chylous reflux syndrome, or both, LSG depicted the enlarged lymphatics and nodes as a fused band or mass. In 3D MRI, the dilated superficial lymphatic collectors and deep lymphatic trunks, as well as the accumulation of chyle and node enlargements, were clearly visualized. In patients with hypoplasia or aplasia of the lymphatics, LSG usually displayed the pattern of dermal backflow in the form of radiotracer filling of the dermal lymphatics or stagnation of the isotope at the injection point. The images obtained by 3D MRI were able to demonstrate the extent of tissue fluid accumulation and distinguish edema fluid from subcutaneous fat.

Conclusions.—In patients with peripheral and central lymphatic malformations, LSG provided images representative of the function of the lymphatic vessels but failed to give detailed information regarding its anatomy. 3D MRI provided extensive information on the anatomy of the lymph stagnated vasculature as well as on the effects of lymphatic dysfunction on local structures and tissue composition (Fig 2).

▶ The magnetic resonance (MR) images detected in this article are every bit as good as one could expect from lymphangiography and are certainly more dramatic and detailed than the "fuzzy" grains of lymphoscintigraphy. I am still not sure how to use this information in clinical practice. Can these MR studies really be used to select patients who will benefit from interventions and to guide interventions?

G. L. Moneta, MD

MRI Versus Helical CT for Endoleak Detection After Endovascular Aneurysm Repair
Pitton MB, Schweitzer H, Herber S, et al (Univ Hosp of Mainz, Germany)
AJR 185:1275-1281, 2005   2–21

Objective.—The objective of our study was to investigate the diagnostic accuracy of MRI and helical CT for endoleak detection.

Subjects and Methods.—Fifty two patients underwent endovascular aneurysm repair with nitinol stent-grafts. Follow-up data sets included contrast-enhanced biphasic CT and MRI within 48 hr after the intervention; at 3, 6, and 12 months; and yearly thereafter. The endoleak size was categorized as $\leq 3\%$, $>3\% \leq 10\%$, $> 10\% \leq 30\%$, or $> 30\%$ of the maximum

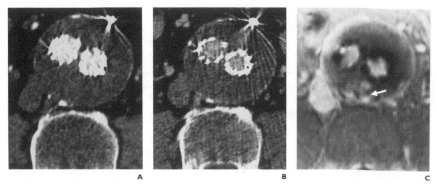

A   B   C

FIGURE 3.—Type II endoleak-size C, > 10% but ≤ 30% of cross-sectional aneurysm area in 71-year-old man. **A** and **B**, Endoleak is not visualized on biphasic scans: arterial phase, **A**; late phase, **B**. **C**, Contrast-enhanced MR image clearly shows endoleak (*arrow*) dorsal in aneurysm sac. (Courtesy of Pitton MB, Schweitzer H, Herber S, et al: MRI versus helical CT for endoleak detection after endovascular aneurysm repair. *AJR* 185:1275-1281, 2005. Reprinted with permission from the *American Journal of Roentgenology.*)

cross-sectional aneurysm area. A consensus interpretation of CT and MRI was defined as the standard of reference.

Results.—Of 252 data sets, 141 showed evidence for endoleaks. The incidence of types I, II, and III endoleaks and complex endoleaks was 3.2%, 40.1%, 8.7%, and 4.0%, respectively. The sensitivity for endoleak detection was 92.9%, 44.0%, 34.8%, and 38.3% for MRI, biphasic CT, uniphasic arterial CT, and uniphasic late CT, respectively. The corresponding negative predictive values were 91.7%, 58.4%, 54.7%, and 56.1%, respectively. The overall accuracy of endoleak detection and correct sizing was 95.2%, 58.3%, 55.6%, and 57.1% for MRI, biphasic CT, uniphasic arterial CT, and uniphasic late CT, respectively.

Conclusion.—MRI is significantly superior to biphasic CT for endoleak detection and rating of endoleak size, followed by uniphasic late and uniphasic arterial CT scans. MRI shows a significant number of endoleaks in cases with negative CT findings and may help illuminate the phenomenon of endotension. Endoleak rates reported after endovascular aneurysm repair substantially depend on the imaging techniques used (Fig 3).

▶ The data clearly imply that endoleak rates after endovascular aneurysm repair are dependent upon the imaging modality used to detect the endoleak. MRI appears to detect more endoleaks than CT. It is interesting to speculate whether unexplained endotension after endovascular aneurysm repair may in many cases reflect undetected endoleak. Perhaps unexplained endotension would be explained more often if MRI rather than CT was used routinely in the evaluation of endoleaks after endovascular aneurysm repair?

G. L. Moneta, MD

Noninvasive Detection of Steno-Occlusive Disease of the Supra-Aortic Arteries With Three-Dimensional Contrast-Enhanced Magnetic Resonance Angiography: A Prospective, Intra-Individual Comparative Analysis With Digital Subtraction Angiography

Willinek WA, von Falkenhausen M, Born M, et al (Univ of Bonn, Germany)
Stroke 36:38-43, 2005   2–22

Background and Purpose.—Concomitant disease of the supra-aortic arteries can influence the outcome of surgical treatment of carotid artery stenosis. However, sensitivity and specificity data of noninvasive contrast-enhanced 3-dimensional (3D) magnetic resonance angiography (CE MRA) for the detection of steno-occlusive disease of the entire supra-aortic arteries including the circle of Willis remain unclear. We aimed to intra-individually compare high-spatial-resolution CE 3D MRA and digital subtraction angiography (DSA) for the assessment of steno-occlusive vascular disease of the supra-aortic arteries.

Methods.—CE MRA and DSA of the supra-aortic arteries were prospectively performed in 50 consecutive patients. Intra-individual comparison of CE MRA and DSA was available in 833 arteries. High-spatial-resolution CE MRA comprised a measured voxel size of 0.81 mm × 0.81 mm × 1 mm (0.66 mm³). Steno-occlusive vascular disease of the 833 arteries was assessed independently by 2 radiologists according to the NASCET criteria.

Results.—CE MRA had a sensitivity of 100% (73/73), a specificity of 99.3% (760/765), a positive predictive value of 93.6% (73/78), and a negative predictive value of 100% (760/760) by using a 70% to 99% threshold of arterial diameter stenosis. For detection of occlusion, sensitivity, specificity, PPV, and NPV value of CE MRA were 100%, respectively.

Conclusions.—Noninvasive high-spatial-resolution CE MRA is suited to replace diagnostic DSA for the detection of steno-occlusive disease of the supra-aortic arteries.

► These are excellent results. The usual proclivity of MRA to exaggerate stenosis was not really seen here. Most importantly, negative predictive value was essentially perfect. Therefore, if the MRA is negative, one has adequate inflow for the reconstruction.

G. L. Moneta, MD

3 Perioperative Considerations

Is abdominal aortic aneurysm repair appropriate in oxygen-dependent chronic obstructive pulmonary disease patients?
Compton CN, Dillavou ED, Sheehan MK, et al (Univ of Pittsburgh, Pa)
J Vasc Surg 42:650-653, 2005   3–1

Background.—The life expectancy of patients with oxygen-dependent chronic obstructive pulmonary disease (COPD) is significantly reduced, but the risk of any intervention is considered prohibitive. However, severe COPD may increase the risk of abdominal aortic aneurysm (AAA) rupture. We reviewed our experience with AAA repair in oxygen-dependent patients to determine whether operative risk and expected long-term survival justify surgical intervention.

Methods.—A retrospective review of 44 consecutive patients with oxygen-dependent COPD undergoing AAA repair over an 8-year period was performed. Information was recorded for survival, length of follow-up, patient age, medical comorbidities, pulmonary function tests, and operative approach. Survival data were analyzed by Kaplan-Meier curves and compared with published cohorts of oxygen-dependent patients and the natural history of untreated aneurysms.

Results.—Twenty-four patients underwent endovascular aneurysm repair (EVAR), and 20 underwent open procedures (14 retroperitoneal and 6 transabdominal). The mean AAA diameter was 6.1 cm (range, 5-9.5 cm). The mean age was 71.4 years, and 82% of patients were male. Operative mortality was 0%. The mean length of stay was 11.2 days for open procedures and 4.3 days for EVAR (significantly longer than that for standard-risk patients). The mean survival time was 37.9 months (range, 2-91 months). Preoperative medical comorbidities, type of repair, and pulmonary function tests were not predictive of survival. Postoperative morbidity was significantly higher with open repair. Long term survival was comparable to historical series of the natural history of O2 dependent patients without AAA but better than untreated 6 cm AAA cohorts. At 42 months, almost 50% of patients in our study group were still alive, compared to 20% survival at 34 months for those with untreated 6 cm AAAs.

Conclusions.—It is reasonable to continue to offer AAA repair to home oxygen-dependent COPD patients who are ambulatory and medically optimized and who are without untreated coronary artery disease. Although EVAR may be the most suitable treatment for oxygen-dependent COPD patients, our results show that even open repair may be safely performed in this population, with acceptable results.

▶ It is important to consider what is not in this article as well as to consider what is in the article. There is no information on renal function, liver function, current tobacco use, ejection fraction, need for supraceliac clamping, etc. It is best to remember that risk factors are additive. With bad lungs, AAA repair is safely possible, but for safety sake it should be assumed that the patients in this series may have had COPD as their only major risk factor.

G. L. Moneta, MD

Perioperative Beta-Blocker Therapy and Mortality after Major Noncardiac Surgery

Lindenauer PK, Pekow P, Wang K, et al (Baystate Med Ctr, Springfield, Mass; Tufts Univ, Boston; Univ of Massachusetts at Amherst; et al)
N Engl J Med 353:349-361, 2005   3–2

Background.—Despite limited evidence from randomized trials, perioperative treatment with beta-blockers is now widely advocated. We assessed the use of perioperative beta-blockers and their association with in-hospital mortality in routine clinical practice.

Methods.—We conducted a retrospective cohort study of patients 18 years of age or older who underwent major noncardiac surgery in 2000 and 2001 at 329 hospitals throughout the United States. We used propensity-score matching to adjust for differences between patients who received perioperative beta-blockers and those who did not receive such therapy and compared in-hospital mortality using multivariable logistic modeling.

Results.—Of 782,969 patients, 663,635 (85 percent) had no recorded contraindications to beta-blockers, 122,338 of whom (18 percent) received such treatment during the first two hospital days, including 14 percent of patients with a Revised Cardiac Risk Index (RCRI) score of 0 and 44 percent with a score of 4 or higher. The relationship between perioperative beta-blocker treatment and the risk of death varied directly with cardiac risk; among the 580,665 patients with an RCRI score of 0 or 1, treatment was associated with no benefit and possible harm, whereas among the patients with an RCRI score of 2, 3, or 4 or more, the adjusted odds ratios for death in the hospital were 0.88 (95 percent confidence interval, 0.80 to 0.98), 0.71 (95 percent confidence interval, 0.63 to 0.80), and 0.58 (95 percent confidence interval, 0.50 to 0.67), respectively.

Conclusions.—Perioperative beta-blocker therapy is associated with a reduced risk of in-hospital death among high-risk, but not low-risk, patients

Propensity-Matched Cohort

RCRI score 0		1.43 (1.29–1.58)
RCRI score 1		1.13 (0.99–1.30)
RCRI score 2		0.90 (0.75–1.08)
RCRI score 3		0.71 (0.56–0.91)
RCRI score ≥4		0.57 (0.42–0.76)
Entire Study Cohort		
RCRI score 0		1.36 (1.27–1.45)
Hypertension		0.96 (0.82–1.13)
RCRI score 1		1.09 (1.01–1.19)
Diabetes		1.28 (1.10–1.50)
Ischemic heart disease		1.12 (0.95–1.31)
Renal insufficiency		1.03 (0.82–1.23)
Cerebrovascular disease		1.01 (0.76–1.35)
High-risk surgery		0.94 (0.84–1.05)
RCRI score 2		0.88 (0.80–0.98)
RCRI score 3		0.71 (0.63–0.80)
RCRI score ≥4		0.58 (0.50–0.67)

0.4   0.6   0.8   1.0   2.0

Odds Ratio for Death in the Hospital
(95% confidence interval)

FIGURE 1.—Adjusted Odds Ratio for In-Hospital Death Associated with Perioperative Beta-Blocker Therapy among Patients Undergoing Major Noncardiac Surgery, According to the RCRI Score and the Presence of Other Risk Factors in the Propensity-Matched Cohort and the Entire Study Cohort. *Open boxes* represent patient subgroups within the listed RCRI category. (Reprinted by permission of *The New England Journal of Medicine* from Lindenauer PK, Pekow P, Want K, et al: Perioperative beta-blocker therapy and mortality after major noncardiac surgery. *N Engl J Med* 353:349-361, 2005. Copyright 2005, Massachusetts Medical Society. All rights reserved.)

undergoing major noncardiac surgery. Patient safety may be enhanced by increasing the use of beta-blockers in high-risk patients (Fig 1).

▶ Only approximately 51,000 of the 700,000 patients analyzed in this study underwent a vascular surgical procedure. Nevertheless, vascular patients generally have increased cardiac risk, and the results of this study strongly support the use of β-blockers in patients with high cardiac risk. There is no question that routine perioperative use of β-blockers in vascular surgical patients without contraindications to β-blocker therapy should be standard practice.

G. L. Moneta, MD

Cardiac troponin I predicts outcome after ruptured adominal aortic aneurysm repair

Tambyraja AL, Dawson ARW, Murie JA, et al (Univ of Edinburgh, Scotland)
Br J Surg 92:824-827, 2005   3–3

Background.—Cardiac troponin I (cTnI) is a highly sensitive and specific marker for myocardial injury that predicts mortality in patients with acute coronary syndromes. This study examined the relationship between perioperative cTnI levels and clinical outcome in patients with ruptured abdominal aortic aneurysm (AAA).

Methods.—Consecutive patients who underwent operative repair of a ruptured AAA over a 22-month interval and survived for more than 24 h were entered into a prospective observational cohort study. Levels of cTnI were measured immediately before, and at 24 and 48 h after surgery, and related to clinical outcome.

Results.—Of 62 patients who underwent attempted operative repair of ruptured AAA, 50 (81 per cent) survived for more than 24 h and were included in this study. Twenty-three (46 per cent) of the 50 had a detectable cTnI level at one or more time points during the first 48 h. Of these, 11 patients had clinical or electrocardiographic evidence of an acute cardiac event and 12 did not; five patients in each of these two groups died. Of 27 patients with no increase in cTnI in the first 48 h, only three died ($P = 0.031$ and $P = 0.043$ respectively, relative to the groups with detectable cTnI).

Conclusion.—Approximately half of patients who survived repair of ruptured AAA for more than 24 h sustained a detectable myocardial injury within the first 48 h. A perioperative increase in the level of cTnI, with or without clinically apparent cardiac dysfunction, was associated with postoperative death.

▶ It is difficult to know what to do with information such as this. It certainly can be one element of a complex decision process in deciding how aggressive to be in caring for the patient with ruptured AAA. A single blood test, however, will never be enough for me to suggest withdrawal of support from a critically ill patient.

G. L. Moneta, MD

Randomized Trial of Lifestyle Modification and Pharmacotherapy for Obesity

Wadden TA, Berkowitz RI, Womble LG, et al (Univ of Pennsylvania, Philadelphia; Children's Hosp of Philadelphia; Brown Med School, Providence, RI; et al)
N Engl J Med 353:2111-2120, 2005   3–4

Background.—Weight-loss medications are recommended as an adjunct to a comprehensive program of diet, exercise, and behavior therapy but are

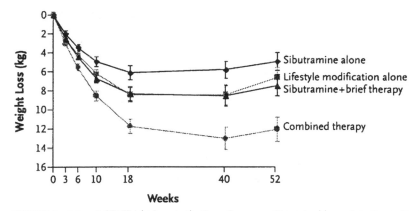

FIGURE 2.—Mean (±SE) Weight Loss in the Four Groups, as Determined by an Intention-to-Treat Analysis (Panel A). Subjects who received combined therapy lost significantly more weight at all times than subjects in the other three groups. Subjects treated with lifestyle modification along and those treated with sibutramine plus brief therapy lost significantly more weight at week 18 than those who received sibutramine alone, with no other significant differences at any other time. (Reprinted by permission of *The New England Journal of Medicine* from Wadden TA, Berkowitz RI, Womble LG, et al: Randomized trial of lifestyle modification and pharmacotherapy for obesity. *N Engl J Med* 353:2111-2120, 2005. Copyright 2005, Massachusetts Medical Society. All rights reserved.)

typically prescribed with minimal or no lifestyle modification. This practice is likely to limit therapeutic benefits.

Methods.—In this one-year trial, we randomly assigned 224 obese adults to receive 15 mg of sibutramine per day alone, delivered by a primary care provider in eight visits of 10 to 15 minutes each; lifestyle-modification counseling alone, delivered in 30 group sessions; sibutramine plus 30 group sessions of lifestyle-modification counseling (i.e., combined therapy); or sibutramine plus brief lifestyle-modification counseling delivered by a primary care provider in eight visits of 10 to 15 minutes each. All subjects were prescribed a diet of 1200 to 1500 kcal per day and the same exercise regimen.

Results.—At one year, subjects who received combined therapy lost a mean (±SD) of 12.1±9.8 kg, whereas those receiving sibutramine alone lost 5.0±7.4 kg, those treated by lifestyle modification alone lost 6.7±7.9 kg, and those receiving sibutramine plus brief therapy lost 7.5±8.0 kg (P<0.001). Those in the combined-therapy group who frequently recorded their food intake lost more weight than those who did so infrequently (18.1±9.8 kg vs. 7.7±7.5 kg, P−0.04).

Conclusions.—The combination of medication and group lifestyle modification resulted in more weight loss than either medication or lifestyle modification alone. The results underscore the importance of prescribing weight-loss medications in combination with, rather than in lieu of, lifestyle modification (Fig 2).

▶ Obesity appears to have many of the elements of other addictive conditions such as tobacco and drug abuse. The best medicine is prevention. But a combination of medication and lifestyle modification (or psychotherapy) works better than drugs alone. Medications help but the patient needs to change their entire approach to life. Physicians will do best to encourage the obese in their attempts to lose weight. Little is to be gained by ridicule.

G. L. Moneta, MD

Obstructive Sleep Apnea as a Risk Factor for Stroke and Death

Yaggi HK, Concato J, Kernan WN, et al (Yale Univ, New Haven, Conn; Veterans Affairs Connecticut Healthcare System, West Haven)
N Engl J Med 353:2034-2041, 2005   3–5

Background.—Previous studies have suggested that the obstructive sleep apnea syndrome may be an important risk factor for stroke. It has not been determined, however, whether the syndrome is independently related to the risk of stroke or death from any cause after adjustment for other risk factors, including hypertension.

Methods.—In this observational cohort study, consecutive patients underwent polysomnography, and subsequent events (strokes and deaths) were verified. The diagnosis of the obstructive sleep apnea syndrome was based on an apnea-hypopnea index of 5 or higher (five or more events per hour); patients with an apnea-hypopnea index of less than 5 served as the comparison group. Proportional-hazards analysis was used to determine the

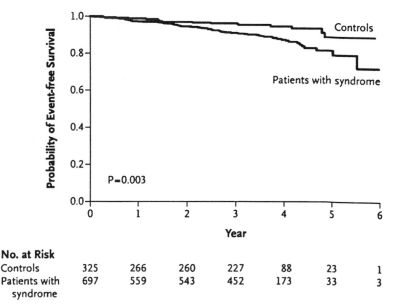

No. at Risk							
	0	1	2	3	4	5	6
Controls	325	266	260	227	88	23	1
Patients with syndrome	697	559	543	452	173	33	3

FIGURE 1.—Kaplan-Meier Estimates of the Probability of Event-free Survival among Patients with the Obstructive Sleep Apnea Syndrome and Controls. (Reprinted by permission of *The New England Journal of Medicine* from Yaggi HK, Concato J, Kernan WN, et al: Obstructive sleep apnea as a risk factor for stroke and death. *N Engl J Med* 353:2034-2041, 2005. Copyright 2005, Massachusetts Medical Society. All rights reserved.)

independent effect of the obstructive sleep apnea syndrome on the composite outcome of stroke or death from any cause.

Results.—Among 1022 enrolled patients, 697 (68 percent) had the obstructive sleep apnea syndrome. At baseline, the mean apnea-hypopnea index in the patients with the syndrome was 35, as compared with a mean apnea-hypopnea index of 2 in the comparison group. In an unadjusted analysis, the obstructive sleep apnea syndrome was associated with stroke or death from any cause (hazard ratio, 2.24; 95 percent confidence interval, 1.30 to 3.86; P=0.004). After adjustment for age, sex, race, smoking status, alcohol-consumption status, body-mass index, and the presence or absence of diabetes mellitus, hyperlipidemia, atrial fibrillation, and hypertension, the obstructive sleep apnea syndrome retained a statistically significant association with stroke or death (hazard ratio, 1.97; 95 percent confidence interval, 1.12 to 3.48; P=0.01). In a trend analysis, increased severity of sleep apnea at baseline was associated with an increased risk of the development of the composite end point (P=0.005).

Conclusions.—The obstructive sleep apnea syndrome significantly increases the risk of stroke or death from any cause, and the increase is independent of other risk factors, including hypertension (Fig 1).

▶ Obstructive sleep apnea (OSA) is associated with vascular risk factors and cardiovascular events. Previously, it was unknown if OSA patients had an increased risk of cardiovascular events secondary to their vascular risk factors or if OSA itself acted independently to increase risk. It now appears that OSA is an independent risk factor for stroke. Since OSA is common in patients with vascular risk factors, vascular surgeons should question their patients about symptoms of OSA and refer patients with symptoms consistent with OSA for treatment of their sleep disorder.

G. L. Moneta, MD

Cystatin C and the Risk of Death and Cardiovascular Events among Elderly Persons
Shlipak MG, Sarnak MJ, Katz R, et al (Univ of California, San Francisco; Tufts-New England Med Ctr, Boston; Collaborative Health Studies Coordinating Ctr, Seattle; et al)
N Engl J Med 352:2049-2060, 2005   3–6

Background.—Cystatin C is a serum measure of renal function that appears to be independent of age, sex, and lean muscle mass. We compared creatinine and cystatin C levels as predictors of mortality from cardiovascular causes and from all causes in the Cardiovascular Health Study, a cohort study of elderly persons living in the community.

Methods.—Creatinine and cystatin C were measured in serum samples collected from 4637 participants at the study visit in 1992 or 1993; follow-up continued until June 30, 2001. For each measure, the study population was divided into quintiles, with the fifth quintile subdivided into thirds (designated 5a, 5b, and 5c).

Results.—Higher cystatin C levels were directly associated, in a dose-response manner, with a higher risk of death from all causes. As compared with the first quintile, the hazard ratios (and 95 percent confidence intervals) for death were as follows: second quintile, 1.08 (0.86 to 1.35); third quintile, 1.23 (1.00 to 1.53); fourth quintile, 1.34 (1.09 to 1.66); quintile 5a, 1.77 (1.34 to 2.26); 5b, 2.18 (1.72 to 2.78); and 5c, 2.58 (2.03 to 3.27). In contrast, the association of creatinine categories with mortality from all causes appeared to be J-shaped. As compared with the two lowest quintiles combined (cystatin C level, ≤0.99 mg per liter), the highest quintile of cystatin C (≥1.29 mg per liter) was associated with a significantly elevated risk of death from cardiovascular causes (hazard ratio, 2.27 [1.73 to 2.97]), myocardial infarction (hazard ratio, 1.48 [1.08 to 2.02]), and stroke (hazard ratio, 1.47 [1.09 to 1.96]) after multivariate adjustment. The fifth quintile of creatinine, as compared with the first quintile, was not independently associated with any of these three outcomes.

Conclusions.—Cystatin C, a serum measure of renal function, is a stronger predictor of the risk of death and cardiovascular events in elderly persons than is creatinine.

▶ It is well known that impaired renal function is associated with adverse cardiovascular outcome. However, creatinine and measurements of glomerular filtration rate are relatively insensitive indicators of renal function and a great deal of renal function must be lost before they become abnormal. Cystatin C may therefore be a marker of cardiovascular risks that can be measured earlier than changes in creatinine or glomerular filtration rate.

However, cystatin C may have other toxic effects that are independent of its correlation with renal function but may contribute to its association with cardiovascular risk and mortality. Also, keep in mind that this study applies only to patients greater than 65 years old.

G. L. Moneta, MD

High prevalence of thrombophilia among young patients with myocardial infarction and few conventional risk factors

Segev A, Ellis MH, Segev F, et al (Tel-Aviv Univ, Israel)
Int J Cardiol 98:421-424, 2005   3–7

Background.—Thrombophilia refers to series of acquired and inherited conditions that confer a tendency to thrombus formation. The exact relationship between thrombophilia and MI is not well established.

Objectives.—To determine the prevalence of thrombophilia in young patients with their first MI and few conventional risk factors.

Methods.—We evaluated the baseline characteristics and the thrombophilia profile, including anti-cardiolipin antibodies, activated protein C resistance (APCR) with the factor V Leiden mutation, prothrombin G20210A

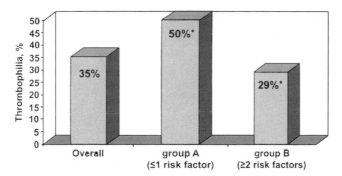

FIGURE 1.—The presence of at least one thrombophilia marker in relation to conventional risk factors. *$p=0.046$. (Reprinted by permission of the publisher from Segev A, Ellis MH, Segev F, et al: High prevalence of thrombophilia among young patients with myocardial infarction and few conventional risk factors. *Int J Cardiol* 98:421-424, 2005. Copyright 2005 by Elsevier Science Inc.)

mutation, protein C, protein S, and antithrombin III levels, among 85 consecutive patients (<50 year old) who were admitted to CCU with their first MI. Patients were divided into two groups: group A—patients with ≤1 risk factor and group B—patients with ≥2 risk factors.

Results.—92% were male and 55% with anterior wall MI. Overall, the risk factor profile was: smoking in 60%, hyperlipidemia in 42%, positive family history in 29%, hypertension in 18%, diabetes mellitus in 13%, and obesity in 8%. Forty-seven percent of patients had ≤1 risk factor ($n40$, group A) and 53% had ≥2 risk factors ($n=45$, group B). The prevalence of the prothrombin mutation was 15% in group A compared to 7% in group B ($p=0.12$). APCR secondary to a heterozygous genotype of factor V Leiden mutation was found in 20% in group A compared to 2% in group B ($p<0.01$). Anti-cardiolipin antibodies were found in 16% in group A compared to 22% in group B ($p=ns$). Finally, we have found that the likelihood of identifying at least one thrombophilia marker was 50% in group A compared to 29% in group B ($p=0.046$).

Conclusions.—The likelihood to detect at least one thrombophilia marker in young patients with MI and few conventional risk factors is significantly high. Thrombophilia may contribute to the development of MI in this specific group of young patients (Fig 1).

▶ The patient without risk factors or with minimal risk factors of cardiovascular disease and who suffers an MI or a cardiovascular event is an enigma. Some of these patients are known to have abnormalities of particle size of low-density lipoprotein cholesterol, and now it appears thrombophilia may also be important. Information such as this indicates that patients with a history of premature cardiovascular disease in their families should have an evaluation that is beyond assessment of traditional risk factors and basic low-density lipoprotein cholesterol, high-density lipoprotein cholesterol, and triglyceride levels.

G. L. Moneta, MD

Suboptimal intensity of risk factor modification in PAD

Oka RK, Umoh E, Szuba A, et al (Univ of California at San Francisco; Stanford Univ, Calif)

Vasc Med 10:91-96, 2005   3-8

This study extends earlier trials indicating that atherosclerosis risk factors are underdetected and undertreated in peripheral arterial disease (PAD) patients. Recognition and treatment of hyperlipidemia and hypertension in PAD patients is suboptimal. Diabetes appears to be detected more frequently although glycemic control is still suboptimal. The use of antiplatelet therapy is particularly underutilized. Additionally, despite the demonstrated efficacy of regular exercise in PAD patients, almost half of the study sample was sedentary. Approximately one third of the current study sample was overweight and nearly one third was obese by ATP-III guidelines. Only 31% of subjects were taking dietary measures to improve their cardiovascular health, and even fewer were physically active. To rectify suboptimal management of risk factors, there is a need for increased public awareness of PAD, reimbursement and implementation of screening programs and more aggressive treatment. Future studies are needed to examine innovative interventions for identification and management of cardiovascular risk factors in patients with PAD.

▶ The study is small and therefore subject to type II statistical error. Nevertheless, the results are similar to the larger national PARTNERS (PAD Awareness, Risk and Treatment) study and indicate suboptimal management of risk factors in patients with PAD. It is clear that one publication, the PARTNERS publication, has not had a dramatic impact on primary care practice with respect to management of PAD.

G. L. Moneta, MD

Intensive Lipid Lowering with Atorvastatin in Patients with Stable Coronary Disease

LaRosa JC, for the Treating to New Targets (TNT) Investigators (State Univ of New York, Brooklyn; et al)

N Engl J Med 352:1425-1435, 2005   3-9

Background.—Previous trials have demonstrated that lowering low-density lipoprotein (LDL) cholesterol levels below currently recommended levels is beneficial in patients with acute coronary syndromes. We prospectively assessed the efficacy and safety of lowering LDL cholesterol levels below 100 mg per deciliter (2.6 mmol per liter) in patients with stable coronary heart disease (CHD).

Methods.—A total of 10,001 patients with clinically evident CHD and LDL cholesterol levels of less than 130 mg per deciliter (3.4 mmol per liter) were randomly assigned to double-blind therapy and received either 10 mg or 80 mg of atorvastatin per day. Patients were followed for a median of 4.9

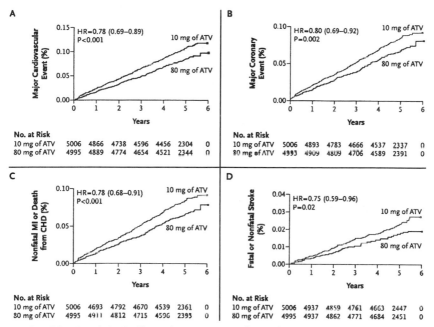

FIGURE 3.—Cumulative Incidence of a First Major Cardiovascular Event (Panel A), a First Major Coronary Event (Panel B), Nonfatal Myocardial Infarction (MI) or Death from CHD (Panel C), and a First Fatal or Nonfatal Stroke (Panel D). The primary end point was a first major cardiovascular event, and a first major coronary event was defined as death from CHD, nonfatal non–procedure-related MI, or resuscitation after cardiac arrest. HR denotes hazard ratio for the group given 80 mg of atorvastatis (ATV) as compared with the group given 10 mg of ATV. (Reprinted by permission of *The New England Journal of Medicine* from LaRosa JC, for the Treating to New Targets (TNT) Investigators. *N Engl J Med* 352:1425-1435, 2005. Copyright 2005, Massachusetts Medical Sociaty. All rights reserved.)

years. The primary end point was the occurrence of a first major cardiovascular event, defined as death from CHD, nonfatal non–procedure-related myocardial infarction, resuscitation after cardiac arrest, or fatal or nonfatal stroke.

Results.—The mean LDL cholesterol levels were 77 mg per deciliter (2.0 mmol per liter) during treatment with 80 mg of atorvastatin and 101 mg per deciliter (2.6 mmol per liter) during treatment with 10 mg of atorvastatin. The incidence of persistent elevations in liver aminotransferase levels was 0.2 percent in the group given 10 mg of atorvastatin and 1.2 percent in the group given 80 mg of atorvastatin (P<0.001). A primary event occurred in 434 patients (8.7 percent) receiving 80 mg of atorvastatin, as compared with 548 patients (10.9 percent) receiving 10 mg of atorvastatin, representing an absolute reduction in the rate of major cardiovascular events of 2.2 percent and a 22 percent relative reduction in risk (hazard ratio, 0.78; 95 percent confidence interval, 0.69 to 0.89; P<0.001). There was no difference between the two treatment groups in overall mortality.

Conclusions.—Intensive lipid-lowering therapy with 80 mg of atorvastatin per day in patients with stable CHD provides significant clinical benefit beyond that afforded by treatment with 10 mg of atorvastatin per day. This

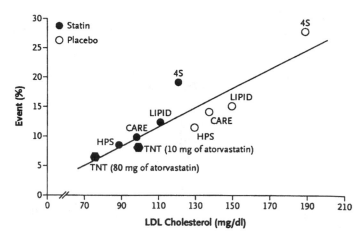

FIGURE 4.—Event Rates Plotted against LDL Cholesterol Levels during Statin Therapy in Secondary-Prevention Studies. HPS denotes Heart Protection Study (Heart Protection Study Collaborative Group. MRC/BHF Heart Protection Study of cholesterol lowering with simvastatin in 20,536 high-risk individuals: A randomized placebo-controlled trial. *Lancet* 360:7-22, 2002); CARE Cholesterol and Recurrent Events Trial (Sacks FM, Pfeffer MA, Moyé LA, et al: The effect of pravastatin on coronary events after myocardial infarction in patients with average cholesterol levels. *N Engl J Med* 335:1001-1009, 1996); LIPID Long-term Intervention with Pravastatin in Ischaemic Disease (The Long-Term Intervention with Pravastatin in Ischaemic Disease [LIPID] Study Group: Prevention of cardiovascular events and death with pravastatin in patients with coronary heart disease and a broad range of initial cholesterol levels. *N Engl J Med* 339:1349-1357, 1998); and 4S Scandinavian Simvastatin Survival Study (Scandinavian Simvastatin Survival Study Group: Randomised trial of cholesterol lowering in 4444 patients with coronary heart disease: The Scandinavian Simvastatin Survival Study (4S). *Lancet* 344:1383-1389, 1994). Event rates for HPS, CARE, and LIPID are for death from CHD and nonfatal myocardial infarction. Event rates for 4S and the TNT Study also include resuscitation after cardiac arrest. To convert values for LDL cholesterol to millimoles per liter, multiply by 0.02586. (Reprinted by permission of *The New England Journal of Medicine* from LaRosa JC, for the Treating to New Targets (TNT) Investigators. *N Engl J Med* 352:1425-1435, 2005. Copyright 2005, Massachusetts Medical Sociaty. All rights reserved.)

occurred with a greater incidence of elevated aminotransferase levels (Figs 3 and 4).

▶ The safety data for the 2 doses of atorvastatin utilized in this trial are consistent with other large-scale trials of this drug.[1,2] The trial was not adequately powered to detect differences in risk of death from any cause. Nevertheless, the study is part of a growing body of evidence suggesting that lowering LDL cholesterol levels significantly below traditionally recommended values has clinical benefit.

G. L. Moneta, MD

References

1. Cannon CP, Braunwald E, McCabe CH, et al: Intensive versus moderate lipid lowering with statins after acute coronary syndromes. *N Engl J Med* 350:1495-1504, 2004.
2. Severs PS, Dahlof B, Poulter NR, et al: Prevention of coronary and stroke events with atorvastatin in hypertensive patients who have average or lower-than-average cholesterol concentrations, in the Anglo-Scandinavian Cardiac Outcomes Trial–Lipid Lowering Arm (ASCOT-LLA): A multicentre randomized controlled trial. *Lancet* 361:1147-1158, 2003.

Cost-effectiveness of simvastatin in people at different levels of vascular disease risk: economic analysis of a randomised trial in 20 536 individuals

Heart Protection Study Collaborative Group (Radcliffe Infirmary, Oxford, England)

Lancet 365:1779-1785, 2005   3–10

Background.—Statin therapy reduces the rates of heart attack, stroke, and revascularisation among a wide range of individuals. Reliable assessment of its cost-effectiveness in different circumstances is needed.

Methods.—20 536 adults (aged 40-80 years) with vascular disease or diabetes were randomly allocated 40 mg simvastatin daily (10 269) or placebo (10 267) for an average of 5 years. Comparisons were made of hospitalisation and statin costs (2001 UK prices) during the scheduled treatment period between all simvastatin-allocated versus all placebo-allocated partici-

	Vascular event costs (£)		Relative cost (95% CI)	Heterogeneity p value
	Simvastatin -allocated	Placebo -allocated		
Prior disease				
Any CHD	2138	2655		0·9
No CHD				
CVD	1258	1630		
PVD	1845	2539		
Diabetes	1070	1430		
Sex				
Male	1896	2448		0·5
Female	1507	1856		
Age (years)				
<65	1560	2044		0·7
≥65 to <70	1937	2352		
≥70	2089	2697		
LDL cholesterol (mmol/L)				
<3·0	1666	1976		0·2
≥3·0 to <3·5	1757	2509		
≥3·5	1930	2436		
Risk group (5-year MVE risk)				
1 (12%)	778	1210		0·4
2 (18%)	1354	1728		
3 (22%)	1753	2097		
4 (28%)	2132	2585		
5 (42%)	2978	3889		
All patients	1800	2301	0·78 (0·73–0·84)	

0·4   0·6   0·8   1·0   1·2   1·4

Simvastatin better | Placebo better

FIGURE 1.—Proportional reductions in vascular event costs with simvastatin allocation by prior disease, sex, age, LDL cholesterol, and multivariate risk subgroups. CHD=coronary heart disease; CVD=cerebrovascular disease; PVD=peripheral vascular disease; MVE=major vascular event. (Courtesy of Heart Protection Study Collaborative Group: Cost-effectiveness of simvastatin in people at different levels of vascular disease risk: Economic analysis of a randomized trial in 20 536 individuals. *Lancet* 365:1779-1785, 2005. Reprinted with permission from Elsevier.)

pants. Cost-effectiveness was estimated among different categories of participant.

Findings.—Allocation to simvastatin was associated with a highly significant 22% (95% CI 16-27; p<0.0001) proportional reduction in hospitalisation costs for all vascular events, with similar proportional reductions in every subcategory of participant studied. During an average of 5 years, estimated absolute reductions in vascular event costs per person allocated 40 mg simvastatin daily ranged from UK£847 (SE 137) in the highest risk quintile studied to £264 (48) in the lowest. Mean excess cost of statin therapy among participants allocated simvastatin was £1497 (8), with similar absolute increases in every subcategory. Costs of preventing a major vascular event with 40 mg simvastatin daily ranged from £4500 (95% CI 2300-7400) among participants with a 42% 5-year major vascular event rate to £31 100 pounds sterling (22 900-42 500) among those with a 12% rate (corresponding to 5-year major coronary event rates of 22% and 4%, respectively).

Interpretation.—Statin therapy is cost effective for a wider range of individuals with vascular disease or diabetes than previously recognised (particularly with lower-priced generics). It would be appropriate to consider reducing the estimated level of vascular event risk at which statin therapy is recommended (Fig 1).

▶ This is among the most compelling studies documenting the favorable pleotropic effects of statins in patients at risk for cardiovascular events. Statins are effective and cost effective in reducing cardiovascular events across a wide range of ages and risks. There seems to be no reason other than drug intolerance to not treat patients with cardiovascular risk factors with a statin medication.

G. L. Moneta, MD

A Randomized Trial of Low-Dose Aspirin in the Primary Prevention of Cardiovascular Disease in Women

Ridker PM, Cook NR, Lee I-M, et al (Harvard Med School, Boston; Harvard School of Public Health, Boston; Veterans Affairs Boston Healthcare System; et al)

N Engl J Med 352:1293-1304, 2005   3–11

Background.—Randomized trials have shown that low-dose aspirin decreases the risk of a first myocardial infarction in men, with little effect on the risk of ischemic stroke. There are few similar data in women.

Methods.—We randomly assigned 39,876 initially healthy women 45 years of age or older to receive 100 mg of aspirin on alternate days or placebo and then monitored them for 10 years for a first major cardiovascular event (i.e., nonfatal myocardial infarction, nonfatal stroke, or death from cardiovascular causes).

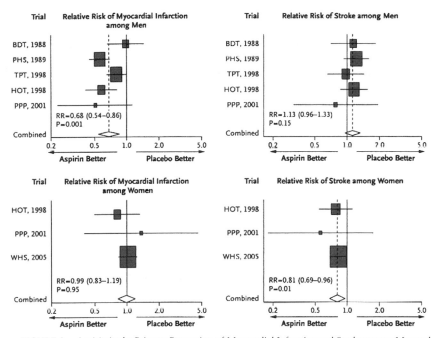

FIGURE 3.—Aspirin in the Primary Prevention of Myocardial Infarction and Stroke among Men and Women. The results of a sex-specific random-effects meta-analysis of data from six trials are shown: the British Doctors' Trial (BDT), the Physicians' Health study (PHS), the Thrombosis Prevention Trial (TPT), the Hypertension Optimal Treatment (HOT) study, the Primary Prevention Project (PPP), and the current Women's Health Study (WHS). The relative risk (RR) and 95 percent confidence interval (in parentheses) are shown for each trial (indicated by the *box* and *horizontal line* through each box, respectively), and the relative risk is shown for the combined results (indicated by the *diamond* and the *dashed line* in each graph). For the relative risk of myocardial infarction among women, the dashed line is coincident with the solid line at 1.00. The size of the box is proportional to the amount of information in the corresponding trial. (Reprinted by permission of *The New England Journal of Medicine* from Ridker PM, Cook NR, Lee I-M, et al: A randomized trial of low-dose aspirin in the primary prevention of cardiovascular disease in women. *N Engl J Med* 352:1293-1304, 2005. Copyright 2005, Massachusetts Medical Society. All rights reserved.)

Results.—During follow-up, 477 major cardiovascular events were confirmed in the aspirin group, as compared with 522 in the placebo group, for a nonsignificant reduction in risk with aspirin of 9 percent (relative risk, 0.91; 95 percent confidence interval, 0.80 to 1.03; P=0.13). With regard to individual end points, there was a 17 percent reduction in the risk of stroke in the aspirin group, as compared with the placebo group (relative risk, 0.83; 95 percent confidence interval, 0.69 to 0.99; P=0.04), owing to a 24 percent reduction in the risk of ischemic stroke (relative risk, 0.76; 95 percent confidence interval, 0.63 to 0.93; P=0.009) and a nonsignificant increase in the risk of hemorrhagic stroke (relative risk, 1.24; 95 percent confidence interval, 0.82 to 1.87; P−0.31). As compared with placebo, aspirin had no significant effect on the risk of fatal or nonfatal myocardial infarction (relative risk, 1.02; 95 percent confidence interval, 0.84 to 1.25; P=0.83) or death from cardiovascular causes (relative risk, 0.95; 95 percent confidence interval, 0.74 to 1.22; P=0.68). Gastrointestinal bleeding requiring transfusion was more frequent in the aspirin group than in the placebo group (relative risk, 1.40; 95 percent confidence interval, 1.07 to 1.83; P=0.02). Subgroup analyses showed that aspirin significantly reduced the risk of major cardiovascular events, ischemic stroke, and myocardial infarction among women 65 years of age or older.

Conclusions.—In this large, primary-prevention trial among women, aspirin lowered the risk of stroke without affecting the risk of myocardial infarction or death from cardiovascular causes, leading to a nonsignificant finding with respect to the primary end point (Fig 3).

▶ It is important to remember that this was a primary prevention trial. The patients were initially healthy, without significant known cardiovascular disease. The trial should in no way influence use of aspirin in patients with established cardiovascular disease or risk factors. Why aspirin is effective in primary prevention of stroke in women but not men is unknown. Perhaps men and women are indeed different.

G. L. Moneta, MD

Intensive Diabetes Treatment and Cardiovascular Disease in Patients with Type 1 Diabetes

Nathan DM, and The Diabetes Control and Complications Trial/Epidemiology of Diabetes Interventions and Complications (DCCT/EDIC) Study Research Group (DCCT/EDIC Research Group, Bethesda, Md)

N Engl J Med 353:2643-2653, 2005   3–12

Background.—Intensive diabetes therapy aimed at achieving near normoglycemia reduces the risk of microvascular and neurologic complications of type 1 diabetes. We studied whether the use of intensive therapy as compared with conventional therapy during the Diabetes Control and Complications Trial (DCCT) affected the long-term incidence of cardiovascular disease.

Methods.—The DCCT randomly assigned 1441 patients with type 1 diabetes to intensive or conventional therapy, treating them for a mean of 6.5 years between 1983 and 1993. Ninety-three percent were subsequently followed until February 1, 2005, during the observational Epidemiology of Diabetes Interventions and Complications study. Cardiovascular disease (defined as nonfatal myocardial infarction, stroke, death from cardiovascular disease, confirmed angina, or the need for coronary-artery revascularization) was assessed with standardized measures and classified by an independent committee.

Results.—During the mean 17 years of follow-up, 46 cardiovascular disease events occurred in 31 patients who had received intensive treatment in the DCCT, as compared with 98 events in 52 patients who had received conventional treatment. Intensive treatment reduced the risk of any cardiovascular disease event by 42 percent (95 percent confidence interval, 9 to 63 percent; P=0.02) and the risk of nonfatal myocardial infarction, stroke, or death from cardiovascular disease by 57 percent (95 percent confidence in-

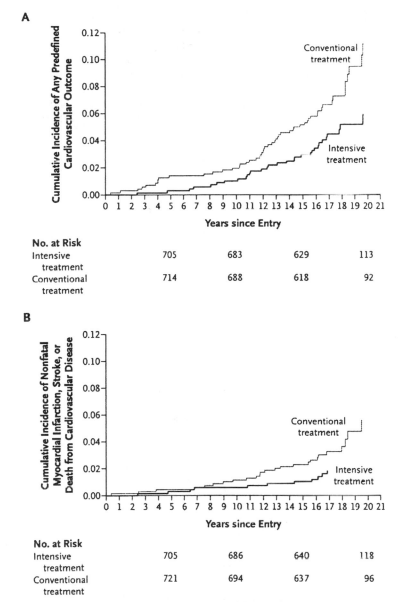

FIGURE 1.—Cumulative Incidence of the First of Any of the Predefined Cardiovascular Disease Outcomes (Panel A) and of the First Occurrence of Nonfatal Myocardial Infarction, Stroke, or Death from Cardiovascular Disease (Panel B). As compared with conventional treatment, intensive treatment reduced the risk of any predefined cardiovascular disease outcome by 42 percent (95 percent confidence interval, 9 to 63 percent; P=0.02) (Panel A) and reduced the risk of the first occurrence of nonfatal myocardial infarction, stroke, or death from cardiovascular disease by 57 percent (95 percent confidence interval, 12 to 79 percent; P=0.02) (Panel B). (Reprinted by permission of *The New England Journal of Medicine* from Nathan DM, and The Diabetes Control and Complications Trial/Epidemiology of Diabetes Interventions and Complications (DCCT/EDIC) Study Research Group: Intensive diabetes treatment and cardiovascular disease in patients with type 1 diabetes. *N Engl J Med* 353:2643-2653, 2005. Copyright 2005, Massachusetts Medical Society. All rights reserved.)

terval, 12 to 79 percent; P=0.02). The decrease in glycosylated hemoglobin values during the DCCT was significantly associated with most of the positive effects of intensive treatment on the risk of cardiovascular disease. Microalbuminuria and albuminuria were associated with a significant increase in the risk of cardiovascular disease, but differences between treatment groups remained significant (P≤0.05) after adjusting for these factors.

Conclusions.—Intensive diabetes therapy has long-term beneficial effects on the risk of cardiovascular disease in patients with type 1 diabetes (Fig 1).

▶ This is an extremely important article for 2 reasons. First, it indicates that much of the cardiovascular risk imparted by type 1 diabetes can be controlled by intensive diabetic therapy. Second, combined with evidence of favorable effects of intensive diabetic therapy on microvascular disease, the culmination of data suggests a common underlying mechanism to the microvascular and macrovascular adverse effects of diabetes.

G. L. Moneta, MD

Antibiotic Treatment of *Chlamydia pneumoniae* after Acute Coronary Syndrome
Cannon CP, for the Pravastatin or Atorvastatin Evaluation and Infection Therapy–Thrombolysis in Myocardial Infarction 22 Investigators (Harvard Med School, Boston; et al)
N Engl J Med 352:1646-1654, 2005 3–13

Background.—*Chlamydia pneumoniae* has been found within atherosclerotic plaques, and elevated titers of antibody to this organism have been

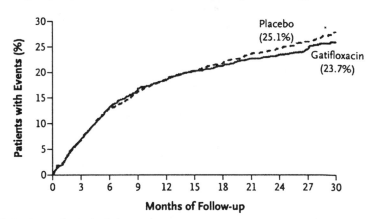

FIGURE 2.—Kaplan-Meier Estimates of Events over Time among Patients Treated with Gatifloxacin or Placebo. Events were defined as deaths or major cardiovascular events, and rates noted were at two years. (Reprinted by permission of *The New England Journal of Medicine* from Cannon CP, for the Pravastatin or Atorvastatin Evaluation and Infection Therapy–Thrombolysis in Myocardial Infarction 22 Investigators: Antibiotic treatment of *Chlamydia pneumoniae* after acute coronary syndrome. *N Engl J Med* 352:1646-1654, 2005. Copyright 2005, Massachusetts Medical Society. All rights reserved.)

Characteristic	of Patients	2-Year Event Rate (%)		
		Gatifloxacin	Placebo	
Sex				
Male	78	23.6	25.7	
Female	22	24.2	23.0	
Diabetes				
Yes	18	32.6	30.5	
No	82	21.6	23.9	
Age				
≥65 yr	30	29.0	28.6	
<65 yr	70	21.5	23.5	
Smoker				
Current	37	22.1	24.2	
Not current	63	24.6	25.6	
Unstable angina	29	29.6	28.4	
Myocardial infarction	71	21.2	23.7	
C-reactive protein				
≥Median	50	25.2	24.9	
<Median	50	21.6	24.4	
Antibody titer				
Negative	36	25.4	25.5	
Positive				
<1:256	47	22.5	24.8	
≥1:256	15	21.9	22.2	

```
        0.50   0.75   1.00   1.25   1.50
            Gatifloxacin      Placebo
              Better           Better
```

FIGURE 4.—Hazard Ratios for Death or a Major Cardiovascular Event, with Two-Year Event Rates, According to Baseline Characteristics. *Squares* denote hazard ratios and *horizontal lines* 95 percent confidence intervals. None of the tests for interaction were significant. The median C-reactive protein level was 12.1 mg per liter. (Reprinted by permission of *The New England Journal of Medicine* from Cannon CP, for the Pravastatin or Atorvastatin Evaluation and Infection Therapy–Thrombolysis in Myocardial Infarction 22 Investigators: Antibiotic treatment of *Chlamydia pneumoniae* after acute coronary syndrome. N Engl J Med 352:1646-1654, 2005. Copyright 2005, Massachusetts Medical Society. All rights reserved.)

linked to a higher risk of coronary events. Pilot studies have suggested that antibiotic treatment may reduce the risk of cardiovascular events.

Methods.—We enrolled 4162 patients who had been hospitalized for an acute coronary syndrome within the preceding 10 days and evaluated the efficacy of long-term treatment with gatifloxacin, a bactericidal antibiotic known to be effective against *C. pneumoniae,* in a double-blind, randomized, placebo-controlled trial. Subjects received 400 mg of gatifloxacin daily during an initial 2-week course of therapy that began 2 weeks after randomization, followed by a 10-day course every month for the duration of the trial (mean duration, 2 years), or placebo. The primary end point was a composite of death from all causes, myocardial infarction, documented unstable angina requiring rehospitalization, revascularization (performed at least 30 days after randomization), and stroke.

Results.—A Kaplan-Meier analysis revealed that the rates of primary-end-point events at two years were 23.7 percent in the gatifloxacin group and 25.1 percent in the placebo group (hazard ratio, 0.95; 95 percent confidence interval, 0.84 to 1.08; P=0.41). No benefit was seen in any of the prespecified secondary end points or in any of the prespecified subgroups, including patients with elevated titers to C. *pneumoniae* or C-reactive protein.

Conclusions.—Despite long-term treatment with a bactericidal antibiotic effective against C. *pneumoniae*, no reduction in the rate of cardiovascular events was observed (Figs 2 and 4).

▶ *C pneumoniae* has been postulated to have a role in development of atherosclerosis. The data, however, have been largely circumstantial, with isolation of *C pneumoniae* from atherosclerotic plaques. No one was sure whether this was a "chicken or egg" phenomenon. The current article does not exclude *C pneumoniae* as an initiator of atherosclerosis. (It may be that other mechanisms promote atherosclerosis once it is initiated.) However, it now appears that treatment of potential *C pneumoniae* infection will be unlikely to alter the course of patients with established atherosclerosis.

G. L. Moneta, MD

Long-Term Outcomes of Coronary-Artery Bypass Grafting Versus Stent Implantation
Hannan EL, Racz MJ, Walford G, et al (State Univ of New York, Albany; St Joseph's Hosp, Syracuse, NY; Duke Univ, Durham, NC; et al)
N Engl J Med 352:2174-2183, 2005   3–14

Background.—Several studies have compared outcomes for coronary-artery bypass grafting (CABG) and percutaneous coronary intervention (PCI), but most were done before the availability of stenting, which has revolutionized the latter approach.

Methods.—We used New York's cardiac registries to identify 37,212 patients with multivessel disease who underwent CABG and 22,102 patients with multivessel disease who underwent PCI from January 1, 1997, to December 31, 2000. We determined the rates of death and subsequent revascularization within three years after the procedure in various groups of patients according to the number of diseased vessels and the presence or absence of involvement of the left anterior descending coronary artery. The rates of adverse outcomes were adjusted by means of proportional-hazards methods to account for differences in patients' severity of illness before revascularization.

Results.—Risk-adjusted survival rates were significantly higher among patients who underwent CABG than among those who received a stent in all of the anatomical subgroups studied. For example, the adjusted hazard ratio for the long-term risk of death after CABG relative to stent implantation was 0.64 (95 percent confidence interval, 0.56 to 0.74) for patients with three-vessel disease with involvement of the proximal left anterior descending coronary artery and 0.76 (95 percent confidence interval, 0.60 to 0.96) for patients with two-vessel disease with involvement of the nonproximal left anterior descending coronary artery. Also, the three-year rates of revascularization were considerably higher in the stenting group than in the CABG group (7.8 percent vs. 0.3 percent for subsequent CABG and 27.3 percent vs. 4.6 percent for subsequent PCI).

Conclusions.—For patients with two or more diseased coronary arteries, CABG is associated with higher adjusted rates of long-term survival than stenting.

▶ What this article tells us is that CABG is a good operation. The data were collected before widespread use of drug eluting stents. The article therefore is unlikely to influence any cardiologist to refer a "stentable" patient for a coronary artery bypass.

G. L. Moneta, MD

Complications of the COX-2 Inhibitors Parecoxib and Valdecoxib after Cardiac Surgery
Nussmeier NA, Whelton AA, Brown MT, et al (St Luke's Episcopal Hosp, Houston; Johns Hopkins Univ, Baltimore, Md; Pfizer, Ann Arbor, Mich; et al)
N Engl J Med 352:1081-1091, 2005   3–15

Background.—Valdecoxib and its intravenous prodrug parecoxib are used to treat postoperative pain but may involve risk after coronary-artery bypass grafting (CABG). We conducted a randomized trial to assess the safety of these drugs after CABG.

Methods.—In this randomized, double-blind study involving 10 days of treatment and 30 days of follow-up, 1671 patients were randomly assigned to receive intravenous parecoxib for at least 3 days, followed by oral valdecoxib through day 10; intravenous placebo followed by oral valdecoxib; or placebo for 10 days. All patients had access to standard opioid medications. The primary end point was the frequency of predefined adverse events, including cardiovascular events, renal failure or dysfunction, gastroduodenal ulceration, and wound-healing complications.

Results.—As compared with the group given placebo alone, both the group given parecoxib and valdecoxib and the group given placebo and valdecoxib had a higher proportion of patients with at least one confirmed adverse event (7.4 percent in each of these two groups vs. 4.0 percent in the placebo group; risk ratio for each comparison, 1.9; 95 percent confidence interval, 1.1 to 3.2; P=0.02 for each comparison with the placebo group). In particular, cardiovascular events (including myocardial infarction, cardiac arrest, stroke, and pulmonary embolism) were more frequent among the patients given parecoxib and valdecoxib than among those given placebo (2.0 percent vs. 0.5 percent; risk ratio, 3.7; 95 percent confidence interval, 1.0 to 13.5; P=0.03).

Conclusions.—The use of parecoxib and valdecoxib after CABG was associated with an increased incidence of cardiovascular events, arousing serious concern about the use of these drugs in such circumstances (Fig 2).

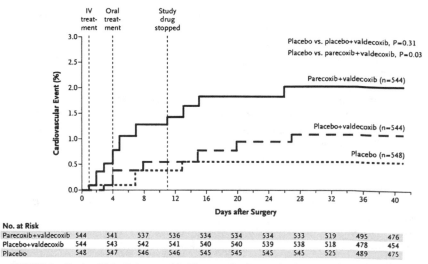

FIGURE 2.—Kaplan-Meier Estimates of the Time to a Cardiovascular Event. Cardiovascular events occurred throughout and after the 10-day period of drug administration in all groups. *IV* denotes intravenous. (Reprinted by permission of *The New England Journal of Medicine* from Nussmeier NA, Whelton AA, Brown MT, et al: Complications of the COX-2 inhibitors parecoxib and valdecoxib after cardiac surgery. *N Engl J Med* 352:1081-1091, 2005. Copyright 2005, Massachusetts Medical Society. All rights reserved.)

▶ Previous data on the adverse effects of COX-2 inhibitors has focused on long-term thromboembolic risk. There has been data to suggest that COX-2 inhibitors could exert significant opiate-sparing effects after surgical procedures. The current study, however, suggests that patients with coronary artery disease who undergo CABG may be adversely impacted by the use of COX-2 inhibitors to control perioperative pain.

While no such data currently exist to implicate COX-2 inhibitors in increased cardiovascular complications after peripheral vascular surgery, the current data certainly suggest that COX-2 inhibitors should be avoided in patients undergoing peripheral vascular surgery.

G. L. Moneta, MD

Paint-Only Is Equivalent to Scrub-and-Paint in Preoperative Preparation of Abdominal Surgery Sites

Ellenhorn JDI, Smith DD, Schwarz RE, et al (City of Hope Natl Med Ctr, Durarte, Calif)
J Am Coll Surg 201:737-741, 2005

3–16

Background.—Antiseptic preoperative skin site preparation is used to prepare the operative site before making a surgical incision. The goal of this preparation is a reduction in postoperative wound infection. The most straightforward technique necessary to achieve this goal remains controversial.

Study Design.—A prospective randomized trial was designed to prove equivalency for two commonly used techniques of surgical skin site preparation. Two hundred thirty-four patients undergoing nonlaparoscopic abdominal operations were consented for the trial. Exclusion criteria included presence of active infection at the time of operation, neutropenia, history of skin reaction to iodine, or anticipated insertion of prosthetic material at the time of operation. Patients were randomized to receive either a vigorous 5-minute scrub with povidone-iodine soap, followed by absorption with a sterile towel, and a paint with aqueous ovidone-iodine or surgical site preparation with a povidone-iodine paint only. The primary end point of the study was wound infection rate at 30 days, defined as presence of clinical signs of infection requiring therapeutic intervention.

Results.—Patients randomized to the scrub-and-paint arm (n − 115) and the paint-only arm (n = 119) matched at baseline with respect to age, comorbidity, wound classification, mean operative time, placement of drains, prophylactic antibiotic use, and surgical procedure (all p > 0.09). Wound infection occurred in 12 (10%) scrub-and-paint patients, and 12 (10%) paint-only patients. Based on our predefined equivalency parameters, we conclude equivalence of infection rates between the two preparations.

Conclusions.—Preoperative preparation of the abdomen with a scrub with povidone-iodine soap followed by a paint with aqueous povidone-iodine can be abandoned in favor of a paint with aqueous povidone-iodine alone. This change will result in reductions in operative times and costs.

▶ These data apply only to clean and clean contaminated cases that do not involve placement of a prosthetic device. While the data are interesting, they do not provide guidance as to the proper surgical site preparation technique for patients undergoing insertion of prosthetic grafts.

G. L. Moneta, MD

Perioperative β-blockade (POBBLE) for patients undergoing infrarenal vascular surgery: Results of a randomized double-blind controlled trial
Powell JT, for the POBBLE Trial Investigators (Imperial College, Charing Cross Campus, London)
J Vasc Surg 41:602-609, 2005   3–17

Objective.—To assess whether a pragmatic policy of perioperative β-blockade, with metoprolol, reduced the 30-day cardiovascular morbidity and mortality and reduced the length of hospital stay in average patients undergoing infrarenal vascular surgery.

Methods.—This was a double-blind randomized placebo-controlled trial that occurred in vascular surgical units in four UK hospitals. Participants were 103 patients without previous myocardial infarction who had infrarenal vascular surgery between July 2001 and March 2004. Interventions were oral metoprolol (50 mg twice daily, supplemented by intravenous doses when necessary) or placebo from admission until 7 days after surgery. Holter monitors were kept in place for 72 hours after surgery.

Results.—Eighty men and 23 women (median age, 73 years) were randomized, 55 to metoprolol and 48 to placebo, and 97 (94%) underwent surgery during the trial. The most common operations were aortic aneurysm repair (38%) and distal bypass (29%). Intraoperative inotropic support was required in 64% and 92% of patients in the placebo and metoprolol groups, respectively. Within 30 days, cardiovascular events occurred in 32 patients, including myocardial infarction (8%), unstable angina (9%), ventricular tachycardia (19%), and stroke (1%). Four (4%) deaths were reported. Cardiovascular events occurred in 15 (34%) and 17 (32%) patients in the placebo and metoprolol groups, respectively (unadjusted relative risk, 0.94; 95% confidence interval, 0.53-1.66; adjusted [for age, sex, statin use, and aortic cross-clamping] relative risk, 0.87; 95% confidence interval, 0.48-1.55). Time from operation to discharge was reduced from a median of 12 days (95% confidence interval, 9-19 days) in the placebo group to 10 days (95% confidence interval, 8-12 days) in the metoprolol group (adjusted hazard ratio, 1.71; 95% confidence interval, 1.09-2.66; $P < .02$).

Conclusions.—Myocardial ischemia was evident in a high proportion (one third) of the patients after surgery. A pragmatic regimen of perioperative β-blockade with metoprolol did not seem to reduce 30-day cardiovascular events, but it did decrease the time from surgery to discharge.

▶ This study was stopped early because of inability to recruit patients. The numbers reported are very small and apply to only a small subset of vascular surgical patients. We will continue to use perioperative β-blockers in our patients. This is an example of a study conceived during a time of clinical equipoise, but then an attempt was made to carry it out when perioperative β-blockade had evolved into standard practice. It is no wonder recruitment was difficult.

G. L. Moneta, MD

4 Grafts and Graft Complications

Rapamycin-coated expanded polytetrafluoroethylene bypass grafts exhibit decreased anastomotic neointimal hyperplasia in a porcine model
Cagiannos C, Abul-Khoudoud ORA, DeRijk W, et al (Univ of Tennessee, Memphis)
J Vasc Surg 42:980-988, 2005   4–1

Objective.—We tested the hypothesis that rapamycin coated onto, and eluted from, expanded polytetrafluoroethylene (ePTFE) grafts would diminish neointimal hyperplasia in a porcine model.

Methods.—Rapamycin (also called sirolimus) was coated onto the luminal surface of 6-mm-internal-diameter thin-walled ePTFE grafts by using an adhesive polymer that allows timed release of the drug. An adhesive polymer that allows timed release of rapamycin from ePTFE was developed with commercially available chemicals and applied on 6-mm ePTFE grafts. Graft integrity was characterized by scanning electron microscopy, and rapamycin levels were quantified by using high-performance liquid chromatography. Twenty-two mongrel pigs were randomized into three groups: untreated ePTFE (n = 6), adhesive-only coated ePTFE (n = 6), or adhesive- and rapamycin-coated ePTFE (n = 10). End-to-side unilateral aortoiliac bypasses were performed by using 6-mm-internal-diameter ePTFE grafts and standardized anastomotic lengths. Unilateral end-to-side aortoiliac ePTFE grafts (6-mm internal diameter) were inserted by using polypropylene sutures, 6-0 proximally and 7-0 distally; all anastomoses were 12 mm long. All animals received aspirin (325 mg orally) daily. All animals were given oral aspirin (325 mg) daily beginning on the day before surgery. At 28 days, the animals were killed, and the grafts were explanted in continuity with the adjacent aortic cuff and the outflow iliac artery. Variables compared between groups included graft patency, distal anastomotic length and cross-sectional narrowing, and intimal thickness at the arterial-graft junction indexed to the adjacent graft thickness. Microscopic analysis was performed with hematoxylin and eosin and Masson trichrome stains on paraffin sections. A pathologist blinded to experimental groups graded sections for collagen deposition, neointima formation, inflammatory cellular infiltrates, medial necrosis, and aneurysmal degeneration.

Results.—All animals survived until they were killed without clinical evidence of limb ischemia or graft infection. Preplanned *t* tests in the context of one-way analysis of variance showed no difference in outcome measures between the untreated ePTFE and adhesive-only coated ePTFE groups; therefore, they were combined in further comparisons with the adhesive- and rapamycin-coated ePTFE group. The Rapamycine eluting expanded polytetrafluoroethylene group had longer anastomoses (85.6% vs 60.6% of the initial anastomotic length maintained; $P < .0001$) and less cross-sectional narrowing in the outflow graft (16.2% vs 28.5%; $P = .0007$) when compared with the other two groups by using two-tailed Student *t* tests. There was no evidence of medial necrosis or aneurysmal degeneration. All patent grafts had complete endothelialization on hematoxylin and eosin sections. Rapamycin was detectable and quantifiable in the arterial wall at 28 days after implantation.

Conclusions.—Rapamycin can be coated onto and eluted from ePTFE by using a nonionic polymer and a simple coating technique. At 4 weeks after implantation, the rapamycin-eluting ePTFE grafts demonstrate gross, pathologic, and morphometric features of diminished neointimal hyperplasia when compared with non-drug-eluting ePTFE. Four weeks after implantation in a porcine model, rapamycin-eluting ePTFE grafts demonstrated gross, pathologic, and morphometric features of diminished neointimal hyperplasia when compared with untreated and adhesive-only coated ePTFE grafts.

▶ These clever investigators in Tennessee have figured out, and submitted for a patent, a method of binding rapamycin (sirolimus) to PTFE. Perhaps this will translate to increased patency of small-caliber PTFE grafts. The "fly in the ointment" is that sirolimus-coated stents have thus far not worked well in the infrainguinal position. It may be that the ability of drugs to limit intimal hyperplasia is specific to the hemodynamics of individual circulatory distributions.

G. L. Moneta, MD

Detection of aortic graft infection by fluorodeoxyglucose positron emission tomography: Comparison with computed tomographic findings
Fukuchi K, Ishida Y, Higashi M, et al (Osaka Med Ctr for Cancer and Cardiovascular Diseases, Japan; Natl Cardiovascular Ctr, Osaka, Japan)
J Vasc Surg 42:919-925, 2005
4–2

Objective.—Radionuclide imaging with fluorodeoxyglucose (FDG) and positron emission tomography (PET) has been proposed for the identification of vascular graft infection; however, its accuracy has not been determined. We performed this prospective study to compare the usefulness of FDG-PET in the assessment of vascular graft infection relative to computed tomography (CT).

Methods.—FDG-PET was performed for 33 consecutive patients with a suspected arterial prosthetic graft infection. The PET images were then as-

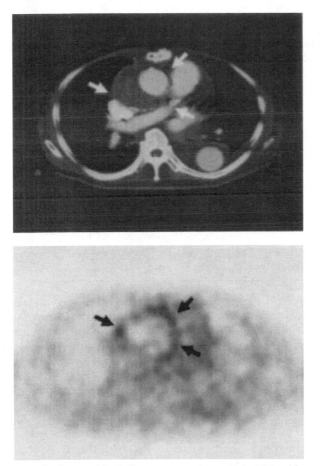

FIGURE 1.—Example of true-positive findings on computed tomography (CT) and fluorodeoxyglucose (FDG) positron emission tomography in a patient with graft infection. The patient had undergone total aortic arch replacement 4 months before the imaging examinations. Focal FDG accumulation in the graft (*black arrows*) is accompanied by fluid collection and extraluminal air on the enhanced CT image (*white arrows*). (Reprinted by permission of the publisher from Fukuchi K, Ishida Y, Higashi M, et al: Detection of aortic graft infection by fluorodeoxyglucose positron emission tomography: Comparison with computed tomographic findings. *J Vasc Surg* 42:919-925, 2005. Copyright 2005 by Elsevier.)

sessed visually in terms of the density of uptake. In cases with positive uptake, the pattern of accumulation was also defined, such as focal or diffuse uptake. We compared the diagnostic efficiency of PET with contemporaneous CT in detection of infection of the arterial prosthetic graft.

Results.—On the basis of the surgical, microbiological, and clinical follow-up findings, the aortic grafts were considered infected in 11 patients and not infected in 22 patients. Although the sensitivity of PET (91%) was higher than that of CT (64%), its specificity (64%) was lower than that of CT (86%). When focal uptake was set as the positive criterion in FDG, the specificity and positive predictive value of PET for the diagnosis of aortic graft infection improved significantly to 95% (P < .05 for both).

Conclusions.—Although both techniques are useful in evaluation of patients with suspected aortic graft infection, using the characteristic FDG uptake pattern described previously as a diagnostic criterion made the efficacy of FDG superior to that of CT in the diagnostic assessment of patients with suspected aortic graft infection (Fig 1).

▶ I doubt PET scanning ever will be clinically useful for sorting out possible prosthetic graft infection. In most cases, it is not difficult to tell whether a prosthetic graft is infected. If there is doubt, allowing a little time to go by will usually settle the issue.

G. L. Moneta, MD

Immediate and One-Year Outcome of Percutaneous Intervention of Saphenous Vein Graft Disease With *Paclitaxel*-Eluting Stents
Tsuchida K, Ong ATL, Aoki J, et al (Erasmus Med Ctr, Rotterdam, The Netherlands)
Am J Cardiol 96:395-398, 2005   4–3

Background.—Dramatic reductions in restenosis have been reported with the use of sirolimus-eluting stents in native coronary arteries. A recent study reported that the use of sirolimus-eluting stents resulted in a low rate of target vessel revascularization in saphenous vein graft disease. Paclitaxel-eluting stents (PESs) have also shown excellent results in reducing restenosis in native vessels. The immediate and 1-year outcome of PES implantation in patients with saphenous vein graft disease were investigated in a study conducted between February and December 2003.

Methods.—Coronary intervention was performed in 50 consecutive patients with 62 vein graft lesions. Eight patients received bare metal stents because PESs were not available in diameters larger than 3.5 mm. Two patients presented with cardiogenic shock after acute myocardial infarction and died of refractory left ventricular failure immediately after the procedure. Thus, 40 consecutive patients with 52 vein graft lesions underwent elective coronary intervention with PESs and were included in the study. All patients were treated with life-long aspirin therapy and received a loading dose of 300 mg clopidogrel followed by 75 mg/d for 6 months. IV heparin was administered during the procedure to maintain an activated clotting time of more than 250 seconds. Angiographic variables were assessed before and after each procedure. Degenerated grafts were defined as grafts with luminal irregularities or ectasia involving more than 50% of its total length. Patients were followed prospectively and evaluated for survival free of major adverse cardiac events, which were defined as death, myocardial infarction, target lesion revascularization, or target vessel revascularization.

Results.—Kaplan-Meier analysis showed that the probability of major adverse cardiac event-free survival for 1 year was 92.5% with PESs (Table 4). One patient had a non–Q-wave myocardial infarction related to the pro-

TABLE 4.—Results of saphenous vein graft stenting-published reports with mid-term follow-up (one year or less)

First Author/ Reference	Years of Enrollment	Follow-up	Patients (n)	Age (yrs)	Graft Age (yrs)	Reference Diameter (mm)	Lesion Length (mm)	MACE* Free (%)
Strumpf[5]	1990-1991	5 mo	26	68	8.8	3.6†	8.2	85
Fenton[16]	1990-1991	1 yr	198	66	8	3.4	8.6	70
Wong[17]	1990-1992	1 yr	582	66	9	3.0-5.0‡	<15‡	76.3
Brener[12]	1990-1992	1 yr	377	66	9	3.6	<15‡	77
Savage[11]	1993-1995	8 mo	108	66	10.1	3.18	9.6	73
Ahmed[18]	1994-1998	1 yr	951 (men)	67	9	3.5	10.1	70-80§
Harekamp[13]	1996-1998	1 yr	77	66.9	11.8	3.33	10.6	76.3
Hoye[3]	2002	1 yr	19	67	NA	2.8	15.6	84
Present study	2003	1 yr	40	70.6	12.7	2.9	19.1	92.5

*MACE included death, myocardial infarction, TLR, or target vessel revascularization.
†Only mean minimum luminal diameter after stenting is available.
‡Only inclusion criteria available.
§Estimated from event-free survival curve.
(Reprinted from Tsuchida K, Ong ATL, Aoki J, et al: Immediate and one-year outcome of percutaneous intervention of saphenous vein graft disease with Paclitaxel-eluting stents, Am J Cardiol 96:395-398, 2005. Copyright 2005 with permission from Excerpta Medica Inc.)

cedure as an in-hospital major adverse cardiac event. During the 1-year follow up, there were no patient deaths.

Conclusions.—The use of paxlitaxel-eluting stents for treatment of saphenous vein graft narrowing is associated with low clinical event rates, including death, myocardial infarction, and the need for repeat revascularization. The use of bare metal stents in vein graft disease has not been shown to decrease morbidity and mortality and is associated with a high 6-month restenosis rate.

▶ It appears coronary vein grafts can be successfully treated with Paclitaxel-eluting stents with associated favorable short term clinical follow up (no angiographic follow up was presented in this study). The different flow characteristics of peripheral saphenous vein grafts versus coronary grafts are obvious. Therefore, these data cannot be used to justify treatment of peripheral saphenous vein grafts with drug eluting stents. However, the results are certainly intriguing and it is only a matter of time before drug eluting stents will be tested in peripheral vein grafts.

G. L. Moneta, MD

Vascular PET Prostheses Surface Modification with Cyclodextrin Coating: Development of a New Drug Delivery System
Blanchemain N, Haulon S, Martel B, et al (Université de Lille, France; CHRU de Lille, France; UPRES, Villeneuve d'Ascq, France)
Eur J Vasc Endovasc Surg 29:628-632, 2005   4–4

Purpose.—Cyclodextrins (CDs) are torus shaped cyclic oligosaccharides with a hydrophobic internal cavity and a hydrophilic external surface. We performed and analysed an antibiotic binding on Dacron (polyethylene-terephtalate, PET) vascular grafts, previously coated with CDs based polymers.

Methods.—The CDs coating process was based on the pad-dry-cure method patented in our laboratory. The Dacron prostheses were immersed into a solution containing a polycarboxylic acid, a cyclodextrin and a catalyst, and placed into a thermofixation oven before impregnation with an antibiotic solution (Vancomycin). Biocompatibility tests were performed with L132 human epithelial cells. The antibiotic release in an aqueous medium was assessed by batch type experiments using UV spectroscopy.

Results.—Viability tests confirmed that the CDs polymers coating the Dacron fibers were not toxic towards L132 cell. Cell proliferation was similar on coated and uncoated grafts. A linear release of Vancomycin was observed over 50 days.

Conclusion.—Our results demonstrate the feasibility of coating CDs onto vascular Dacron grafts. Biological tests show no toxicity of the different cyclodextrins coated. A linear release of antibiotics was depicted over 50 days, demonstrating that cyclodextrin grafting was an efficient drug delivery system (Fig 3).

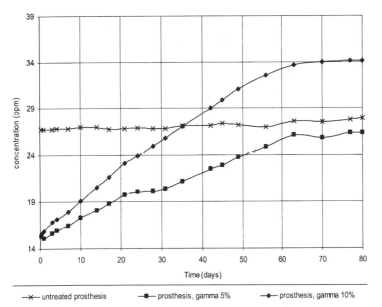

FIGURE 3.—Release of Vancomycin in physiologic medium during 80 days. Results with uncoated and gamma cyclodextrin-coated Dacron prosthesis (coating rate of 5 and 10%). (Reprinted from Blanchemain N, Haulon S, Martel B, et al: Vascular PET prostheses surface modification with cyclodextrin coating: Development of a new drug delivery system. *Eur J Vasc Endovasc Surg* 29:628-632, 2005, by permission of the publisher.)

▶ This study focused on binding of antibiotic to a Dacron graft with use of a "carrier" substance. Obviously, the technique has the potential to be extended to other molecules, enabling vascular grafts to serve as drug delivery systems providing a constant delivery of drug over a prolonged period.

G. L. Moneta, MD

Engineering of fibrin-based functional and implantable small-diameter blood vessels

Swartz DD, Russell JA, Andreadis ST (State Univ of New York, Buffalo)
Am J Physiol Heart Circ Physiol 288:H1451-H1460, 2005   4–5

We engineered implantable small-diameter blood vessels based on ovine smooth muscle and endothelial cells embedded in fibrin gels. Cylindrical tissue constructs remodeled the fibrin matrix and exhibited considerable reactivity in response to receptor- and nonreceptor-mediated vasoconstrictors and dilators. Aprotinin, a protease inhibitor of fibrinolysis, was added at varying concentrations and affected the development and functionality of tissue-engineered blood vessels (TEVs) in a concentration-dependent manner. Interestingly, at moderate concentrations, aprotinin increased mechanical strength but decreased vascular reactivity, indicating a possible relationship between matrix degradation/remodeling, vasoreactivity, and mechanical properties. TEVs developed considerable mechanical strength to withstand interpositional implantation in jugular veins of lambs. Implanted TEVs integrated well with the native vessel and demonstrated patency and similar blood flow rates as the native vessels. At 15 wk postimplantation, TEVs exhibited remarkable matrix remodeling with production of collagen and elastin fibers and orientation of smooth muscle cells perpendicular to the direction of blood flow. Implanted vessels gained significant mechanical strength and reactivity that were comparable to those of native veins. Our work demonstrates that fibrin-based TEVs hold significant promise for treatment of vascular disease and as a biological model for studying vascular development and pathophysiology.

▶ One of the "Holy Grails" of vascular surgery is the development of a commercially available, off-the-shelf, highly effective arterial substitute for a small-caliber vessel. This study indicates that the use of a fibrin scaffold for development of such an arterial substitute is a potentially fertile line of inquiry. These engineered vessels appear to remain patent when implanted, seamlessly integrate into a native vessel, and display vasoreactivity similar to that of normal veins. It is good to know that, even after failure of endothelial seeding of prosthetic grafts, investigators are still pursuing the development of a small-caliber arterial substitute.

G. L. Moneta, MD

5   Aortic Aneurysm

Detection of Abdominal Aortic Aneurysm in Patients with Peripheral Artery Disease
Barba A, Estallo L, Rodríguez L, et al (Hosp de Galdakao, Bizkaia, Spain)
Eur J Vasc Endovasc Surg 30:504-508, 2005   5–1

Objective.—To describe the prevalence of abdominal aortic aneurysms (AAA) in patients with peripheral artery disease (PAD).

Design.—Observational, descriptive, transverse study.

Patients and Methods.—We performed an abdominal ultrasound in 1190 consecutive patients with lower limb chronic ischemia (1/99-12/04). We registered cardiovascular risk factors and clinical data for analysis.

Results.—The ultrasound was inconclusive in 24 (2%) patients; 1166 patients completed the study. They were mostly male (93.7%), with an age mean of 67 ± 9.9 years (37.7-93.4). The main cardiovascular risk factors were: smoking (80.9%), hypertension (41.7%) and hypercholesterolemia (31.4%). The prevalence of AAA was 13% ($n = 151$). Only 1.5% ($n = 17$) of the patients had a large AAA (>5 cm). The AAA was clearly more prevalent in men ($n = 148$; 13.6%) than in women ($n = 3$; 4.1%) (RR 3.47; 95% CI 1.11-10.89; $p = 0.02$). The prevalence significantly increased with age, with a maximum of 17.1% in over 75-year-old men ($p = 0.006$). Patients with

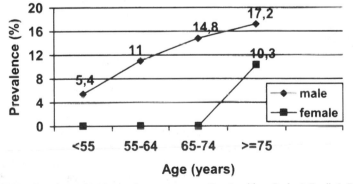

FIGURE 2.—Prevalence of AAA according to age groups. (Reprinted from Barba A, Estallo L, Rodríguez L, et al: Detection of abdominal aortic aneurysm in patients with peripheral artery disease. *Eur J Vasc Endovasc Surg* 30:504-508, 2005, copyright 2005 by permission of the publisher W B Saunders Company Limited London.)

tibial disease had a significantly higher prevalence of AAA than aortoiliac or femoro-popliteal disease ($p = 0.02$).

Conclusions.—The prevalence of AAA in patients with PAD is much higher than that reported in the general population. We recommend that an abdominal ultrasound be routinely included in the study of these patients. Over 75-year-old men are at particularly high-risk (Fig 2).

▶ The yield of screening for AAA appears to be too low to justify screening all patients with PAD. Screening older men does seem reasonable, especially when the PAD is not so severe that the patient's life expectancy appears to be at least 5 years.

G. L. Moneta, MD

Screening for abdominal aortic aneurysms: single centre randomised controlled trial
Lindholt JS, Juul S, Fasting H, et al (Sygehus Viborg, Denmark; Univ of Aarhus, Denmark)
BMJ 330:750-752, 2005   5–2

Objective.—To determine whether screening Danish men aged 65 or more for abdominal aortic aneurysms reduces mortality.

Design.—Single centre randomised controlled trial.

Setting.—All five hospitals in Viborg County, Denmark.

Participants.—All 12,639 men born during 1921-33 and living in Viborg County. In 1994 we included men born 1921-9 (64-73 years). We also included men who became 65 during 1995-8.

Interventions.—Men were randomised to the intervention group (screening by abdominal ultrasonography) or control group. Participants with an abdominal aortic aneurysm > 5 cm were referred for surgical evaluation, and those with smaller aneurysms were offered annual scans

Outcome Measures.—Specific mortality due to abdominal aortic aneurysm, overall mortality, and number of planned and emergency operations for abdominal aortic aneurysms.

Results.—4860 of 6333 men were screened (attendance rate 76.6%). 191 (4.0% of those screened) had abdominal aortic aneurysms. The mean follow-up time was 52 months. The screened group underwent 75% (95% confidence interval 51% to 91%) fewer emergency operations than the control group. Deaths due to abdominal aortic aneurysms occurred in nine patients in the screened group and 27 in the control group. The number needed to screen to save one life was 352. Specific mortality was significantly reduced by 67% (29% to 84%). Mortality due to non-abdominal aortic aneurysms was non-significantly reduced by 8%. The benefits of screening may increase with time.

Conclusion.—Mass screening for abdominal aortic aneurysms in Danish men aged 65 or more reduces mortality (Fig 1).

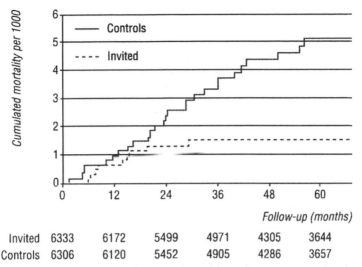

Invited 6333   6172   5499   4971   4305   3644
Controls 6306   6120   5452   4905   4286   3657

FIGURE 1. –Kaplan-Meier estimates of mortality due to abdominal aortic aneurysm in Danish men aged 64-73 years. Difference between screened and control groups is P=0.003 (log rank test). (Courtesy of Lindholt JS, Juul S, Fasting H, et al: Screening for abdominal aortic aneurysms: Single centre randomised controlled trial. *BMJ* 330:750-752, 2005. Reprinted with permission from the BMJ Publishing Group.)

▶ This is one of the 4 major randomized trials evaluating the efficacy of screening for AAA. This trial, along with 2 of the other trials, only evaluated men. This is however, one of the pivotal trials used by the US Preventative Task Force in generating recommendations for screening males for AAA who are, or had been, smokers and are 65 to 74 years old.

G. L. Moneta, MD

Decision-analytical model with lifetime estimation of costs and health outcomes for one-time screening for abdominal aortic aneurysm in 65-year-old men

Henriksson M, Lundgren F (Linköping Univ, Sweden; Univ Hosp, Linköping, Sweden)
Br J Surg 92:976-983, 2005   5–3

Background.—Abdominal aortic aneurysm (AAA) causes about 2 per cent of all deaths in men over the age of 65 years. A major improvement in operative mortality would have little impact on total mortality, so screening for AAA has been recommended as a solution. The cost-effectiveness of a programme that invited 65-year-old men for ultrasonographic screening was compared with current clinical practice in a decision-analytical model.

Methods.—In a probabilistic Markov model, costs and health outcomes of a screening programme and current clinical practice were simulated over a lifetime perspective. To populate the model with the best available evidence, data from published papers, vascular databases and primary research were used.

Results.—The results of the base-case analysis showed that the incremental cost per gained life-year for a screening programme compared with current practice was €7760, and that for a quality-adjusted life-year was €9700. The probability of screening being cost-effective was high.

Conclusion.—A financially and practically feasible screening programme for AAA, in which men are invited for ultrasonography in the year in which they turn 65, appears to yield positive health outcomes at a reasonable cost.

▶ There have now been a number of studies examining the efficacy of screening for AAA (see also Abstract 5–2). The data clearly show screening of elderly men with a history of smoking is effective. Articles such as this indicate that not only will targeted AAA screening save lives, it will do so at a very reasonable cost.

G. L. Moneta, MD

Can Computed Tomography Scan Findings Predict "Impending" Aneurysm Rupture?

Boules TN, Compton CN, Stanziale SF, et al (Univ of Pittsburgh, Pa)
Vasc Endovasc Surg 40:41-47, 2006

5–4

Several findings on computed tomography (CT) scans of intact aneurysms have been taken to suggest "imminent" or "impending" aneurysm rupture. Often these are identified incidentally in asymptomatic patients when an ur-

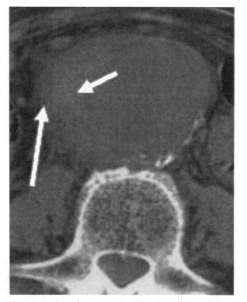

FIGURE 1.—AAA with crescent sign (short arrow) and aortic wall irregularity (long arrow). (Courtesy of Boules TN, Compton CN, Stanziale SF, et al: Can computed tomography scan findings predict "impending" aneurysm rupture? *Vasc Endovasc Surg* 40:41-47, 2006.)

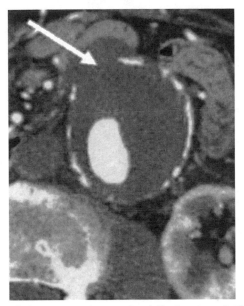

FIGURE 2.—AAA with discontinuous circumaortic calcifications (arrow). (Courtesy of Boules TN, Compton CN, Stanziale SF, et al: Can computed tomography scan findings predict "impending" aneurysm rupture? *Vasc Endovasc Surg* 40:41-47, 2006.)

gent operation was not planned and may even be ill advised. The authors evaluated whether these signs can truly predict short-term aneurysm rupture. A computerized medical archival system was reviewed from August 1994 to August 2004. Patients with aortic aneurysms and official CT scan reports of "impending rupture" were reviewed. CT films and reports were reviewed for aneurysm characteristics, while computerized medical records were reviewed for patient demographics, comorbidities, symptoms, documented subsequent rupture, and operative findings. Signs of "impending rupture" included the crescent sign, discontinuous circumaortic calcification, aortic bulges or blebs, aortic draping, and aortic wall irregularity. Rupture occurring within 2 weeks of the index CT was defined as supporting the "imminent" label. Forty-five patients with aortic aneurysms and CT stigmata of "impending rupture" were identified. Five patients with additional signs of suspicious leak and 1 with an infected previously repaired aneurysm were excluded. Of 39 intact aneurysms, 26 (67%) were infrarenal, 2 (5%) were suprarenal, and the remaining 11 (28%) were thoracoabdominal. The patient group had more women than expected (19/39, 49%) and larger aneurysms (mean diameter, 6.8 ± 1.4 cm). Mean age was 74 years. Ten patients underwent elective repair within the first 2 weeks after the index CT scan (mean, 4 days), precluding adequate observation for early rupture. None had intraoperative signs of rupture. Early rupture: 2 of the 29 remaining patients ruptured within 72 hours of the CT scan, for a positive predictive value of 6.9%. One additional patient ruptured 7 months later after declining an early intervention. No Rupture: 26 patients were observed an average of 246 days (range, 14 days to 3 years) without evidence of rupture. Fourteen were repaired electively 2 weeks to 3 years after the index CT scan, and 12 never underwent repair, mostly because of severe associated comorbidities, and were observed a mean of 394 days without rupture. Although they should be taken seriously, CT signs of "impending rupture" alone are poor predictors of short-term aortic aneurysm rupture, and alternative terminology is needed until better predictors can be identified (Figs 1 and 2).

▶ Every vascular surgeon will at some time be faced with the dilemma of what to do with a patient with a large abdominal aortic aneurysm and a radiologic diagnosis of "impending rupture" but no evidence of leakage from the aneurysm. Actually, the risk of imminent rupture in these patients is quite low. The authors' data suggest that an approach of expedient, but not emergent, operation is reasonable. Nevertheless, the weaknesses of these data are obvious in that only patients who had a diagnosis of "impending rupture" included in their official CT report were used in the database for preparation of this article. The data would have been more complete if the authors had also evaluated all patients with aortic aneurysm rupture and a previous CT scan. Perhaps there were signs of "impending rupture" in some of these patients, but they were not included in the official report.

G. L. Moneta, MD

Age-related increase in wall stress of the human abdominal aorta: An in vivo study
Åstrand H, Rydén-Ahlgren Å, Sandgren T, et al (Univ of Linköping, Sweden; Jönköping Hosp, Sweden; Univ Hosp Malmö, Sweden; et al)
J Vasc Surg 42:926-931, 2005   5–5

Background.—The regulation of wall stress in the abdominal aorta (AA) of humans might be of specific interest, because the AA is the most common site for aneurysm formation in which wall stress seems to be an important pathophysiological factor. We studied the age-related changes in wall stress of the AA in healthy subjects, with the common carotid artery (CCA) as a comparison.

Methods.—A total of 111 healthy subjects were examined with B-mode ultrasonography to determine the lumen diameter and intima-media thickness (IMT) in the AA and the CCA.

Results.—Aortic IMT was affected by age in men and by both age and lumen diameter in women. Carotid IMT was affected by age and pulse pressure in both men and women. Wall stress was higher in the AA than in the CCA ($P < .001$), and men had higher wall stress than women in both the AA ($P < .001$) and the CCA ($P < .05$). Furthermore, wall stress was constant during life in the CCA of men and women and in the AA of women. In the male aorta, however, wall stress increased with age ($P < 0.01$).

Conclusions.—Arterial diameters increase with age, and a compensatory thickening of the arterial wall prevents the circumferential wall stress from increasing. However, this compensatory response is insufficient in the male AA and results in an increase in stress with age. These findings might explain the propensity for aneurysms to develop in the AA of men.

▶ All the subjects of this study were nonsmokers yet virtually everyone with an abdominal aortic aneurysm (AAA) has been a smoker at some point in their life. One therefore cannot conclude that changes in wall stress lead to AAA, as nonsmokers seldom get AAAs and nonsmokers were the only ones investigated in this study.

G. L. Moneta, MD

Increased Growth Rate of Abdominal Aortic Aneurysms in Women. The Tromsø Study

Solberg S, Singh K, Wilsgaard T, et al (Univ of Tromsø, Norway; Rikshospitalet, Oslo, Norway)
Eur J Vasc Endovasc Surg 29:145-149, 2005   5–6

Objectives.—The present study was undertaken in order to assess the effect of gender on the growth rate of abdominal aortic aneurysms (AAAs).

Methods.—One hundred and eighty-five men and 49 women with AAAs were studied, mean follow-up 62 months, giving 14,544 patient-months of follow-up. A mean of 16 ultrasound examinations was performed on each patient.

Results.—The mean growth rate was 1.82; 1.65 and 2.43 mm per year in men and women, respectively. In a weighted linear regression analysis, high initial diameter and female gender were independent and significant ($p < 0.001$ and $p = 0.003$, respectively) predictors for increased growth rate of AAAs. None of the other considered risk factors predicted the growth rate.

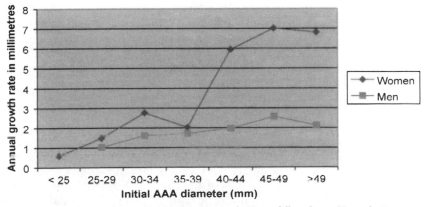

FIGURE 1.—The growth rate of AAA in 49 women and 185 men followed up to 90 months. In a regression analysis, both initial AAA diameter and female gender predicted the growth rate ($p<0.001$ and $p=0.003$, respectively). (Reprinted from Solberg S, Singh K, Wilsgaard T, et al: Increased growth rate of abdominal aortic aneurysms in women. The Tromsø study. *Eur J Vasc Endovasc Surg* 29:145-149, 2005, copyright 2005 by permission of the publisher W B Saunders Company Limited London.)

Conclusions.—This is the first study to report a significantly different growth rate of AAAs in females compared to males. It, thus, adds evidence to the view that AAA is a more malignant condition in females than in males and could have implications for the frequency of follow-up in women (Fig 1).

▶ There is increasing evidence that AAA is a more malignant disease in females, with a propensity of smaller aneurysms to rupture. There is also now evidence, as suggested by this study, that AAAs expand more rapidly in females. This study needs to be confirmed by additional studies and, if corroborated, more frequent follow-up should be prescribed for women with small AAAs.

G. L. Moneta, MD

Risk factors and prevalence of perioperative cognitive dysfunction in abdominal aneurysm patients
Benoit AG, Campbell BI, Tanner JR, et al (Univ of Manitoba, Winnipeg, Canada)
J Vasc Surg 42:884-890, 2005   5–7

Background.—Perioperative delirium is common in high-risk surgery and is associated with age, education, preoperative cognitive functioning, preexisting medical conditions, and postoperative complications. We investigated these factors as well as lifestyle and demographic variables by using cognitive measures that were more sensitive than those used in previous studies.

Methods.—Extensive medical and demographic data were collected on 102 patients between 41 and 88 years of age to identify comorbidities and lifestyle considerations preoperatively. Elective abdominal aortic aneurysm surgery was performed under combined general/epidural anesthesia with postoperative epidural analgesia. A battery of sensitive, cognitive measures was administered preoperatively, at the time of discharge from hospital, and 3 months postoperatively. Symptoms of delirium were assessed during the first 6 postoperative days using *Diagnostic and Statistical Manual of Mental Disorders-4th Edition* criteria. Intraoperative and postoperative data, including medications, vital signs, conduct of the surgery and anesthesia, complications, and details of pain control, were collected.

Results.—Delirium occurred in 33% of the patients during the first 6 days after surgery. Longer duration of delirium was related to lower education, preoperative depression, and greater preoperative psychoactive medication use. Characteristics of the surgery and hospital stay were unrelated to the development of delirium. Patients who were diagnosed with delirium had lower cognitive scores during each of the three assessment periods, even when controlling for age and education. Logistic regression analysis indicated that the most powerful preoperative predictors of delirium were number of pack years smoked ($P = .001$), mental status scores ($P = .003$), and number of psychoactive medications ($P = .005$).

Conclusion.—A significant proportion of patients undergoing elective abdominal aortic aneurysm repair are susceptible to the development of delirium and are at risk for cognitive dysfunction after surgery. Our findings have implications for promoting long-term lifestyle changes, including smoking cessation and improved management of mental health as risk-reduction strategies.

▶ The confused patient places a great strain on physicians, nurses, and most of all, on the patient's family. This article is very useful in that it can help the surgeon counsel patients and their families about what to expect postoperatively. It has been my experience that if families are made aware of the likelihood of postoperative confusion, then they will not be as frightened when faced with a confused relative in the postoperative period.

G. L. Moneta, MD

Infrarenal Abdominal Aortic Aneurysm Repair via Endovascular Versus Open Retroperitoneal Approach

Mehta M, Roddy SP, Darling C III, et al (Albany Med College, NY)
Ann Vasc Surg 19:374-378, 2005   5–8

The beneficial effects of open surgical abdominal aortic aneurysm (AAA) repair via a left retroperitoneal approach have been established. We compared the short-term outcome of infrarenal AAA repair via an endovascular approach with that of an open retroperitoneal approach. From October 2001 to April 2003, patients with infrarenal AAA >5 cm were offered repair via an endovascular approach (group I) with a variety of industry-made stent grafts or with an open retroperitoneal surgical approach (group II). Data were prospectively collected in the vascular registry and complications were analyzed. Data comparison between the two groups was done by using chi-squared analysis and two-tailed Students t-test. Statistical significance was identified at $p < 0.05$. Over an 18-month period, 492 patients underwent evaluation for AAA. Of these, 446 patients had infrarenal AAA and underwent either endovascular (group I: $n = 175$, male 85%, female 15%) or open surgical repair (group II: $n = 232$, male 74%, female 26%) via a left retroperitoneal approach. Group I patients had a higher incidence of coronary artery disease (66% vs. 35%, $p < 0.05$), hypertension (74% vs. 43%, $p < 0.05$), chronic obstructed pulmonary disease (29% vs. 12%, $p < 0.05$), and diabetes mellitus (20% vs. 7%, $p < 0.05$), a lower mean amount of intraoperative blood loss (277 cc vs. 1452 cc, $p < 0.05$), and shorter length of stay in the hospital (1.7 days vs., 7.3 days, $p < 0.05$). Group I also had fewer complications of myocardial infarction (1.7% vs. 5.2%, $p =$ NS), renal failure (0% vs. 2.6%, $p < 0.05$), pulmonary failure (1.7% vs. 2.6%, $p =$ NS), ischemic colitis requiring colectomy (0.6% vs. 2.6%, $p < 0.05$), multisystem organ failure (0% vs. 1.3%, p = NS), and death (0.6% vs. 1.3%, $p < 0.05$). Despite increased preexisting comorbidities, patients undergoing endovascular aneurysm repair had less morbidity, mortality, and blood loss and a shorter in-hospital length of stay than patients undergoing open surgical aneurysm repair via a left retroperitoneal approach.

▶ It is interesting that many investigators are now comparing various open approaches to AAA repair (mini-lap, standard midline approach, retroperitoneal approach) to endovascular repair thus suggesting that endovascular repair is now the de facto "standard." By and large, all comparisons like this one are retrospective and uncontrolled. All document higher systemic risk in endovascular patients and less morbidity and mortality with endovascular repair despite higher risk. The Albany surgeons are very experienced with the retroperitoneal approach to the aorta. If retroperitoneal aortic aneurysm repair cannot beat endovascular AAA repair in Albany, it is not likely to do so anywhere else either.

G. L. Moneta, MD

Genetic analysis of polymorphisms in biologically relevant candidate genes in patients with abdominal aortic aneurysms
Ogata T, Shibamura H, Tromp G, et al (Applied Genomics Technology Ctr, Detroit, Mich; Wayne State Univ, Cleveland, Ohio; Case Western Reserve Univ, Clevevland, Ohio; et al)
J Vasc Surg 41:1036-1042, 2005   5–9

Background.—Abdominal aortic aneurysms (AAAs) are characterized by histologic signs of chronic inflammation, destructive remodeling of extracellular matrix, and depletion of vascular smooth muscle cells. We investigated the process of extracellular matrix remodeling by performing a genetic association study with polymorphisms in the genes for matrix metalloproteinases (MMPs), tissue inhibitors of metalloproteinases (TIMPs), and structural extracellular matrix molecules in AAA. Our hypothesis was that genetic variations in one or more of these genes contribute to greater or lesser activity of these gene products, and thereby contribute to susceptibility for developing AAAs.

Methods.—DNA samples from 812 unrelated white subject (AAA, n = 387; controls, n = 425) were genotyped for 14 polymorphisms in 13 different candidate genes: MMP1(nt−1607), MMP2(nt−955), MMP3 (nt−1612), MMP9(nt−1562), MMP10(nt+180), MMP12(nt−82), MMP13(nt−77), TIMP1(nt+434), TIMP1(rs2070584), TIMP2 (rs2009196), TIMP3(nt−1296), TGFB1(nt−509), ELN(nt+422), and COL3A1(nt+581). Odds ratios and P values adjusted for gender and country of origin using logistic regression and stratified by family history of AAA were calculated to test for association between genotype and disease status. Haplotype analysis was carried out for the two TIMP1 polymorphisms in male subjects.

Results.—Analyses with one polymorphism per test without interactions showed an association with the two TIMP1 gene polymorphisms (nt+434, P = .0047; rs2070584, P = .015) in male subjects without a family history of

AAA. The association remained significant when analyzing TIMP1 haplotypes (χ^2 $P = .014$ and empirical $P = .009$). In addition, we found a significant interaction between the polymorphism and gender for MMP10 ($P = .037$) in cases without a family history of AAA, as well as between the polymorphism and country of origin for ELN ($P = 0169$) and TIMP3 ($P = .0023$) in cases with a family history of AAA.

Conclusions.—These findings suggest that genetic variations in TIMP1, TIMP3, MMP10, and ELN genes may contribute to the pathogenesis of AAAs. Further work is needed to confirm the findings in an independent set of samples and to study the functional role of these variants in AAA. It is noteworthy that contrary to a previous study, we did not find an association between the MMP9 (nt−1562) polymorphism and AAA, suggesting genetic heterogeneity of the disease.

Clinical Relevance.—Abdominal aortic aneurysms (AAAs) are an important cardiovascular disease, but the genetic and environmental risk factors, which contribute to individual's risk to develop an aneurysm, are poorly understood. Histologically, AAAs are characterized by signs of chronic inflammation, destructive remodeling of the extracellular matrix, and depletion of vascular smooth muscle cells. We hypothesized that genes involved in these events could harbor changes that make individuals more susceptible to developing aneurysms. This study identified significant genetic associations between DNA sequence changes in tissue inhibitor of metalloproteinase 1 (TIMP1), TIMP3, matrix metalloproteinase 10 (MMP10) and elastin (ELN) genes, and AAA. The results will require confirmation using an independent set of samples. After replication it is possible that these sequence changes in combination with other risk factors could be used in the future to identify individuals who are at increased risk for developing an AAA.

▶ Epidemiologic studies have previously confirmed at least a partial genetic basis to development of AAA. Investigators are now zeroing in on specific genes and gene products. Much work obviously remains to be done. Even in this data set, only a single polymorphism of most genes was investigated. Other potentially important polymorphisms could have been missed.

G. L. Moneta, MD

Functional outcome after open repair of ruptured abdominal aortic aneurysm

Tambyraja AL, Fraser SCA, Murie JA, et al (Univ of Edinburgh, England)

J Vasc Surg 41:758-761, 2005   5–10

Background.—Outcome after operative repair of ruptured abdominal aortic aneurysm (AAA) has traditionally been assessed in terms of survival. This study examines the functional outcome of patients who survive operation.

Methods.—Consecutive patients who survived open repair over an 18-month period were entered into a prospective case-control study. Age- and sex-matched controls were identified from patients undergoing elective AAA repair. The Short Form-36 health survey was administered to both groups of patients at 6 months after operation. Results were compared with the expected scores for an age- and sex-matched normal UK population.

Results.—Fifty-seven patients underwent open repair of a ruptured AAA, and 30 survived; no patient was lost to follow-up. There were no significant differences in quality of life between patients who had an emergency repair and those who had an elective repair. Both of these groups had poorer health-related quality of life outcomes than the matched normal population. Surprisingly, compared with the normal population, patients after elective repair had poorer outcomes in more health domains than patients who survived emergency operation.

Conclusions.—Survivors of ruptured AAA repair have a good functional outcome within 6 months of operation.

▶ This study surprised me. It had been my impression that patients surviving repair of ruptured AAA often did so with great difficulty and considerable perceived decreased quality of life. The results of this study may reflect selection bias in which patients with ruptured AAAs were actually operated, poor outcomes in the elective patients, or diminished expectations among the survivors of ruptured AAAs versus those having elective repair. Clearly, however, some patients survive ruptured AAA with good functional outcome.

G. L. Moneta, MD

6 Abdominal Aortic Endografting

What imaging studies are necessary for abdominal aortic endograft sizing? A prospective blinded study using conventional computed tomography, aortography, and three-dimensional computed tomography
Parker MV, O'Donnell SD, Chang AS, et al (Walter Reed Army Med Ctr, Washington, DC; Uniformed Services Univ of the Health Sciences, Bethesda, Md)
J Vasc Surg 41:199-205, 2005   6–1

Objective—Preoperative imaging modalities for endovascular abdominal aortic aneurysm repair (EVAR) include conventional computed tomography (CT), aortography with a marking catheter, and three-dimensional computed tomography (3D CT). Although each technique has advantages, to date no study has compared in a prospective manner the reproducibility of measurements and impact on graft selection of all three modalities. The objective of this study was to determine the most useful imaging studies in planning EVAR.

Methods.—Twenty patients being considered for EVAR were enrolled prospectively to undergo a conventional CT scan and aortography. The CT scans were then reconstructed into 3D images using Preview Treatment Planning Software (Medical Media Systems, West Lebanon, NH). Four measurements of diameter and six of length were made from each modality in determining the proper graft for EVAR (Fig 2).

Results.—Measurements from all three modalities were reproducible with intraobserver correlation coefficients of 0.79 to 1.0 for aortography, 0.87 to 1.0 for CT, and 0.96 to 1.0 for 3D CT. Measurements between observers were also similar from each modality; interobserver correlations were 0.70 to 0.97 for aortography, 0.76 to 0.97 for CT, and 0.73 to 0.99 for 3D CT. Significant differences ($P < .01$) in diameter measurements were noted at D2 with aortography compared with 3D CT, whereas differences in length measurements were found between CT and 3D CT at L4 (nonaneurysmal right iliac) ($P < .01$). The correlation between CT and 3D CT for most length measurements was acceptable (0.63 to 1.0). Aortography for diameters correlated poorly (0.35 to 0.67) with 3D CT. When the endograft selected by aortography/CT or 3D CT alone was compared with the actual

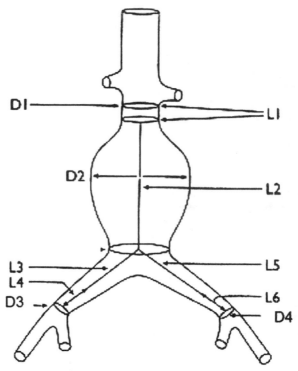

FIGURE 2.—Drawing demonstrates the locations of the 4 measurements of diameter and 6 measurements of length used in this study with reference to the abdominal aortic aneurysm. *D1*, aortic diameter at lowest renal; *D2* maximal aneurysm diameter; *D3*, diameter at right iliac landing zone; *D4*, diameter at left iliac landing zone; *L1*, length of aortic neck below renals; *L2*, length of aorta from beginning of aneurysm to bifurcation; *L3*, length of aneurysmal right iliac; *L4*, length of nonaneurysmal right iliac; *L5*, length of aneurysmal left iliac; *L6*, length of nonaneurysmal left iliac. (Reprinted by permission of the publisher from Parker MV, O'Donnell SD, Chang AS, et al: What imaging studies are necessary for abdominal aortic endograft sizing? A prospective blinded study using conventional computed tomography, aortography, and three-dimensional computed tomography. *J Vasc Surg* 41:199-205, 2005. Copyright 2005 by Elsevier.)

endograft used, there was agreement in 11 of 11 patients when adjusted for ± one size in diameter or length.

Conclusion—Reproducible and comparable measures of diameter and length can be obtained by each of three imaging modalities available for endograft sizing. As a single imaging modality, 3D CT appears to have the best correlation for both diameters and lengths; however, the difference is not sufficient enough to alter endograft selection. Three-dimensional CT may be reserved for challenging aortic anatomy where small differences in measurements would affect patient or graft selection for EVAR.

▶ The authors found a good correlation for abdominal aortic aneurysm endograft sizing when comparing standard CT/angiography with 3D reconstructions using Medical Media Systems software. Since most patients had a suitable neck the study may not have been powered sufficiently to demonstrate a difference. I have often found neck measurements exceedingly difficult in the presence of significant angulation. I do believe 3D reconstructions provide better preoperative planning in this patient subset.

K. Kasirajan, MD

Endovascular aneurysm repair and outcome in patients unfit for open repair of abdominal aortic aneurysm (EVAR trial 2): randomised controlled trial
Greenhalgh RM, for the EVAR Trial Participants (Imperial College London; et al)
Lancet 365:2187-2192, 2005   6 2

Background.—Endovascular aneurysm repair (EVAR) to exclude abdominal aortic aneurysm (AAA) was introduced for patients of poor health status considered unfit for major surgery. We instigated EVAR trial 2 to identify whether EVAR improves survival compared with no intervention in patients unfit for open repair of aortic aneurysm.

Methods.—We did a randomised controlled trial of 338 patients aged 60 years or older who had aneurysms of at least 5.5 cm in diameter and who had been referred to one of 31 hospitals in the UK. We assigned patients to receive either EVAR (n=166) or no intervention (n=172). Our primary endpoint was all-cause mortality, with secondary endpoints of aneurysm-related mortality, health-related quality of life (HRQL), postoperative complications, and hospital costs. Analyses were by intention to treat.

Findings.—197 patients underwent aneurysm repair (47 assigned no intervention) and 80% of patients adhered to protocol. The 30-day operative mortality in the EVAR group was 9% (13 of 150, 95% CI 5–15) and the no intervention group had a rupture rate of 9.0 per 100 person years (95% CI 6.0–13.5). By end of follow up 142 patients had died, 42 of aneurysm-related factors; overall mortality after 4 years was 64%. There was no significant difference between the EVAR group and the no intervention group for all-cause mortality (hazard ratio 1.21, 95% CI 0.87–1.69, p=0.25). There was no difference in aneurysm-related mortality. The mean hospital costs per patient over 4 years were UK£13,632 in the EVAR group and £4983 in the no intervention group (mean difference £8649, SE 1248), with no difference in HRQL scores.

Interpretation.—EVAR had a considerable 30-day operative mortality in patients already unfit for open repair of their aneurysm. EVAR did not improve survival over no intervention and was associated with a need for continued surveillance and reinterventions, at substantially increased cost. Ongoing follow-up and improved fitness of these patients is a priority.

▶ The data suggest that patients unfit for open AAA repair are approaching the end of life. The combination of high perioperative mortality rates for the EVAR patients along with other sources of mortality renders EVAR ineffective in prolonging survival in this patient group. This study brings into serious question the concept that EVAR should be offered to patients with large AAA who are unfit for open repair.

G. L. Moneta, MD

Early outcomes of endovascular versus open abdominal aortic aneurysm repair in the National Surgical Quality Improvement Program–Private Sector (NSQIP–PS)

Hua HT, Cambria RP, Chuang SK, et al (Harvard Med School, Boston; VA Boston Healthcare System; Univ of Colorado, Denver)
J Vasc Surg 41:382-389, 2005   6–3

Background.—There remains no consensus on the appropriate application of endovascular abdominal aortic aneurysm repair (EVAR). Information from administrative databases, industry-sponsored trials, and single institutions has inherent deficiencies. This study was designed to compare early outcomes of open (OPEN) versus EVAR in a contemporary (2000 to 2003) large, multicenter prospective cohort.

Methods.—Fourteen academic medical centers contributed data to the National Surgical Quality Improvement Program-Private Sector (NSQIP-PS), which ensures uniform, comprehensive, prospective, and previously validated data entry by trained, independent nurse reviewers. A battery of clinical and demographic features was assessed with multivariate analysis for association with the principal study end points of 30-day operative mortality and morbidity.

Results.—One thousand forty-two patients underwent elective infrarenal abdominal aortic aneurysm (AAA) repairs: 460 EVAR and 582 OPEN. EVAR patients were older (74 vs 71 years, $P < .0001$), included more men (84.6% vs 79.6%, $P < .05$), and had a higher incidence of chronic obstructive pulmonary disease (25.4% vs 17.9%, $P < .01$). EVAR resulted in significantly reduced overall morbidity (24% vs 35%, $P < .0001$) and hospital stay (4 vs 9 days, $P < .0001$). Cardiopulmonary and renal function-related comorbidities had the expected significant impact on mortality for both procedures at univariate analysis ($P < .05$) While crude mortality rates between EVAR and OPEN did not differ significantly (2.8% vs 4.0%) ($P = 0.32$). After multivariate analysis, correlates of operative mortality included OPEN (odds ratio [OR], 2.44; 95% confidence interval [CI], 1.03 to 5.78; $P < .05$), advanced age (OR, 1.11; $P < .001$), history of angina (OR, 5.54; $P < .01$), poor functional status (OR, 5.78; $P < .001$), history of weight loss (OR, 7.42; $P < .01$), and preoperative dialysis (OR, 51.4; $P < .0001$). EVAR also compared favorably to OPEN (OR, 2.14; 95% CI, 1.58 to 2.89; $P < .0001$) for overall morbidity.

Conclusion.—Significant morbidity accompanies AAA repair, even at major academic medical centers. These data strongly endorse EVAR as the preferred approach in the presence of significant cardiopulmonary or renal comorbidities, or poor preoperative functional status.

▶ There is not a lot different here from other studies examining 30-day morbidity and mortality rates for open repair versus EVAR. Even given generally higher risk factors in the EVAR patients, the 30-day morbidity and mortality rate is lower than with open repair. The NSQIP data do show the mortality rate overall for AAA repair is increased 51 times in patients on dialysis. Anyone who repairs an AAA on a dialysis patient needs a very, very good reason to do so or should rightfully expect a visit from the sheriff!

G. L. Moneta, MD

Lifeline registry of endovascular aneurysm repair: Long-term primary outcome measures
Siami FS, for the Lifeline Registry of EVAR Publications Committee (New England Research Insts, Inc, Watertown, Mass; et al)
J Vasc Surg 42:1-10, 2005   6–4

Purpose.—To determine the long-term outcome after endovascular aneurysm repair (EVAR) of infrarenal abdominal aortic aneurysms (AAA).

Methods.—Review the primary outcome measures of patients treated with endovascular grafts (EG) in the Lifeline Registry of EVAR. The registry contains data on 2,664 EG patients and 334 open surgical control (SC) patients collected under four multicenter Investigational Device Exemption (IDE) clinical trials that lead to United States Food and Drug Administration (FDA) approval with mandatory 5-year follow-up. Primary outcome measures include operative mortality, AAA-related death, all-cause mortality, aneurysm rupture, and surgical conversion.

Results.—Pooled data from IDE clinical trials revealed that EG patients were 3 years older (73 ± 8 years) than SC patients (70 ± 8 years, $P < .01$) and had significantly more cardiac comorbidities before treatment. However, there was no difference in 30-day operative mortality between EG (1.7%) and SC (1.4%) ($P = .72$). Both EG and SC were successful in preventing rupture, with freedom from aneurysm rupture in 99.8% of EG and 100% of SC patients at 1 year ($P = .51$). Freedom from rupture remained at 99% in years 1 to 6 after EG, with no increasing risk of late rupture. There was no significant difference in the AAA-related death rate at 1 year between EG (98.2%) and SC (98.6%) ($P = .64$). Freedom from AAA-related death remained at 98% in years 1 to 6 after EG, with no increasing risk of late AAA-related death. Kaplan-Meier analysis at 6 years revealed freedom from aneurysm rupture in 99%, freedom from AAA-related death in 98%, and freedom from surgical conversion in 95% of EG patients. There was no difference in survival at 4 years between EG (74%) and SC (71%) ($P = .49$). Overall EG patient survival at 5 years was 66% and at 6 years was 52%. Women had a higher risk of rupture (2.4%) than men (1.2%) ($P = .01$) and a higher rate of surgical conversion (8.3%) than men (3.8%) ($P < .01$) but had the same low AAA-related death rate (3.5%) as men (2.1%) ($P = 16$) at 5 years. Most secondary interventional procedures (85%) were performed ≤30 days after

All-cause Mortality	N	Events
EG-IDE	2664	603
SC	334	42
K-M Log-rank	p-value	0.4587

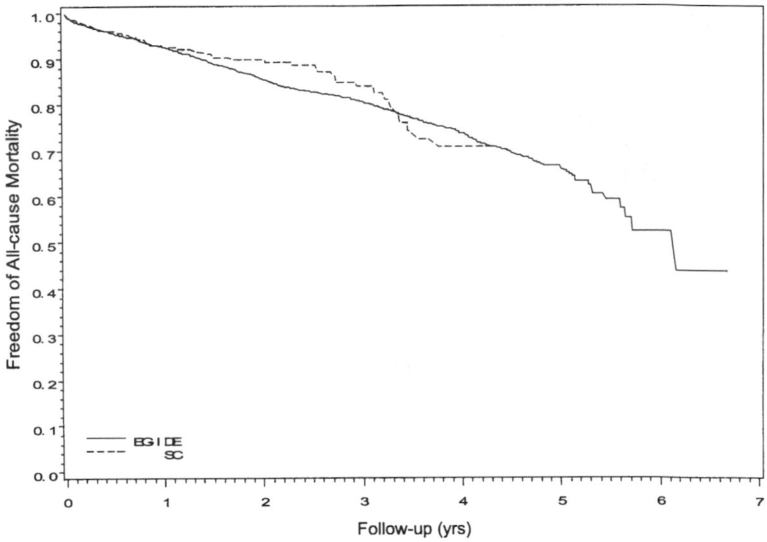

		0 to 30D	30d to 6m	6m to 1yr	1 to 2yr	2 to 3yr	3 to 4yr	4 to 5yr	5 to 6yr
EG-IDE	# at risk	2664	2577	2471	2230	1752	1366	819	289
	# of events	45	71	76	154	91	94	56	15
	# censored	42	35	165	324	295	453	474	265
	K-M est	0.9830	0.9557	0.9259	0.8552	0.8063	0.7376	0.6628	0.5243
	Std Err	0.00252	0.00403	0.00515	0.00725	0.00847	0.0103	0.0134	0.0439
SC	# at risk	334	270	255	219	167	97	32	
	# of events	4	7	9	6	8	8	0	
	# censored	60	8	27	46	62	57	32	
	K-M est	0.9862	0.9601	0.9251	0.8973	0.8391	0.7072	0.7072	
	Std Err	0.00690	0.0118	0.0162	0.0192	0.0269	0.0487	0.0487	

FIGURE 2.—Kaplan-Meier (K-M) analysis of all-cause mortality of endograft-Investigational Device Exemption (EG-IDE) group versus surgical controls (SC). (Reprinted by permission of the publisher from Siami FS, for the Lifeline Registry of EVAR Publications Committee: Lifeline registry of endovascular aneurysm repair: Long-term primary outcome measures. J Vasc Surg 42:1-10, 2005. Copyright 2005 by Elsevier.)

EVAR. Freedom from secondary intervention was 84% at 1 year and 78% at 5 years.

Conclusions.—Endovascular aneurysm repair using FDA-approved devices is a safe, effective, and durable treatment for anatomically suited patients with infrarenal abdominal aortic aneurysms (Fig 2).

▶ Endovascular AAA repair is a durable procedure at 6 years. In older patients with an ideal anatomy for endovascular repair, most physicians would preferentially offer an endovascular procedure. However, the question that all of us get asked is about the 50-year-old man with an AAA. In the presence of an ideal anatomy, I recommend an endovascular procedure, as complications during follow-up are uncommon in patients with good seal zones, especially with grafts using positive fixation. It is, however, certainly possible to perform an open repair with comparable operative mortality rates to endovascular procedures, as demonstrated by the Lifeline Registry.

K. Kasirajan, MD

Endovascular repair of abdominal aortic aneurysm in octogenarians: An analysis based on EUROSTAR data
Lange C, for the EUROSTAR collaborators (Univ Hosp of Trondheim, Norway; et al)
J Vasc Surg 42:624-630, 2005   6–5

Purpose.—To investigate the early and late outcome after endovascular treatment of abdominal aortic aneurysm (EVAR) in octogenarians compared with patients aged <80 years.

Methods.—Patients treated for abdominal aortic aneurysm (AAA) with endovascular repair during the period 1996 to 2004 were collated in the EUROSTAR registry. This study group consisted of 697 patients aged ≥80 years. Comparison was made with 4198 patients aged <80 years with regard to the incidence of preoperative characteristics and outcomes of the procedure.

Results.—The proportion of octogenarians treated by EVAR increased during the study period, from 11% in the first year to 18% in the last year. Octogenarians more frequently had cardiac disease, impaired renal function, and pulmonary disease ($P = .03$, $P < .0001$ and $P = .0001$). Thirty-two percent of the octogenarians were recorded unfit for open surgery as opposed to 22% in younger patients ($P < .0001$); they also had a larger aneurysm diameter (62 vs 58 mm, respectively; $P < .0001$). The 30-day and in-hospital mortality in octogenarians was 5% vs 2% in the younger group ($P < .0001$). More device-related complications and systemic complications, including cardiac disease, were noted in octogenarians (7% vs 5% and 19% vs 11%, $P = .03$ and $P < .0001$, respectively). This group of patients also had a higher incidence of postoperative hemorrhagic complications, including hematoma (7% vs 3%, $P < .0001$, respectively). No differences in conversion to open repair and post-EVAR rupture rate were observed. Aneurysm-related mortality and late all-cause mortality was 7% vs 3% and 10% vs 7%, both $P < .0001$.

Conclusion.—Our study supports that EVAR might be considered when treating elderly patients, provided their aneurysms are anatomically suited for the endovascular technique. The risk for late complications compared with open repair may be outweighed by a lower early mortality as well as a shorter time for physical recovery (Fig 2).

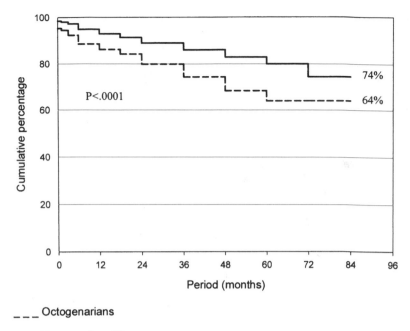

___ Octogenarians

___ Younger than 80 years

FIGURE 2.—Kaplan-Meier graph represents long-term survival after endovascular repair of abdominal aortic aneurysm in octogenarians and patients aged <80 years (Reprinted by permission of the publisher from Lange C, for the EUROSTAR collaborators: Endovascular repair of abdominal aortic aneurysm in octogenarians: An analysis based on EUROSTAR data. *J Vasc Surg* 42:624-630, 2005. Copyright 2005 by Elsevier.)

▶ Every time vascular surgeons look at the results of vascular procedures in the elderly, the results are predictably the same. Older patients don't do as well as younger patients, but they don't do so badly as to make the operation prohibitive in the more fit older patient. Such is the case with EVAR as well.

G. L. Moneta, MD

Endovascular Repair or Surveillance of Patients with Small AAA
Zarins CK, Crabtree T, Arko FR, et al (Stanford Univ, Calif; Cleveland Clinic, Ohio; Harbor UCLA, Torrance, Calif)
Eur J Vasc Endovasc Surg 29:496-503, 2005   6–6

Objective.—To compare the outcome of patients with small abdominal aortic aneurysms (AAA) treated in a prospective trial of endovascular aneurysm repair (EVAR) to patients randomized to the surveillance arm of the UK Small Aneurysm Trial.

Method.—All patients with small AAA (≤5.5 cm diameter) treated with a stent graft (EVARsmall) in the multicenter AneuRx clinical trial from 1997 to 1999 were reviewed with follow up through 2003. A subgroup of patients (EVARmatch) who met the age (60–76 years) and aneurysm size (4.0–5.5 cm diameter) inclusion criteria of the UK Small Aneurysm Trial were compared to the published results of the surveillance patient cohort (UKsurveil) of the UK Small Aneurysm Trial (NEJM 346:1445, 2002). Endpoints of comparison were aneurysm rupture, fatal aneurysm rupture, operative mortality, aneurysm related death and overall mortality. The total patient years of follow-up for EVAR patients was 1369 years and for UK patients was 3048 years. Statistical comparisons of EVARmatch and UKsurveil patients were made for rates per 100 patient years of follow up (/100 years) to adjust for differences in follow-up time.

Results.—The EVARsmall group of 478 patients comprised 40% of the total number of patients treated during the course of the AneuRx clinical trial. The EVARmatch group of 312 patients excluded 151 patients for age < 60 or > 76 years and 15 patients for AAA diameter <4 cm. With the exception of age, there were no significant differences between EVARsmall and EVARmatch in pre-operative factors or post-operative outcomes. In comparison to the UKsurveil group of 527 patients, the EVARmatch group was slightly older (70 ± 4 vs. 69 ± 4 years, $p = 0.009$), had larger aneurysms (5.0 ± 0.3 vs. 4.6 ± 0.4 cm, $p < 0.001$), fewer women (7 vs. 18%, $p < 0.001$), and had a higher prevalence of diabetes and hypertension and a lower prevalence of smoking at baseline. Ruptures occurred in 1.6% of EVARmatch patients and 5.1% of UKsurveil patients; this difference was not significant when adjusted for the difference in length of follow up. Fatal aneurysm rupture rate, adjusted for follow up time, was four times higher in UKsurveil (0.8/100 patient years) than in EVARmatch (0.2/100 patient years, $p < 0.001$); this difference remained significant when adjusted for difference in gender mix. Elective operative mortality rate was significantly lower in EVARmatch (1.9%) than in UKsurveil (5.9%, $p < 0.01$). Aneurysm-related death rate was two times higher in UKsurveil (1.6/100 patient years) than in EVARmatch (0.8/100 patient years, $p = 0.03$). All-cause mortality rate was significantly higher in UKsurveil (8.3/100 patient years) than in EVARmatch (6.4/100 patient years, $p = 0.02$).

Conclusions.—It appears that endovascular repair of small abdominal aortic aneurysms (4.0–5.5 cm) significantly reduces the risk of fatal aneurysm rupture and aneurysm-related death and improves overall patient survival compared to an ultrasound surveillance strategy with selective open surgical repair.

▶ This article was accompanied by invited commentaries. Commentaries indicate 2 polar views of "interesting" manipulation of statistics presented in the study. Dr Brunkwall argues that the "article strongly supports the need for trials of EVAR versus surveillance in small aneurysms." Dr Powell states "there is just a suspicion that Zarins and colleagues are using inappropriate comparisons in an attempt to find new markets for endovascular devices." As in most cases of widely disparate opinions there is probably some truth to both points of view.

G. L. Moneta, MD

Fenestrated endovascular grafting: The renal side of the story

Haddad F, Greenberg RK, Walker E, et al (Cleveland Clinic Found, Ohio)
J Vasc Surg 41:181-190, 2005
6–7

Background.—Fenestrated endovascular aneurysm repair uses the visceral aortic segment, in the setting of a suboptimal proximal neck, for sealing and fixation. This technique requires the placement of visceral stents and might be hampered by the deleterious effects of such interventions. This study was performed to define outcomes related to renal events.

Materials and Methods.—Consecutive clinical records and radiographic studies of patients treated primarily with an endovascular approach with a fenestrated endograft were reviewed. The population was divided into groups with and without baseline renal dysfunction based on the National Kidney Foundation definition of chronic kidney disease. Morphologic measurements and the detection of postoperative renal events such as renal artery stenosis or occlusion, need for dialysis, deterioration of renal function by using estimated glomerular filtration rate (GFR), and secondary interventions related to the renal arteries were assessed. Preoperative and postprocedural factors predictive for the development of renal dysfunction were assessed by using a Fisher exact test, t test, and logistic regression.

Results.—A total of 72 patients were treated between 2001 and 2004 with a mean age, aneurysm size, and follow-up of 75 years, 6.2 cm, and 6 months (range, 1 to 24 months), respectively. No ruptures and five deaths (two procedure-related) were observed (Fig 3). There were 23 patients with baseline

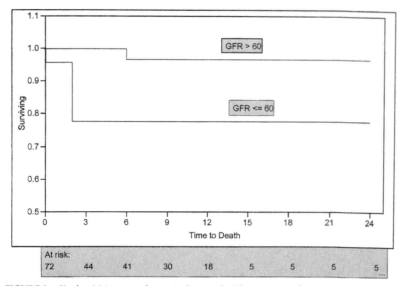

FIGURE 3.—Kaplan-Meier curves for survival in months. The *top curve* is for patients without renal dysfunction at baseline. The *bottom curve* is for patients with renal dysfunction at baseline. The total patients at risk is given at the *bottom* of the figure. Survival in the two groups is statistically different ($P = .02$). (Reprinted by permission of the publisher from Haddad F, Greenberg RK, Walker E, et al: Fenestrated endovascular grafting: The renal side of the story. *J Vasc Surg* 41:181-190, 2005. Copyright 2005 by Elsevier.)

renal insufficiency and 49 patients without insufficiency. Twenty-four patients had deterioration in GFR >30% during the follow-up period, and 17 patients experienced 19 renal-related events (more common in patients with baseline insufficiency, 39% vs 16.3%; $P = .04$; relative risk, 2.4). Four patients required dialysis (two permanent), and all had preoperative renal dysfunction ($P = .002$); similarly, death was also more common in this group (17.4% vs 2%; $P = .02$; relative risk, 8.52). Renal events in most patients occurred within the first postoperative month (59%). However, mean GFR stabilized after 6 months.

Conclusion.—Aneurysm repair with fenestrated endovascular grafts is associated with a significant risk for adverse renal events (16% in those without renal dysfunction, although none developed a creatinine >2 mg/dL, and 39% for patients with preoperative renal dysfunction). These patients must be meticulously followed, particularly within the first month after such a procedure. When renal artery restenosis is suspected or diagnosed, aggressive approach might be warranted to limit the extent of late renal dysfunction.

▶ It has been demonstrated by the Cleveland Clinic group that preexisting renal dysfunction is one of the most powerful predictors of poor early and late outcomes after open abdominal aortic aneurysm repair. The authors evaluated first-generation fenestrated devices used to include the renal artery as a proximal seal zone. Despite the short follow-up (mean, 6 months) 10 renal artery stenoses, 5 renal artery occlusions, and 4 patients requiring dialysis were noted. I suspect with longer follow-up and a higher incidence of graft migration with time, there will be a significant problem with renal stent occlusions/stenosis. I wonder if hybrid renal bypass procedures combined with endografts as championed by the group from University of North Carolina may be a more durable technique?

K. Kasirajan, MD

Cost-effectiveness of endovascular abdominal aortic aneurysm repair
Michaels JA, Drury D, Thomas SM (Northern Gen Hosp, Sheffield, England)
Br J Surg 92:960-967, 2005   6–8

Background.—The rapid introduction of endovascular abdominal aortic aneurysm repair (EVAR) has considerable implications for the management of abdominal aortic aneurysm (AAA). This study was undertaken to determine an optimal strategy for the use of EVAR based on the best currently available evidence.

Methods.—Economic modelling and probabilistic sensitivity analysis considered reference cases representing a fit 70-year-old (Fig 2) with a 5.5-cm diameter AAA (RC1) and an 80-year-old (Fig 3) with a 65-cm AAA unfit for open surgery (RC2). Results were assessed as incremental cost-effectiveness ratio (ICER) compared with open repair (RC1) or conservative management (RC2).

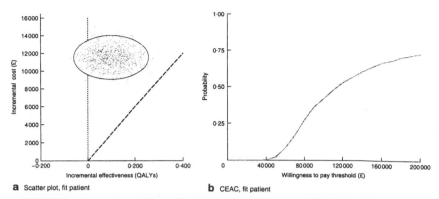

a Scatter plot, fit patient **b** CEAC, fit patient

FIGURE 2.—a Scatter plot and b cost-effectiveness acceptability curve (CEAC) derived from probabilistic sensitivity analysis (1000 simulations) for reference case 1 (fit 70-year-old). The scatter plot in a shows the results of 1000 simulations with the incremental effectiveness plotted on the horizontal axis and the incremental cost on the vertical axis. The ellipse contains 95 per cent of the simulations. Points above and to the left of the dashed line have a cost per quality-adjusted life year (QALY) of over £30 000 and those to the left of the vertical dotted line have a net loss of effectiveness. The CEDAC in b shows the proportion of simulations that would be acceptable given differing willingness to pay thresholds (equivalent to changing the slope of the dashed line in a). (Courtesy of Michaels JA, Drury D, Thomas SM: Cost-effectiveness of endovascular abdominal aortic aneurysm repair. *Br J Surg* 92:960-967, 2005. Reprinted by permission of Blackwell Publishing.)

Results.—In RC1 EVAR produced a gain of 0.10 quality-adjusted life years (QALYs) for an estimated cost of £11 449, giving an ICER of £110 000 per QALY. EVAR consistently had an ICER above £30 000 per QALY over a range of sensitivity analyses and alternative scenarios. In RC2 EVAR produced an estimated benefit of 1.64 QALYs for an incremental cost of £14 077 giving an incremental cost per QALY of £8579.

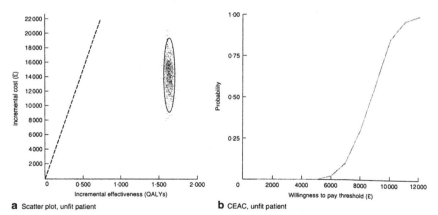

a Scatter plot, unfit patient **b** CEAC, unfit patient

FIGURE 3.—a Scatter plot and b cost-effectiveness acceptability curve (CEAC) (b) derived from probabilistic sensitivity analysis (1000 simulations) for reference case 2 (80-year-old unfit for surgery). The dotted line represents a willingness to pay threshold of £30 000 per quality-adjusted life year (QALY) (see footnote to *Fig 2* for further explanation). (Courtesy of Michaels JA, Drury D, Thomas SM: Cost-effectiveness of endovascular abdominal aortic aneurysm repair. *Br J Surg* 92:960-967, 2005. Reprinted by permission of Blackwell Publishing.)

Conclusion.—It is unlikely that EVAR for fit patients suitable for open repair is within the commonly accepted range of cost-effectiveness for a new technology. For those unfit for conventional open repair it is likely to be a cost-effective alternative to non-operative management. Sensitivity analysis suggests that research efforts should concentrate on determining accurate rates for late complications and reintervention, particularly in patients with high operative risks.

▶ The data suggest that in patients suitable for both EVAR and open repair, EVAR is not cost effective, but that it may be cost effective in patients unsuitable for open repair but only if they have what is basically a prohibitive projected operative mortality.

Economic modeling is a means of trying to help guide introduction of new technology into the health care system. It is obviously a surrogate, and a relatively poor surrogate, for well-conducted randomized trials. This type of data will be of some interest to health care policymakers. However, the field of endovascular aneurysm repair is evolving so rapidly that I doubt either patients or physicians will permit what is essentially speculation to drive the availability of EVAR.

G. L. Moneta, MD

Follow-up costs increase the cost disparity between endovascular and open abdominal aortic aneurysm repair
Hayter CL, Bradshaw SR, Allen RJ, et al (Canberra Hosp, Australia; Australian Natl Univ, Canberra)
J Vasc Surg 42:912-918, 2005   6–9

Objective.—This study compared the hospital and follow-up costs of patients who have undergone endovascular (EVAR) or open (OR) elective abdominal aortic aneurysm repair.

Methods.—The records of 195 patients (EVAR, n = 55; OR, n = 140) who underwent elective aortic aneurysm repair between 1995 and 2004 were reviewed. Primary costing data were analyzed for 54 EVAR and 135 OR patients. Hospital costs were divided into preoperative, operative, and postoperative costs. Follow-up costs for EVAR patients were recorded, with a median follow-up time of 12 months.

Results.—Mean preoperative costs were slightly higher in the EVAR group (AU $961/US $733 vs AU $869/US $663; not significant). Operative costs were significantly higher in the EVAR group (AU $16,124/US $12,297 vs AU $6077/US $4635; $P < .001$); this was entirely due to the increased cost of the endograft (AU $10,181/US $7,765 for EVAR vs AU $476/US $363 for OR). Postoperative costs were significantly reduced in the EVAR group (AU $4719/US $3599 vs AU $11,491/US $8,764; $P < .001$). Total hospital costs were significantly greater in the EVAR group (AU $21,804/US $16,631 vs AU $18,437/US $14,063; $P < .001$). The increase in total hospital costs was due to a significant difference in graft costs, which was not offset by reduced postoperative costs. The average follow-up cost per year after EVAR was AU $1316/US $999. At 1 year of follow-up, EVAR remained significantly more expensive than OR (AU $23,120/US $17,640 vs AU $18,510/US $14,122; $P < .001$); this cost discrepancy increased with a longer follow-up.

Conclusions.—EVAR results in significantly greater hospital costs compared with OR, despite reduced hospital and intensive care unit stays. The inclusion of follow-up costs further increases the cost disparity between EVAR and OR. Because EVAR requires lifelong surveillance and has a high rate of reintervention, follow-up costs must be included in any cost comparison of EVAR and OR. The economic cost, as well as the efficacy, of new technologies such as EVAR must be addressed before their widespread use is advocated.

▶ The study demonstrates higher in-hospital and follow-up costs for EVAR compared with OR abdominal aortic aneurysm repair. However, 20% of EVAR repair patients spent time in the ICU, and the mean length of stay for EVAR patients was 6 days. Most EVAR patients currently do not have an ICU stay and many are discharged home on postoperative day 1. Despite the cost of grafts, follow-up CT scans add significant cost to EVAR. We have been able to significantly decrease the follow-up costs by eliminating the 1-month CT scan and 6-month CT scan in patients with ideal anatomy and no intraoperative endoleaks. Also, the use of duplex studies and pressure sensor devices may completely eliminate the use of follow-up CT scans. However, the cost of EVAR may never be comparable to OR unless the cost of EVAR devices is drastically reduced.

K. Kasirajan, MD

Abdominal aortic aneurysm sac shrinkage after endovascular aneurysm repair: Correlation with chronic sac pressure measurement
Ellozy SH, Carroccio A, Lookstein RA, et al (Mount Sinai School of Medicine, New York)
J Vasc Surg 43:2-7, 2006   6–10

Objectives.—Abdominal aortic aneurysm (AAA) sac shrinkage after endovascular aneurysm repair (EVAR) is considered to be evidence of clinical success. Exclusion of the sac from systemic pressure is the likely cause of shrinkage. We report our continuing clinical experience with the use of a permanently implantable, ultrasound-activated remote pressure transducer to measure intrasac pressure and its correlation with changes in sac diameter over time (Fig 1).

Methods.—Over a 22-month period, 21 patients underwent EVAR of an infrarenal AAA with implantation of an ultrasound-activated remote pressure transducer fixed to the outside of the stent-graft and exposed to the excluded aortic sac. Intrasac pressures were measured directly with an intravascular catheter and by the remote sensor at the time of stent-graft deployment. Follow-up sac pressures were measured by remote sensor and

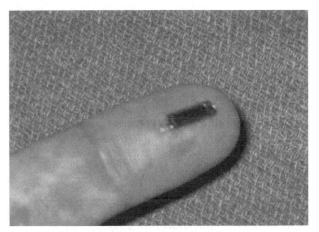

FIGURE 1.—The Remon Impressure AAA Sac Pressure Transducer (Remon Medical, Cesaria, Israel). (Reprinted by permission of the publisher from Ellozy SH, Carroccio A, Lookstein RA, et al: Abdominal aortic aneurysm sac shrinkage after endovascular aneurysm repair: Correlation with chronic sac pressure measurement. *J Vasc Surg* 43:2-7, 2006. Copyright 2006 by Elsevier.)

compared with systemic arterial pressure at every follow-up visit. Mean follow-up was 11.4 ± 5.0 months (range, 1 to 26 months). Twenty patients had follow-up of ≥6 months. Mean pressure index (MPI) was calculated as the ratio of mean sac pressure to mean systemic pressure.

Results.—Pressures could be obtained at all visits in 15 of the 21 patients. Fourteen of these 15 patients had follow-up of at least 6 months. Aneurysm sac shrinkage of >5 mm was seen in seven (50%) of these 14 patients. No aneurysm enlargement was observed in any patient. The MPI was significantly lower in patients with sac shrinkage at 6 months and at final follow-up.

Conclusions.—Endovascular aneurysm repair results in marked reduction of sac pressure in most patients. Patients with aneurysm shrinkage after EVAR have significantly lower MPI; however, the absence of sac shrinkage does not imply persistent pressurization of the sac. Further clinical follow-up will delineate the role of long-term sac pressure monitoring in surveillance after EVAR.

▶ This is a novel device to measure intrasac pressures noninvasively with excellent correlation between the presence of endoleaks, sac shrinkage, and intrasac pressure measurements. (One such device is currently on the market and FDA approved.) Despite this, use of this technology is not widespread. I suspect this is due to the cost of the device, no current reimbursement codes, and the additional time it adds to an endograft procedure.

K. Kasirajan, MD

Aneurysm Sac Thrombus Load Predicts Type II Endoleaks after Endovascular Aneurysm Repair

Sampaio SM, Panneton JM, Mozes GI, et al (Mayo Clinic, Rochester, Minn)
Ann Vasc Surg 19:302-309, 2005   6–11

Type II endoleaks are associated with the absence of aneurysm shrinkage after endovascular abdominal aortic aneurysm repair (EVAR). This study aims at determining the predictability of this complication, whose potential risk factors have been the subject of conflicting reports. Preoperative computed tomography (CT) scans of 178 patients who underwent EVAR for true infrarenal abdominal aortic aneurysms between January 20, and April 17, 2003, with a minimum follow-up of 30 days, were reviewed. The following information was retrieved: maximum aneurysm diameter, aneurysm thrombus load (maximum thickness, percentage of sac circumference wall coverage, percentage of maximum sac area occupancy); number, diameter, and nature (lumbar, inferior mesenteric, accessory renal, middle sacral) of patent aortic side-branch arteries; thrombus thickness at each aortic branch ostium, and aneurysm diameter at that level. Postoperative CT and duplex scans supplemented with angiography in selected cases were reviewed for the presence of a type II endoleak observable beyond the 30th postoperative day. Logistic regression was used to assess the association of each variable with this outcome. There were 38 (21.3%) patients with type II endoleaks

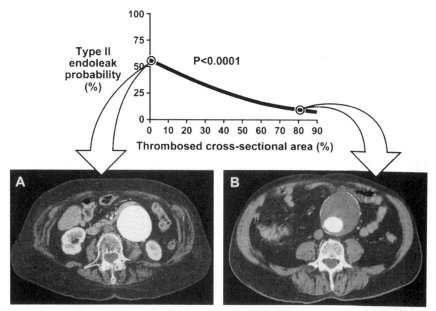

FIGURE 3.—Percentage of thrombosed cross-sectional area and type II endoleak probability. Cumulative logistic probability plot. A With 0% thrombosed area, there is 52.2% probability of a type II endoleak. B With 83.9% thrombosed area, there is 6.8% probability of a type II endoleak. (Courtesy of Sampaio SM, Panneton JM, Mozes GI, et al: Aneurysm sac thrombus load predicts type II endoleaks after endovascular aneurysm repair. Ann Vasc Surg 19:302-309, 2005.)

after the 30th postoperative day. The median follow-up was 12 months (range 1–65 months). By univariate analysis, the following variables significantly decreased the risk of a type II endoleak: thrombus maximum thickness [odds ratio (OR) 0.77 for a 5 mm increase, $p = 0009$], mean thrombus thickness at aortic side-branches ostia (OR 0.65 for a 1 mm increase, $p = 0.0006$), thrombus-occupied percentage of maximum aneurysm area (OR 0.72 for a 10% increase, $p < 0.0001$), percentage of thrombus-lined aneurysm wall (OR 0.53 for a 25% increase, $p < 0.0001$). The presence of a patent inferior mesenteric artery (OR 6.84, $p < 0.01$) and the number of patent aortic side-branches (OR 1.37 for each additional vessel, $p = 0.002$) significantly increased the risk of detecting a late type II endoleak. Aneurysm and aortic side-branch diameters did not have any impact. In a multiple logistic regression model (whole model $p < 0.0001$), the thrombus-occupied percentage of maximum aneurysm area (OR 0.74 for a 10% increase, $p < 0.0005$) and the number of patent aortic side-branches (OR 1.31 for each additional vessel, $p = 0.009$) remained independent predictors of type II endoleaks. The simple measure of the proportion of maximum aneurysm area occupied by thrombus may be a useful way to identify patients at high risk of a persistent type II endoleak. Patients with low preoperative sac thrombus load should be followed with a high degree of suspicion for this complication (Fig 3).

▶ The authors studied several aneurysm sac features and were able to correlate the appearance of type II endoleaks with volume of sac thrombus. I am not sure this is clinically important. Most type II endoleaks are now considered harmless unless associated with sac expansion. The presence of sac thrombus is not protective of aneurysm rupture. This report will not change follow-up requirements or current clinical practice.

K. Kasirajan, MD

Aortic Neck Attachment Failure and the AneuRx Graft: Incidence, Treatment Options, and Early Results

Azizzadeh A, Sanchez LA, Rubin BG, et al (Washington Univ, St Louis)
Ann Vasc Surg 19:516-521, 2005   6–12

Some investigators have reported that proximal attachment failure is a long-term complication of endovascular abdominal aortic aneurysm repair (EVAR) with the AneuRx (Medtronic, Santa Rosa, CA) device. We evaluated the need for an intervention in patients with suboptimal proximal fixation as well as the feasibility and early success of a variety of treatment strategies. From October 1999 to October 2003, we performed 365 EVARs using the AneuRx graft. At a mean follow-up of 23.7 ± 14.8 months, 20 patients (5.5%) with suboptimal outcomes (14 with a type I endoleak, one with a type III endoleak, and 5 with an inadequate seal zone <1 cm) were considered for treatment. Characteristics of each patient's aortic neck anatomy that could be associated with proximal attachment failure were evaluated.

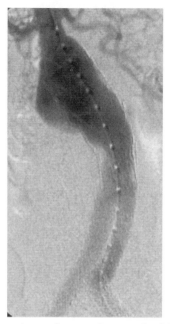

FIGURE 2.—Intraoperative arteriogram demonstrating a type I endoleak. (Courtesy of Azizzadeh A, Sanchez LA, Rubin BG, et al: Aortic neck attachment failure and the AneuRx graft: Incidence, treatment options, and early results. *Ann Vasc Surg* 19:516-521, 2005.)

Eighteen patients (90%) underwent successful treatment (9 AneuRx cuffs, 6 Talent cuffs, 5 aortic stents, one redo endograft, and two surgical conversions) without major perioperative complications, one patient had a persistent type I endoleak despite endovascular treatment, and one patient refused treatment, ultimately leading to aneurysm rupture. There have been no further endoleaks or graft migrations noted since the secondary intervention at a mean follow-up of 13.9 ± 11.8 months. In our experience, proximal attachment failure associated with the AneuRx graft is relatively uncommon and usually associated with unfavorable neck anatomy. Despite this, most cases are treatable by endovascular means. Long-term follow-up is needed to assess the ultimate frequency of these combined device reconstructions (Fig 2).

▶ Follow-up periods in this study are relatively short, with a mean follow-up of 23.7 ± 14.8 months after initial placement of the AneuRx stent graft and a mean follow-up of only 13.9 ± 11.8 months after secondary interventions in 20 patients with suboptimal proximal fixation. Likely there will be more proximal attachment site failures as time goes by. The follow-up periods presented here are simply too short to suggest either continued use, or immediate abandonment, of the AneuRx graft system. Longer-term data are required. A comparison of rates of proximal site attachment failure with other types of aortic stent grafts is also required.

G. L. Moneta, MD

AneuRx Device Migration: Incidence, Risk Factors, and Consequences
Sampaio SM, Panneton JM, Mozes G, et al (Mayo Clinic, Rochester, Minn)
Ann Vasc Surg 19:178-185, 2005   6–13

Success after endovascular abdominal aortic aneurysm repair (EVAR) is dependent on device positional stability. The quest for such stability has motivated different endograft designs, and the risk factors entailed remain the subject of debate. This study aims at defining the incidence, risk factors, and clinical implications of device migration after EVAR with the AneuRx® endograft. In this study we included all consecutive 109 patients submitted to primary AneuRx placement for infrarenal aortic or aortoiliac aneurysms. Preoperative computed tomography (CT) scans were reviewed for the following anatomic characteristics: neck length, diameter, angulation, calcification, and thrombus load; and sac diameter and thrombus load. Percentage of device oversizing relative to the proximal neck diameter was determined. All postoperative CT scans were reviewed, and the distance between the lowest renal artery and the craniad end of the device was measured. A ≥ 5-mm increase in such distance was considered indicative of device migration. Migration cumulative incidence was estimated by the Kaplan-Meier method, and its association with any of the preoperative anatomical characteristics was tested using Cox proportional hazards models. Median follow-up time was 9 (range, 1-31) months. Migration occurred in nine patients, corresponding to a 15.6% estimated probability of migration at 30 months (SE = 5.1%) (Figs 2 and 4). Migration was associated with the risk of proximal type I endoleak (hazard ratio = 3.39, 95% confidence interval = 1.46-7.87; $p = 0.007$). This type of endoleak occurred in three of the migration-affected patients (33.3%); all of them were resolved by additional cuff

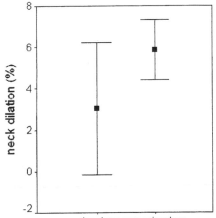

FIGURE 2.—Mean proportion of neck dilation at first postoperative diameter, relative to preoperative diameter, among migrators and nonmigrators. Whiskers represent SEM, $p = 0.365$, Wilcoxon rank-sum test. (Courtesy of Sampaio SM, Panneton JM, Mozes G, et al: AneuRx device migration: Incidence, risk factors, and consequences. *Ann Vasc Surg* 19:178-185, 2005)

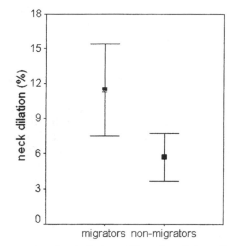

FIGURE 4.—Mean proportion of neck dilation at 18 months, relative to first postoperative diameter, among migrators and nonmigrators. Whiskers represent SEM, $p = 0.077$, Wilcoxon rank-sum test. (Courtesy of Sampaio SM, Panneton JM, Mozes G, et al: AneuRx device migration: Incidence, risk factors, and consequences. *Ann Vasc Surg* 19:178-185, 2005.)

placement at the proximal landing zone. No other migration-related reinterventions were performed. The only significant associations between anatomic factors and device migration probability were the protective effects of longer necks (odds ratio [OR] = 0.71 for each additional 5 mm, $p = 0.045$) and longer overlapped portions of neck and device (OR = 0.56 for each additional 5 mm, $p = 0.003$). There was a trend toward higher probability of migration among reverse-tapered necks (OR = 1.75, $p = 0.109$). Percentage of device oversizing correlated with early neck dilation (between preoperative and first postoperative diameters, correlation coefficient = 0.4, $p < 0.0001$), but not with late neck dilatation (between first postoperative and 1.5-year scan diameters, correlation coefficient = 0.29, $p = 0.112$). There was a trend toward higher mean percentage of late dilation among migrators (11.4%, standard error of the mean [SEM] 2.6) than nonmigrators (5.7%, SEM = 1) ($p = 0.08$), but both groups had similar mean percentages of early dilation (3%, SEM = 1.6%, vs. 5.5%, SEM = 0.6%; $p = 0.365$). This result indicates that device migration is not a rare event after AneuRx implantation. This phenomenon is associated with proximal type I endoleaks. Deployment of the endograft immediately below the renal arteries might help to prevent migration, since use of greater lengths of overlapped device relative to the proximal neck has a protective effect. Migration seems to be independent of the degree of device oversizing.

▶ There was a significant incidence of neck migration with the AneuRx device despite a mean neck length coverage of 27.7 mm. This correlated with type I endoleaks. Mistakes have been corrected with additional proximal cuffs. In our experience, this will fail. The main body of the device will continue to migrate on the proximal cuff. The preferable technique to correct this is the use of an aortomonoiliac device or conversion to open repair. The use of positive fixation with use of barbs, hooks, and suprarenal stents hopefully will decrease the incidence of graft migration. Among the current devices in use, the AneuRx has the longest follow-up; hence, meaningful comparisons to other devices do not exist. Unfortunately, based on currently available data, continued use of the AneuRx device in its current design may not be justified.

K. Kasirajan, MD

Prediction of altered endograft path during endovascular abdominal aortic aneurysm repair with the Gore Excluder
Whittaker DR, Dwyer J, Fillinger MF (Dartmouth-Hitchcock Med Ctr, Lebanon, NH)
J Vasc Surg 41:575-583, 2005   6–14

Objective.—During endovascular abdominal aortic aneurysm (AAA) repair (EVAR), the rapid deployment of the Gore Excluder endograft may be associated with anatomic shortening of the endograft path. This shortened path may result in coverage of the hypogastric artery origin or overly conservative graft length selection that may lead to unnecessary extensions. We quantified the degree of path alteration with this endograft and developed an algorithm to predict it.

Methods.—Preoperative and postoperative three-dimensional (3D) computed tomographic (CT) scans were evaluated for 50 consecutive patients with Gore Excluder endografts by using 21 anatomic measurements and 6 calculated indices (Fig 2). Measurements were evaluated as if only 3D lumen centerline measurements were available, rather than complete 3D computer-aided measurement and "virtual graft" simulation. Tortuosity was quantitated from the renal artery to the hypogastric origin, using the difference between a straight line and the lumen centerline.

Results.—The endograft was deployed successfully in all cases. The graft end points were typically quite close to the preoperative plan: mean renal artery-to-graft distance was within $2.0 \pm .5$ mm, and the limb end point-to-hypogastric origin differed by an average of only 1.8 ± 1.6 mm. Although accurate in most cases, the actual graft path shortened 1 cm or more relative to the centerline in 11% of limbs. On univariate analysis, determinants of alteration of >1 cm in the graft deployment path were (1) aortoiliac tortuosity (renal-to-hypogastric artery, $P < .002$), (2) the degree of planned graft rotation (73% of cases altered >10 mm were in the rotated position, $P < .05$), and (3) the insertion side (73% of alterations >10 mm were ipsilateral to the main device, $P < .05$). On multivariate analysis, the renal-to-hypogastric artery tortuosity index (RHTI) was significant ($P < .004$), and device type and rotation approached significance ($P < .08$). We developed a classification scheme based on RHTI to predict the risk of alteration of the graft path ≥ 1 cm (low risk, 0%; medium risk, 10%; high risk, 25%) and an algorithm to predict the degree of alteration of the anatomy that reduced the number of cases shortening ≥ 1 cm to zero.

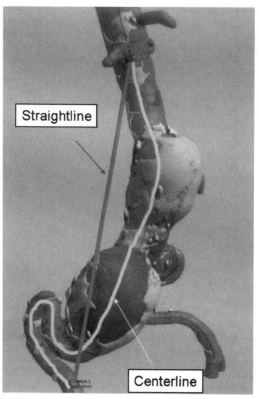

FIGURE 2.—Example of measurements used to evaluate tortuosity. Shown here are 3D measurements for the renal artery-to-hypogastric artery tortuosity index (RHTI), where RHTI = (lumen centerline length − straight line length) as measured from the center of the aorta just below the lowest renal artery to the center of the common iliac artery just proximal to the hypogastric artery origin. The other tortuosity indices are calculated in similar fashion as described in Table I. (Reprinted by permission of the publisher from Whittaker DR, Dwyer J, Fillinger MF: Prediction of altered endograft path during endovascular abdominal aortic aneurysm repair with the Gore Excluder. *J Vasc Surg* 41:575-583, 2005. Copyright 2005 by Elsevier.)

Conclusions.—The graft deployment path will be altered significantly in a minority of cases with the Gore Excluder endograft, but this can cause hypogastric occlusion or other problems. Anatomic shortening is predictable from morphologic features such as tortuosity, graft insertion side, and rotation. We developed an algorithm based on a tortuosity index that quantitates the risk and degree of shortening associated with endograft deployment.

▶ Centerline measurements from 3D CT scan reconstruction were used to determine in situ graft position. In the majority of patients, graft deployment was as predicted and was not altered except in the presence of significant iliac tortuosity. I suspect deployment accuracy would be even greater with grafts with controlled deployment, such as the Zenith or AneuRx. Graft maldeployment is more a factor of poor intraoperative technique and improper gantry position than a factor of poor preoperative planning.

K. Kasirajan, MD

Secondary conversion of the Gore Excluder to operative abdominal aortic aneurysm repair

Kong LS, MacMillan D, Kasirajan K, et al (Emory Univ, Atlanta, Ga)
J Vasc Surg 42:631-638, 2005   6–15

Objective.—Reports continue to document the occurrence of major adverse events after endovascular aortic aneurysm repair. Although many of these problems can be successfully managed through endovascular salvage, operative conversion with explantation of the endoprosthesis remains necessary in some patients. We report herein a review of all patients initially enrolled in multicenter US clinical trials of the Excluder endograft who underwent secondary conversion to open surgical repair.

Methods.—Clinical data and relevant medical records of patients enrolled in phase I and II multicenter US clinical trials of the Excluder endograft were retrospectively reviewed for adverse events and further narrowed to those patients who underwent secondary operative conversion. Hospital records, operative and anesthesia reports, and all imaging studies were analyzed at initial implantation and at the time of subsequent open surgical repair.

Results.—Late open conversion was performed in 16 (2.7%) of the 594 patients enrolled in the Excluder clinical trials. Presumed endotension accounted for 8 of 16 of secondary conversions. In two of these patients, however, an endoleak was identified at the time of open surgical repair. Of the remaining eight patients, two underwent conversion for device infection, five for persistent endoleak, and one for aneurysm rupture. The overall 30-day mortality was 6.25% (1/16), with one death occurring in a patient with a ruptured aneurysm. Of patients who underwent conversion because of endotension, the maximal abdominal aortic aneurysm diameter (mean ± SD) at the time of initial implantation and subsequent graft removal was 61 ± 11 mm and 70 ± 10 mm, respectively. The mean time to open conversion for treatment of endotension was 37 ± 12 months (range, 20-50 months; median, 42 months). Freedom from conversion was 98.6% and 96.7% at 24 and 48 months, respectively.

Conclusions.—Endotension in the absence of a demonstrable endoleak has been a major indication for late surgical conversion in patients treated with the Excluder endograft. Given the potential presence of an undetected endoleak and the possible effects of progressive sac enlargement on long-term device stability, continued close surveillance of patients with assumed endotension is required. Should changes in device design eliminate endotension, a further reduction in the already low incidence of late open conversion of the Excluder endograft can be anticipated.

▶ Half the open conversions performed for the Gore device were due to endotension, and 75% of these were associated with accumulation of gelatinase material within the aneurysm sac. This is presumably secondary to transgraft filtration of plasma components of some sort. The current Gore device has been redesigned with lower porosity to address this problem, but any positive effect of this design change is not completely known at this point. According to the authors, there have been no ruptures associated with seroma-induced endotension. Overall, vascular surgeons are obviously pleased with the Gore device. In its relatively short time in the US market, it has achieved the majority share of the AAA endograft market.

G. L. Moneta, MD

A prospective study of subclinical myocardial damage in endovascular versus open repair of infrarenal abdominal aortic aneurysms
Abraham N, Lemech L, Sandroussi C, et al (Royal Prince Alfred Hosp, Camperdown, Australia; Univ of Sydney)
J Vasc Surg 41:377-381, 2005   6–16

Background.—Endovascular repair of abdominal aortic aneurysms (AAAs) is considered to be less invasive and better tolerated by the cardiovascular system than open repair. Our aim was to assess the true incidence of perioperative myocardial damage associated with endovascular vs open infrarenal AAA repair.

Methods.—Between July 1999 and June 2001, preoperative and postoperative serum troponin T (TnT) levels were measured in all patients presenting for elective AAA repair at Royal Prince Alfred Hospital. The incidence of myocardial damage was recorded on the basis of standard clinical, biochemical, and electrocardiographic changes or a subclinical increase of 50% or more in serum TnT. Patients were excluded if the TnT increase was associated with a significant increase of serum creatinine ($\geq 50\%$) with no other evidence of myocardial ischemia. The differences between the two groups were analyzed with the χ^2 test and odds ratios.

Results.—A total of 35 open and 112 endovascular AAA repairs were included in the study. There was no significant difference in age, sex, preoperative serum creatinine, or preoperative serum TnT between the two treatment groups. Seventeen patients had biochemical evidence of myocardial damage, which was clinically obvious in only one patient. Even though the incidence of previous myocardial infarction was significantly higher in patients undergoing endovascular repair (41%) than open repair (22%; $P < .05$), the overall incidence of myocardial damage (clinical or subclinical) was significantly higher in the open group compared with the endovascular group (8 [25%] of 32 vs 9 [8%] of 109, respectively; odds ratio, 3.7; 95% confidence interval, 1.28-10.49; $P < .02$).

Conclusions.—There is a previously underestimated incidence of subclinical myocardial damage associated with surgery for infrarenal AAA which is lower after endovascular than open repair.

▶ At Dr May's hospital, endovascular aneurysm repair is preferred over open repair in all patients independent of age and risk factors. Open repair is performed only when endovascular repair is not possible. Therefore, as the authors acknowledge, the open patients in this series may be the ones at higher risk for complication. The long-term significance of asymptomatic perioperative troponin increases in the open and endovascular repair patients is unknown.

G. L. Moneta, MD

Midterm outcome of endovascular repair of ruptured abdominal aortic aneurysms
Hechelhammer L, Lachat ML, Wildermuth S, et al (Univ Hosp of Zurich, Switzerland)
J Vasc Surg 41:752-757, 2005   6–17

Purpose.—We sought to analyze the clinical and morphologic outcomes of bifurcated stent grafts in patients with ruptured aortoiliac aneurysms at midterm follow-up.

Methods.—Thirty-seven patients (4 women; mean age, 73 years; mean abdominal aortic aneurysm [AAA] diameter, 77 mm) underwent endovascular abdominal aneurysm repair between June 1997 and July 2003 for ruptured AAA. Devices inserted were as follows: Vanguard (Boston Scientific, Natick, Mass; n = 7), Excluder (WL. Gore, Flagstaff, Ariz; n = 25), Talent (Medtronic Vascular, Santa Rosa, Calif; n = 2), and Zenith (Cook Inc, Bloomington, Ind; n = 3). Except for the adjunct postimplantation computed tomographic scanning, the imaging follow-up was the same as for nonruptured AAAs.

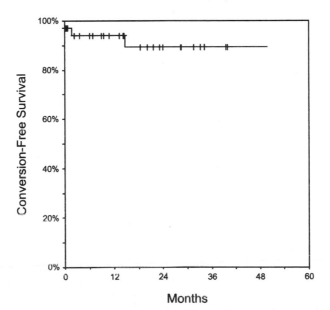

FIGURE 2—Kaplan-Meier curve of conversion-free follow-up. (Reprinted by permission of the publisher from Hechelhammer L, Lachat ML, Wildermuth S, et al: Midterm outcome of endovascular repair of ruptured abdominal aortic aneurysms. *J Vasc Surg* 41:752-757, 2005. Copyright 2005 by Elsevier.)

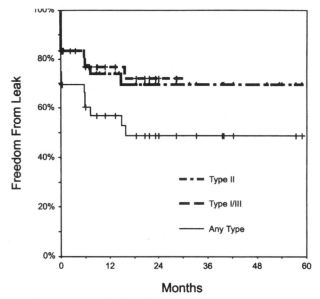

Months

FIGURE 3.—Kaplan-Meier curve of freedom from endoleak over follow-up. (Reprinted by permission of the publisher from Hechelhammer L, Lachat ML, Wildermuth S, et al: Midterm outcome of endovascular repair of ruptured abdominal aortic aneurysms. *J Vasc Surg* 41:752-757, 2005. Copyright 2005 by Elsevier.)

Results.—The mean follow-up period was 24 months (range, 1-59) months. Thirty-day mortality was 10.8%. Three patients died during the follow-up of non-AAA-related causes. One patient was converted early for presumed renal overstenting. The late conversion rate was 9% because of stent graft migration (n = 2) or infection (n = 1). Freedom from endoleak was 57% ± 8.5% and 48.8% ± 9% at 2 and 4 years, respectively (Figs 2 and 3). Seventeen secondary interventions were performed during the follow-up period, 41% of these within 1 month of stent graft placement. Endoleaks, primary or secondary, were responsible for 58.8% of these interventions. The cumulative risk of a secondary intervention was 35.3% ± 9% at 2 years and 44.6% ± 11% at 3 years. Aneurysmal sac shrinkage was observed in 30.8% ± 9.1% and sac enlargement was observed in 15.3% ± 10.8% at 2 years.

Conclusion.—Endoluminal devices are able to convert the acute life-threatening situation of ruptured AAA to a controlled situation that results in good patient survival at midterm follow-up.

▶ The authors have achieved a remarkable low mortality rate (10.8%) for ruptured AAAs with the use of endografts. There maybe a bias toward the treatment of stable ruptures, as all patients had time for a preprocedural CT scan. Hence, these results may not be directly comparable to open surgical mortality rates associated with ruptured AAAs. A unique complication described by the authors is a retroperitoneal compartment syndrome with renal failure secondary to ureter compression. I routinely used ureteric stents when endografts are deployed in the presence of a large retroperitoneal hematoma.

K. Kasirajan, MD

Factors associated with abdominal compartment syndrome complicating endovascular repair of ruptured abdominal aortic aneurysms
Mehta M, Darling RC III, Roddy SP, et al (Inst for Vascular Health and Disease, Albany, NY)
J Vasc Surg 42:1047-1051, 2005   6–18

Background.—Endovascular treatment of ruptured abdominal aortic aneurysms (r-AAAs) has the potential to offer improved outcomes. As our experience with endovascular repair of r-AAA evolved, we recognized that the development of abdominal compartment syndrome (ACS) led to an increase in morbidity and mortality. We therefore reviewed our experience to identify risk factors associated with the development of ACS.

Methods.—From January 2002 to December 2004, 30 patients underwent emergent endovascular repair of r-AAA by using commercially available stent grafts. All patients who developed ACS underwent emergent laparotomy. Physiological and clinical parameters were analyzed between patients with and without ACS after endovascular r-AAA repair.

Results.—Over the past 3 years, 30 patients underwent endovascular r-AAA repair, and 6 (20%) patients developed ACS. Patients with ACS had a higher incidence of the need for aortic occlusion balloon (67% vs 12%; P = .01), a markedly longer activated partial thromboplastin time (128 ± 84 seconds vs 49 ± 31 seconds; P = .01), a greater need for blood transfusion (8 ± 2.5 units vs 1.8 ± 1.7 units; P = .08), and a higher incidence of conversion to aortouni-iliac devices because of ongoing hemodynamic instability and an inability to expeditiously cannulate the contralateral gate (67% vs 8%) when compared with patients without ACS. The mortality was significantly higher in the patients with ACS (67%; 4 of 6) compared with patients without ACS (13%; 3 of 24; P = .01).

Conclusions.—ACS is a potential complication of endovascular repair of r-AAA and negatively affects survival. Factors associated with the development of ACS include (1) use of an aortic occlusion balloon, (2) coagulopathy, (3) massive transfusion requirements, and (4) conversion of bifurcated stent grafts into aortouni-iliac devices. We recommend that, after endovascular repair of r-AAA, these patients undergo vigilant monitoring for the development of ACS.

▶ ACS after repair of r-AAA results from the same things as ACS after any sort of trauma (bowel swelling, hematoma, ongoing bleeding, coagulopathy). Note that when ACS occurs after endovascular repair of r-AAA, the mortality rate is as high as that expected with open repair. However, when there is no ACS after endovascular repair for r-AAA, the mortality rate is low. When possible, endovascular repair is an excellent treatment for r-AAA.

G. L. Moneta, MD

Results of Endovascular Repair of Inflammatory Abdominal Aortic Aneurysms: A Report from the EUROSTAR Database
Lange C, for the EUROSTAR Collaborators (Univ Hosp, Trondheim, Norway; et al)
Eur J Vasc Endovasc Surg 29:363-370, 2005   6–19

Objectives.—To investigate the results following endovascular treatment of patients with inflammatory abdominal aortic aneurysms (IAAA).

Design.—Retrospective study based on the EUROSTAR registry.

Material and Methods.—Patients included in the EUROSTAR registry with IAAA ($n = 52$, 1.4%) were compared to those having aneurysms without aortic fibrosis ($n = 3613$, 98.6%). The mean follow-up period in patients with IAAA was 23 months (range 1–60). In 11 of the patients detailed information on the effect of endovascular repair and perianeurysmal fibrosis and ureteral entrapment was obtained by a dedicated questionnaire.

Results.—Twelve patients (23%) with IAAA had preoperative impairment of renal function and five had known hydronephrosis. Variables that were significantly associated with IAAA included younger age ($p < .0001$,

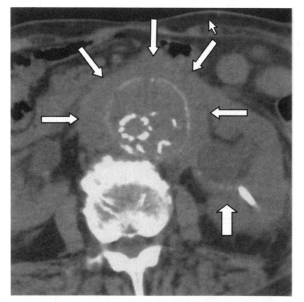

FIGURE 1.—CT examination 4 months after stentgraft repair of an IAAA. Note thick layer of perianeurysmal fibrosis (arrows). The left ureteric system became dilated after the procedure and needed drainage (larger arrow). (Reprinted from Lange C, for the EUROSTAR Collaborators: Results of endovascular repair of inflammatory abdominal aortic aneurysms: A report from the EUROSTAR database. *Eur J Vasc Endovasc Surg* 29:363-370, 2005, by permission of the publisher.)

mean difference 5.9, CI 3.7–7.9) and lower pulmonary risks score (OR 0.38, CI 0.19–0.74). At completion of the endovascular procedure, device stenosis was more frequently observed in patients with IAAA (OR 18.1, CI 3.52–93.0). There were no differences with regard to the rates of mortality, rupture or conversion in patients with IAAA and controls. In the majority, the aneurysm size regressed irrespective of nature of aneurysm. Of the 11 patients with a detailed assessment three had deterioration of renal function and three still had ureteral entrapment during follow-up.

Conclusion.—Despite persistence of perianeurysmal inflammation in a proportion of patients operative and midterm results of endovascular repair were comparable in the patients with inflammatory and standard AAA (Fig 1).

▶ The data indicate that an inflammatory AAA can be repaired with endovascular techniques with overall similar results to that of a standard AAA endovascular repair. The effect of endovascular aneurysm repair on resolution of retroperitoneal fibrosis and ureter entrapment appears similar to that with open repair of inflammatory AAA. This study is limited by its retrospective nature and by the fact that the EUROSTAR registry was not designed for analysis of the pathology associated with inflammatory aneurysms. Nevertheless, the data, such as they are, suggest reasonable results with endovascular repair of inflammatory aortic aneurysms.

G. L. Moneta, MD

Midterm Follow-up of Inflammatory Abdominal Aortic Aneurysms Following Endovascular Repair
Faizer R, DeRose G, Forbes TL, et al (Univ of Western Ontario, London, Canada)
Ann Vasc Surg 19:636-640, 2005   6–20

The role of endovascular therapy in the management of inflammatory aneurysms of the infrarenal abdominal aorta has been controversial. Review of our endovascular database identified six patients who have undergone treatment for preoperatively diagnosed inflammatory abdominal aortic aneurysms. Outcomes measured were primary success of the procedure, variation in computed tomographic (CT) scan-defined perianeurysmal fibrosis, change in aneurysm size, development of endoleak, requirement of reintervention, aneurysm rupture, and progression or resolution of symptoms. At a median follow-up of 20 months (range 4-56 months), endovascular repair has been successful in all six patients. All patients demonstrated CT reduction of perianeurysmal fibrosis, with a median of 47% absolute reduction (range 33–69%, $p = 0.014$) (Fig 2). All patients had aneurysm sac shrinkage, with a mean of 41% (range 6–86%, $p = 0.04$). There were no aneurysm ruptures or persistent endoleaks. Of the three patients who presented with abdominal or back pain, all are now symptom-free. One patient required reintervention for limb thrombosis of a bifurcated graft after 2 years. In

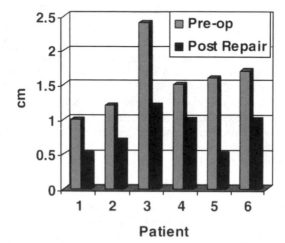

FIGURE 2.—Change in maximal radial extent of perianeurysmal fibrosis. (Courtesy of Faizer R, DeRose G, Forbes TL, et al: Midterm follow-up of inflammatory abdominal aortic aneurysms following endovascular repair. *Ann Vasc Surg* 19:636-640, 2005.)

conclusion, endovascular treatment of an inflammatory abdominal aortic aneurysm is safe and effective and the treatment of choice in anatomically suitable patients.

▶ Favorable results are obtained with endograft treatment of inflammatory aneurysms in this series. Unfortunately, not all publications have had favorable results. Patients with significant compression of the ureters appear to have the least favorable response in our experience.

K. Kasirajan, MD

7 Visceral Renal Disease

Prospective Evaluation of Aggressive Medical Therapy for Atherosclerotic Renal Artery Stenosis, With Renal Artery Stenting Reserved for Previously Injured Heart, Brain, or Kidney
Hanzel G, Balon H, Wong O, et al (William Beaumont Hosp, Royal Oak, Mich; Lenox Hill Hosp, New York; Michigan Cardiovascular Inst, Saginaw)
Am J Cardiol 96:1322-1327, 2005   7–1

Sixty-six patients with atherosclerotic renal artery stenosis (RAS) and serum creatinine ≤2.0 mg/dl were treated with antihypertensive therapy, a statin, and aspirin. Renal stenting was reserved for patients with injuries to the heart, brain, or kidneys. The primary end point was stenotic kidney glomerular filtration rate (GFR) at 21 months; secondary end points included major adverse clinical events, serum creatinine, total GFR, and blood pressure (BP). After baseline evaluation, 26 of 66 patients underwent renal stent-

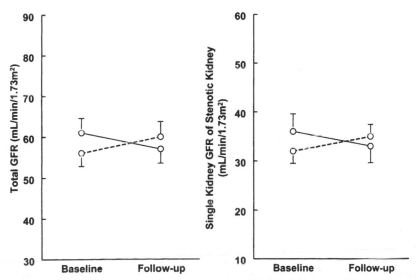

FIGURE 4.—Total kidney (**left panel**) and stenotic kidney (**right panel**) GFR at baseline and follow-up. *Solid lines,* the medical group (p = 0.03 for total GFR, p <0.01 for single kidney GFR); *dashed lines,* the stent group (p = NS for total GFR, p = 0.07 for single-kidney GFR. (Reprinted from Hanzel G, Balon H, Wong O, et al: Prospective evaluation of aggressive medical therapy for atherosclerotic renal artery stenosis, with renal artery stenting reserved for previously injured heart, brain, of kidney. *Am J Cardiol* 96:1322-1327, 2005. Copyright 2005 with permission from Excerpta Medica Inc.)

ing because of injuries to the heart, brain, or kidneys. After 21 months, 6 medical patients required renal stenting, and 5 patients experienced late clinical events (2 medical patients, 3 stent patients). There was no difference in final BP between groups. Whereas medical patients experienced 6% and 8% decreases in total and stenotic kidney GFR, stent patients experienced 7% and 11% increases in total kidney (p = 0.006) and stenotic kidney (p = 0.02) GFR. There was no difference in final serum creatinine. In conclusion, patients with atherosclerotic RAS and baseline creatinine ≤2.0 mg/dl can be safely managed with aggressive medical therapy, with a small decrease in GFR. For patients who develop injuries to the heart, brain, or kidneys, renal artery stenting may further reduce hypertension and improve renal function (Fig 4).

▶ This small study indicates that patients with atherosclerotic RAS and a serum creatinine < 2.0 mg/dL can be managed with medical therapy. The price will be a decrease in GFR, but there will be no change in serum creatinine or severity of hypertension, at least within the limitations imposed by the length of follow-up of this study.

This is clearly a "glass is half full" versus "glass is half empty" article. It will be interpreted by individuals favoring an aggressive policy of renal artery stenting as showing benefit from stenting. Simultaneously, it will be interpreted by individuals favoring a more conservative approach as showing that a more selective approach to renal artery stenting is warranted.

G. L. Moneta, MD

Evaluation of the Safety and Effectiveness of Renal Artery Stenting After Unsuccessful Balloon Angioplasty: The ASPIRE-2 Study

Rocha-Singh K, for the ASPIRE-2 Trial Investigators (Prairie Heart Inst, Springfield, Ill; et al)

J Am Coll Cardiol 46:776-783, 2005   7–2

Objectives.—This study sought to define the safety and durability of renal stenting after suboptimal/failed renal artery angioplasty in patients with suspected renovascular hypertension.

Background.—Few prospective multicenter studies have detailed the safety, efficacy, and long-term clinical benefits of renal artery stent revascularization in hypertensive patients with aorto-ostial atherosclerotic renal artery lesions.

Methods.—This non-randomized study enrolled 208 patients with de novo or restenotic ≥70% aorto-ostial renal artery stenoses, who underwent implantation of a balloon-expandable stent after unsuccessful percutaneous transluminal renal angioplasty (PTRA), which was defined as a ≥50% residual stenosis, persistent translesional pressure gradient, or a flow-limiting dissection. The primary end point was the nine-month quantitative angiographic or duplex ultrasonography restenosis rate adjudicated by core laboratory analysis. Secondary end points included renal function, blood pressure, and cumulative incidence of major adverse events and target lesion revascularization at 24 months.

Results.—The stent procedure was immediately successful in 182 of 227 (80.2%) lesions treated. The nine-month restenosis rate was 17.4%. Systolic/diastolic blood pressure decreased from $168 \pm 25/82 \pm 13$ mm Hg (mean ± standard deviation) at baseline to $149 \pm 24/77 \pm 12$ mm Hg at 9 months (p < 0.001 vs. baseline), and $149 \pm 25/77 \pm 12$ mm Hg at 24 months (p < 0.001 vs. baseline). Mean serum creatinine concentration was unchanged from baseline values at 9 and 24 months. The 24-month cumulative rate of major adverse events was 19.7%.

Conclusions.—In hypertensive patients with aorto-ostial atherosclerotic renal artery stenosis in whom PTRA is unsuccessful, Palmaz (Cordis Corp., Warren, New Jersey) balloon-expandable stents provide a safe and durable revascularization strategy, with a beneficial impact on hypertension.

▶ This study is limited by its retrospective nature and lack of controls in that no patients treated with medical therapy alone or simple balloon angioplasty were included. In addition, primary stenting of renal artery ostial lesions is currently routine. There is reasonable information here with respect to recurrent stenosis in a subgroup of patients undergoing renal artery stenting. Overall, however, there is little relevance to modern practice.

G. L. Moneta, MD

Renovascular disease in children and adolescents

Piercy KT, Hundley JC, Stafford JM, et al (Wake Forest Univ, Winston-Salem, NC)
J Vasc Surg 41:973-982, 2005   7–3

Purpose.—This retrospective review describes the surgical management of renovascular disease in 25 consecutive children and adolescents with severe hypertension.

Methods.—Patients ≤21 years of age (mean age, 11.6 ± 5.4 years; 12 females, 13 males) underwent repair of 34 renal arteries (RAs), and their management forms the basis of this report. Early and late blood pressure responses were adjusted for gender, age, and height. RA repair was evaluated by angiography, renal duplex sonography (RDS) scanning, or both. Primary patency and survival were estimated by product-limit methods.

Results.—Thirty-four RAs among 32 kidneys were repaired. Bilateral renal RA disease to a solitary kidney was present in nine patients. RA lesions included dysplasia (44%), RA hypoplasia (20%), midaortic syndrome (12%), RA aneurysm (12%), dissection (8%), and arteritis (4%). All patients had severe hypertension (>95th percentile systolic or diastolic pressure adjusted for gender, age, and height). RA repair comprised 25 bypasses (73%) consisting of 28% saphenous vein, 60% hypogastric artery, and 12% polytetrafluoroethylene; 2 patch angioplasties (6%), and 7 reimplantations (21%). Branch RA exposure was required in 28 kidneys (88%), and branch

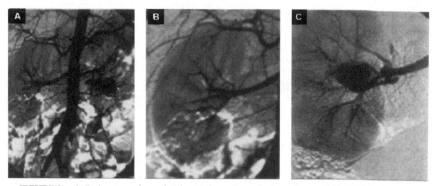

FIGURE 2.—**A, B,** Aortography and right renal arteriography in an 8-year-old boy with an arteritis of unknown etiology (English WP, Edwards MS, Pearce JD, et al: Multiple aneurysms in childhood. *J Vasc Surg* 39:254-259, 2004) demonstrating a left renal artery (RA) aneurysm with normal right RA. **C,** Repeat renal arteriography 5 years later demonstrated branch left RA occlusion and interval development of a 4.5 cm right RA aneurysm. (Reprinted by permission of the publisher from Piercy KT, Hundley JC, Stafford JM, et al: Renovascular disease in children and adolescents. *J Vasc Surg* 41:973-982, 2005. Copyright 2005 by Elsevier.)

reconstruction was required in 61%. Warm in situ repair was used in 53%, in situ cold perfusion in 24%, and ex vivo cold perfusion in 23%. Of six bilateral RA repairs, one was staged and two patients are awaiting a staged repair. Combined aortic reconstruction was required in three patients. No unplanned nephrectomy was performed. There were no perioperative deaths. Hypertension was cured in 36%, improved in 56%, and failed in 8% at mean follow-up of 46.4 ± 7.8 months. The mean calculated glomerular filtration rate increased from 82.0 mL/min/1.73 m² preoperatively to 98.2 mL/min/1.73 m² postoperatively. The postoperative patency of 30 RA re-

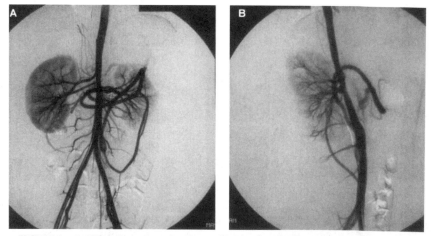

FIGURE 3.—**A,** Midaortic syndrome in a 7-year-old girl with orificial stenoses of two left renal arteries (RAs) and one right RA. **B,** These lesions coexisted in combination with occlusion of the celiac axis and superior mesenteric artery compensated by a larger meandering mesenteric artery. (Reprinted by permission of the publisher from Piercy KT, Hundley JC, Stafford JM, et al: Renovascular disease in children and adolescents. *J Vasc Surg* 41:973-982, 2005. Copyright 2005 by Elsevier.)

constructions was evaluated by angiography, RDS scanning, or both. At mean follow-up of 32.8 months (median, 21.2 months), primary RA patency was 91%. No failures were observed after 2 months follow-up. Estimated survival was 100% at 60 months, with one death 9 years after surgery.

Conclusions.—Renovascular hypertension in children and adolescents was caused by a heterogeneous group of lesions. All patients had RA repair, with arterial autografts in most of the RA bypasses. Cold perfusion preservation was used in half of the complex branch RA repairs. These strategies provided 91% primary patency at mean follow-up of 32.8 months, with beneficial blood pressure response in 92%. Surgical repair of clinically significant renovascular disease in children and adolescents is supported by these results (Figs 2 and 3).

▶ Several points are obvious here. One is that these are rare patients, with only 25 patients at a major referral center in almost 18 years (less than 2 patients per year). Two, the operations are demanding with a high percentage of branch artery and ex vivo repairs required. Three, the Wake Forest surgeons are good, with excellent technical results. Finally, and unfortunately, the patients really don't do all that well with only about one third cured of their hypertension. One would have hoped for better in this age group.

G. L. Moneta, MD

Surgical Management of Renal Fibromuscular Dysplasia: Challenges in the Endovascular Era

Carmo M, Bower TC, Mozes G, et al (Mayo Clinic, Rochester, Minn)
Ann Vasc Surg 19:208-217, 2005   7–4

Percutaneous transluminal renal angioplasty (PTRA) is the primary treatment for renal fibromuscular dysplasia (RFMD). Surgical revascularization is limited to patients who fail or are unsuitable for PTRA. All patients who were operated on with RFMD since the indications for renal PTRA were expanded in our institution were retrospectively reviewed. Outcome included patency, hypertension, and renal function. Twenty-six patients had reconstruction of 32 renal arteries between 1998 and 2004. The mean age was 47.1 ± 14 years; the majority (81%) were female. Six patients had bilateral disease and three had a solitary kidney. Operations were done for hypertension in 25 patients, renal artery aneurysm in 8, and chronic dissection in 1, alone or in combination. Six patients had a failed PTRA and 20 were unsuitable for it. Aortorenal bypass was done most often ($n - 28$) and saphenous vein was the preferred conduit ($n = 25$). The distal anastomosis was to the main renal artery in 13 patients and to the branch arteries in 19. Ex vivo repair was needed in five patients. Five intraoperative revisions were done because of abnormalities on duplex scan. One patient died unexpectedly 42 days after operation from myocardial infarction. Extrarenal complications occurred in five patients. Median follow-up was 2.4 (range, 42 days to 6.3) years and was available in all but one patient (96%). Two bypasses occluded

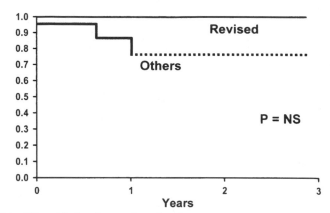

FIGURE 5.—Effect of duplex ultrasound scan-based revision on primary patency. (Courtesy of Carmo M, Bower TC, Mozes G, et al: Surgical management of renal fibromuscular dysplasia: Challenges in the endovascular era. *Ann Vasc Surg* 19(2):208-217, 2005.)

at 3 and 376 days, which resulted in loss of the kidneys. One graft stenosis was treated successfully with PTRA at 239 days. All failures occurred in men. One-year cumulative primary patency was 89 ± 8% and was not adversely affected by prior PTRA or complex repair. Hypertension at 1 year was cured in 27% of the patients and improved in 60%. No patient developed acute or chronic renal failure. Surgical reconstruction for RFMD has excellent short-term patency. Failed PTRA or complex reconstructions did not adversely affect outcome. (Fig 5).

▶ This is another series of interesting and complex renal artery operations (see Abstract 7–3) with excellent technical results and a poor cure rate for hypertension (27%). Clearly, the challenge in renal revascularization is to get better at picking the patients.

G. L. Moneta, MD

Percutaneous Management of Chronic Mesenteric Ischemia: Outcomes after Intervention
Landis MS, Rajan DK, Simons ME, et al (Univ of Toronto; Toronto Gen Hosp)
J Vasc Interv Radiol 16:1319-1325, 2005   7–5

Purpose.—To assess the efficacy and durability of percutaneous transluminal angioplasty (PTA)/stent placement for treatment of chronic mesenteric ischemia (CMI).
Materials and Methods.—A retrospective review of patients treated from January 1986 to August 2003 was conducted. Twenty-nine patients (mean age, 62 years) were treated for clinical symptoms consistent with CMI. Clinical diagnosis was verified with angiographic assessment and PTA with or without stent placement was performed based on angiographic and/or pres-

sure gradient findings. Outcomes were estimated with the Kaplan-Meier method.

Results.—A total of 63 interventions were performed in 29 patients during the study period. Of these 63 interventions, 46 PTA and 17 stent implantation procedures were performed. Thirty-four interventions were performed for SMA stenosis/occlusion, 17 interventions for celiac artery stenosis/occlusion, and four interventions were performed on aorto-mesenteric graft stenoses. Technical success was 97%, and clinical success (defined as clinical resolution of symptoms) was 90% (26 of 29 patients). Mean duration of follow-up was 28.3 months. Primary patency for all interventions at 3, 6, and 12 months was 82.7% (95% CI: 68.7-96.7), 78.9% (66.7-91.1), and 70.1% (55.1-85.6), respectively. Primary assisted patency for all interventions at 3, 6, and 12 months was 87.9% (79.0-95.3), 87.9% (79.2-95.1), and 87.9% (77.3-98.3), respectively. An average of 1.9 interventions per patient was required. One major complication occurred (3.4%). There were three minor complications (10.3%).

Conclusions.—Percutaneous intervention for CMI is safe with durable early and midterm clinical success. However, repeated intervention is often required for improved primary assisted patency.

▶ There are accumulating data detailing the expected results of percutaneous interventions for mesenteric artery stenosis. Excellent initial technical success can be anticipated. The need for repeat intervention to maintain long-term patency should be expected.

G. L. Moneta, MD

Mesenteric stenting for chronic mesenteric ischemia
Brown DJ, Schermerhorn ML, Powell RJ, et al (Dartmouth-Hitchcock Med Ctr, Lebanon, NH; Beth Israel Deaconess Med Ctr, Boston)
J Vasc Surg 42:268-274, 2005   7–6

Background.—Mesenteric stenting has not been widely adopted for the treatment of chronic mesenteric ischemia (CMI). The recent availability of embolic protection and low-profile devices with the theoretical ability to decrease perioperative bowel necrosis, led us to begin using mesenteric stenting for patients with CMI. We review our initial experience to examine short-term outcomes.

Methods.—We performed a retrospective analysis of all patients who were treated by vascular surgeons with mesenteric stenting for CMI. Patients with acute mesenteric ischemia were excluded. We evaluated perioperative morbidity and mortality, restenosis, recurrent symptoms, and re-intervention. Kaplan-Meier methods were used to assess events during follow-up. We also compared these outcomes with a historical control group of patients treated with open surgical revascularization.

Results.—Fourteen patients underwent mesenteric stenting over the past 3 years. Mean age was 73, and 64% were women. There was no periopera-

Chronic Mesenteric Vascular Disease Treated with PTA/Stent: Outcome at 13 Months

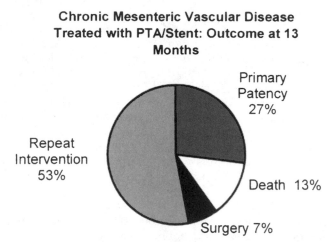

FIGURE 1.—Outcomes in patients undergoing stenting for chronic mesenteric ischemia at a mean follow-up of 13 months. (Reprinted by permission of the publisher from Brown DJ, Schermerhorn ML, Powell RJ, et al: Mesenteric stenting for chronic mesenteric ischemia. *J Vasc Surg* 42:268-274, 2005. Copyright 2005 by Elsevier.)

tive or 30-day mortality or major morbidity. Early restenosis and recurrent symptoms occurred in 10% and 9% of patients at 6 months. At a mean follow-up of 13 months, 53% of patients underwent reintervention. However, 93% were symptom-free at their last follow-up. Compared with open surgery, stent patients had lower perioperative major morbidity (30% vs 0%, $P < .01$) and shorter hospital and intensive care unit length of stay (median 10 days vs 2 days, and 3 days vs 0 days, respectively, $P < .01$ for both). However, stent patients were seven times as likely to develop restenosis ($P < 01$), four times more likely to develop recurrent symptoms ($P < .01$), and 15 times more likely to undergo reintervention ($P < .01$). There was one death 13 months after stenting due to mesenteric infarction in a patient lost to follow-up. One patient was successfully converted to open surgery after a second restenosis. He had regained 20 pounds and was determined to be a better operative candidate than at his initial presentation. There was no perioperative or 30-day mortality or major morbidity with reintervention after mesenteric stenting.

Conclusion.—Mesenteric stenting for CMI can be performed with low perioperative risk. However, stenting is associated with early restenosis and recurrent symptoms requiring secondary procedures. Patients with severe nutritional depletion or high surgical risk may benefit from mesenteric stenting for CMI, but close follow-up is required. Later open surgery can be performed for restenosis if nutritional status and surgical risk are improved, or repeat angioplasty and stenting can be effectively performed if operative risk remains high (Fig 1).

▶ This is another study of a small series of stents placed for mesenteric ischemia. As in the previous abstract (Abstract 7–5), repeat interventions were common, but overall the approach was successful with over 90% of patients remaining symptom free. We have tended to avoid celiac stents at our institution as they have, in our hands, tended to be compressed or dislodged, presumably by external pressure from the median arcuate ligament.

G. L. Moneta, MD

Use of the ascending aorta as bypass inflow for treatment of chronic intestinal ischemia
Chiche L, Kieffer E (Pitié-Salpêtrière Univ, Paris)
J Vasc Surg 41:457-461, 2005   7–7

Purpose.—Surgical revascularization of intestinal arteries is an effective long-term treatment for chronic intestinal ischemia (CII) regardless of the technique used. Conventional antegrade or retrograde bypass techniques are the most common modalities for extensive lesions that cannot be treated by endarterectomy or transposition. In this report, we describe our experience with an antegrade bypass technique from the ascending aorta in patients with no other available inflow.

Methods.—From April 1990 to May 2004, we performed antegrade bypass from the ascending aorta to the celiac artery, superior mesenteric artery (SMA), or both in five patients. These cases accounted for 2.4% of the 211 patients who underwent surgery on intestinal arteries during the study period. Results: Four patients presented with symptomatic CII, and one patient had no intestinal ischemic symptoms. The underlying disease was Takayasu disease in two cases, Erdheim-Chester disease in one case, chronic aortic dissection in one case, and atherosclerosis in one case. Two patients had already undergone an unsuccessful revascularization attempt with another technique. Bypass was performed alone in three cases in association with revascularization of the ascending aorta, aortic arch, and proximal descending thoracic aorta in one case and in association with revascularization of the ascending aorta and proximal aortic arch and renal autotransplantation in one case. Recovery was uneventful in all cases. One venous graft occluded because of technical defects and required reoperation for prosthetic graft replacement on the 10th postoperative day. Symptoms of CII resolved in all cases. Four months after the procedure, one patient underwent dilatation of an asymptomatic stenosis of the SMA distal to the bypass. During the 50th month after the procedure, a new re-stenosis of the SMA appeared. Left untreated, this stenosis led to asymptomatic occlusion of the mesenteric segment of a sequential aortoceliomesenteric bypass 13 months later. This aortoceliac bypass and the other four bypasses were patent after 4, 31, 16, 52, and 120 months of follow-up.

Conclusion.—Antegrade intestinal artery bypass from the ascending aorta is an effective alternative for patients who have no other available inflow for conventional antegrade or retrograde bypass and for patients in whom major technical difficulties are likely after multiple exposures of the thoracoabdominal aorta. Although indications are uncommon, antegrade

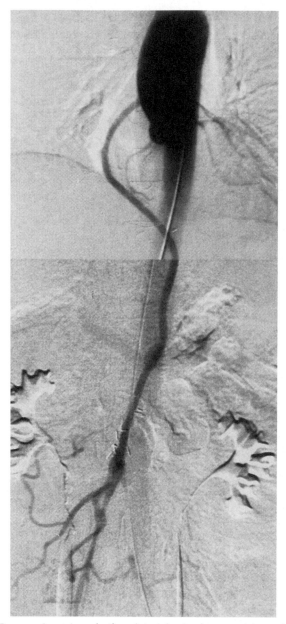

FIGURE 1.—Postoperative angiography (frontal view) showing the antegrade bypass from the ascending aorta to the superior mesenteric artery. (Reprinted by permission of the publisher from Chiche L, Kieffer E: Use of the ascending aorta as bypass inflow for treatment of chronic intestinal ischemia. *J Vasc Surg* 41:457-461, 2005. Copyright 2005 by Elsevier.)

intestinal artery bypass can provide durable revascularization of the intestine (Fig 1).

▶ I have used this technique one time to revascularize the SMA. The graft can be routed either intrapleurally or intrapericardially and passes behind the stomach and pancreas. The article reminds us to keep the ascending aorta in mind as a potential last ditch or near last ditch inflow site for reconstruction of abdominal or lower extremity arteries.

G. L. Moneta, MD

Arcuate ligament vascular compression syndrome in infants and children

Schweizer P, Berger S, Schweizer M, et al (Univ of Tübingen, Germany; Hosp Universitaire Bern, Switzerland; Kinderkrankenhaus Kath, Hamburg, Germany)
J Pediatr Surg 40:1616-1622, 2005   7–8

Background.—Arcuate ligament vascular compression syndrome has not been described previously in the pediatric or pediatric surgical literature. However, it is mentioned in the literature of vascular and general surgery and in journals of radiology and orthopedics. In this review, the intraoperative pathological anatomy and the principles of treatment for 8 children will be presented.

Methods.—The chart records and the anatomical sketches that were documented by the surgeon immediately after each procedure were analyzed retrospectively. In addition, preoperative courses and long-term follow-up (range, 3-18 years) were evaluated by a defined program.

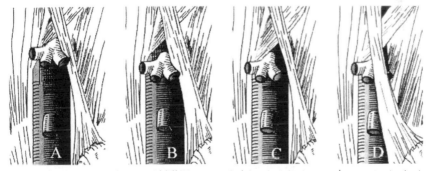

FIGURE 2.—Schematic drawings of different anatomical situations causing vascular compression by the arcuate ligament. A, Median arcuate ligament causes compression of CA if the ligament crosses the celiac trunk more caudal than usual or if celiac trunk exits the aorta more cranial than usual. B, Suspensory duodenal ligament crossing the celiac trunk and SMA more medial than usual, compressing the vessels from the left side. C, Right diaphragmatic crus running more medial than usual, compressing the CA from the right side. D, Both suspensory duodenal ligament and right diaphragmatic crus run more medial than usual, compressing the CA from both sides. (Courtesy of Schweizer P, Berger S, Schweizer M, et al: Arcuate ligament vascular compression syndrome in infants and children. *J Pediatr Surg* 40:1616-1622, 2005.)

Results.—The diagnosis of celiac artery compression by an arcuate ligament was suspected in children presenting with a history of several years of recurrent acute abdominal pain associated with a typical arterial bruit in the midline of the epigastric region.

Conclusions.—Other diseases with recurrent abdominal pain and an arterial bruit must be excluded before making the decision for an operative intervention. Duplex ultrasound and angiography are possibly helpful tools to establish the respective diagnosis, but in the patients of the present series, these techniques neither confirmed compression of the celiac axis nor demonstrated decreased perfusion of the superior mesenteric artery. However, as the clinical symptoms clearly announce the disease, these diagnostic measures are not mandatory (Fig 2).

▶ Median arcuate ligament syndrome as a cause of abdominal pain has basically died a quiet and well-deserved death in the adult vascular surgical literature. However, there appears to be a pocket of believers remaining in Germany. I suppose somewhere out there some patient has had symptoms secondary to median arcuate ligament compression of the celiac axis.

However, until someone can explain why the huge majority of patients with celiac compression do not have symptoms, I am going to continue to doubt the validity of median arcuate ligament syndrome as a source of abdominal pain. This is the abdominal equivalent of neurogenic thoracic outlet syndrome: You either believe or you do not. Thankfully, most do not.

G. L. Moneta, MD

8 Thoracic Aorta

Acute Intramural Hematoma of the Aorta: A Mystery in Evolution

Evangelista A, for the International Registry of Aortic Dissection (IRAD) Investigators (Universitari Vall d'Hebron, Barcelona; et al)
Circulation 111:1063-1070, 2005
8–1

Background.—The definition, prevalence, outcomes, and appropriate treatment strategies for acute intramural hematoma (IMH) continue to be debated.

Method and Results.—We studied 1010 patients with acute aortic syndromes who were enrolled in the International Registry of Aortic Dissection (IRAD) to delineate the prevalence, presentation, management, and outcomes of acute IMH by comparing these patients with those with classic aortic dissection (AD). Fifty-eight (5.7%) patients had IMH, and this cohort tended to be older (68.7 versus 61.7 years; $P<0.001$) and more likely to have distal aortic involvement (60.3% versus 35.3%; $P<0.001$) compared with 952 patients with AD. Patients with IMH described more severe initial pain than did those with AD but were less likely to have ischemic leg pain, pulse deficits, or aortic valve insufficiency; moreover, they required a longer time to diagnosis and more diagnostic tests. Overall mortality of IMH was similar to that of classic AD (20.7% versus 23.9%; $P=0.57$), as was mortality in patients with IMH of the descending aorta (8.3% versus 13.1%; $P=0.60$) and the ascending aorta (39.1% versus 29.9%; $P=0.34$) compared with AD. IMH limited to the aortic arch was seen in 7 patients, with no deaths, despite medical therapy in only 6 of the 7 individuals. Among the 51 patients whose initial diagnostic study showed IMH only, 8 (16%) progressed to AD on a serial imaging study.

Conclusions.—The IRAD data demonstrate a 5.7% prevalence of IMH in patients with acute aortic syndromes. Like classic AD, IMH is a highly lethal condition when it involves the ascending aorta and surgical therapy should be considered, but this condition is less critical when limited to the arch or descending aorta. Fully 16% of patients have evidence of evolution to dissection on serial imaging.

▶ The natural history of acute intramural hematoma (IMH) of the aorta is difficult to determine. Overall, this study and others do suggest that, despite the more limited aortic involvement of IMH and the absence of true dissection flaps at initial presentation, the overall natural history of the disease is similar to that of classic aortic dissection. At this point, treatment and follow-up of IMH should be similar to that for aortic dissection.

G. L. Moneta, MD

Acute Aortic Dissection Presenting with Primarily Abdominal Pain: A Rare Manifestation of a Deadly Disease
Upchurch GR Jr, for the IRAD Investigators (Univ of Michigan, Ann Arbor; et al)
Ann Vasc Surg 19:367-373, 2005   8–2

The objective of this study was to determine the morbidity and mortality of patients with acute thoracic aortic dissections who present primarily with abdominal pain. Nine hundred ninety-two patients (mean age, 62.1 years ± 14.1; 68% male) encountered from 1996 to 2001 with acute thoracic aortic dissections from the International Registry of acute Aortic Dissection were studied. Patient demographics, presenting symptoms, signs of aortic dissection, aortic pathology, and mortality were compared in patients presenting primarily with abdominal pain (group I, 46 patients, 4.6%) versus all others (group II). Demographics were similar between the two groups. When signs of aortic dissection were examined, 63% of patients in group I presented with hypertension compared to only 47% of patients in group II ($p = 0.04$). Patients in group I were less likely to present with evidence of end-organ malperfusion. Importantly, mortality in patients with a type B dissection, specifically following surgery for the dissection, was significantly increased in patients who presented primarily with abdominal pain (group I, 28% mortality vs. group II, 10.2% mortality; $p = 0.02$). This study documented

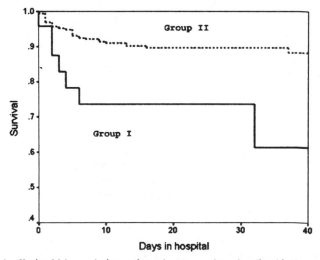

FIGURE 1.—Kaplan-Meier survival curve for patients presenting primarily with (Group I) or without (Group II) abdominal pain in the setting of acute type B thoracic aortic dissections. Log-rank test, $p = 0.003$. (Courtesy of Upchurch GR Jr, for the IRAD Investigators: Acute aortic dissection presenting with primarily abdominal pain: A rare manifestation of a deadly disease. *Ann Vasc Surg* 19:367-373, 2005.)

increased mortality in patients with acute thoracic aortic dissections who present primarily with abdominal pain, underscoring the importance of maintaining a high index of suspicion for an aortic dissection in patients who have appropriate risk factors (Fig 1).

▶ The study indicates a high mortality rate in patients with thoracic aortic dissection who present with primarily abdominal pain. Even in the absence of back pain, one should consider thoracic aortic dissection as an etiology for abdominal pain in patients with appropriate risk factors for dissection. We have seen 2 such cases in the past year.

G. L. Moneta, MD

Outcome of Medical and Surgical Treatment in Patients With Acute Type B Aortic Dissection
Hsu R-B, Ho Y-L, Chen RJ, et al (Natl Taiwan Univ, Taipei, ROC)
Ann Thorac Surg 79:790-795, 2005   8–3

Background.—Optimal treatment of acute type B aortic dissection remains unclear. The aim of this study was to assess the clinical outcome of acute type B aortic dissection.

Methods.—In the last 8 years, 107 patients were admitted for acute type B aortic dissection. We medically treated patients at the time of onset with antihypertensives. Surgery was considered if there is intractable pain, uncontrolled hypertension, severe aortic branch malperfusion, or aneurysm expansion.

Results.—Twenty-nine patients had pleural effusion (27%), 9 patients had leg ischemia (8%), 5 patients had impending rupture, and 2 patients had aneurysm enlargement exceeding 60 mm on repeated imaging studies. A total of 16 patients (15%) underwent surgical intervention: 8 extra-anatomical bypass for leg ischemia, 1 in situ infrarenal aortoiliac bypass for distal aortic obstruction, and 7 thoracic aortic graft replacement. Of the 8 patients with extra-anatomic bypass, 3 patients died: 2 patients died of catastrophic aortic rupture 2 and 9 days after bypass, and 1 patient died of dissection progression to type A lesion 9 days after bypass. There was no in-hospital death in 92 medically treated patients. Follow-up was 92% complete. The mean follow-up duration was 36.1 months (range, 2 to 96 months). The 6-month, 1-year, and 5-year survival rates of all patients were 96.2 ± 1.9%, 95.2% ± 2.1%, and 95.2% ± 2.1%.

Conclusions.—Medical treatment of acute type B aortic dissection produced good outcomes. Central aortic procedures such as aortic fenestration and endovascular stenting should be the preferred methods to treat patients with acute type B aortic dissection and leg ischemia because there was high risk of central aortic complications after extra-anatomic bypass.

▶ Viewed from an intent-to-treat basis, medical treatment of a thoracic dissection is successful in 85% of patients. With development of thoracic stent grafts and their increasing availability, there will surely be a push for a proactive approach for treating acute type B dissection. The results of proactive treatment of type B dissection with thoracic stent grafts will have to be extraordinary to match the standards set by this article. At this point, given the poor outcomes of extra-anatomic bypass in the patients requiring surgical intervention, it would appear that the most reasonable approach for patients with type B dissection is initial medical management followed by some sort of central aortic procedure, whether it be fenestration or stent graft placement, for patients who fail medical management.

G. L. Moneta, MD

Usefulness of Preoperative Detection of Artery of Adamkiewicz with Dynamic Contrast-enhanced MR Angiography

Hyodoh H, Kawaharada N, Akiba H, et al (Sapporo Med Univ, Japan)
Radiology 236:1004-1009, 2005   8–4

Purpose.—To prospectively evaluate the detection of the artery of Adamkiewicz at magnetic resonance (MR) angiography and the effect such detection has on outcome after surgical graft placement in a series of patients with thoracoabdominal aortic disease.

Materials and Methods.—This study had ethics committee approval, and written informed consent was obtained from all patients. Fifty patients (38 men, 12 women; age range, 47-83 years; mean age, 67.2 years) who were scheduled to undergo thoracoabdominal aortic surgery for treatment of thoracoabdominal aortic aneurysm ($n = 42$) or thoracoabdominal aortic dissection ($n = 8$) were enrolled in the study. MR angiography was performed with a 1.5-T system by using dynamic three-dimensional fast spoiled gradient-recalled acquisition in the steady state with a bolus of contrast material and saline injection (4 mL/sec). Differences in the cross-clamping time, bypass time, total surgery time, and spinal complication rate between patients in whom the artery of Adamkiewicz was identified (group A) and those in whom the artery was not identified (group B) were evaluated with χ^2 or Mann-Whitney U testing.

Results.—In 42 of the 50 patients (84% [group A]), at least one artery of Adamkiewicz was seen to arise from an intercostal artery. Two arteries of Adamkiewicz were identified in four of the patients (8%). The artery of Adamkiewicz could not be detected with MR angiography in eight patients (group B). The ranges of cross-clamping, bypass, and total surgery times, respectively, were 30–199 minutes (mean, 78.4 minutes ± 39.1 [standard deviation]), 30–298 minutes (mean, 96.9 minutes ± 60.0), and 135–665 minutes (mean, 354.9 minutes ± 133.9) in group A and 53–124 minutes (mean, 72.8 minutes ± 29.8), 10–124 minutes (mean, 66.0 minutes ± 41.0), and 220–405 minutes (mean, 315.6 minutes ± 68.8) in group B. Spinal complications occurred in two patients in group B but in none of the patients in group A ($P < .001$).

Conclusion.—The artery of Adamkiewicz was detected in a large percentage of patients in whom there were no spinal complications, unlike the spinal complications that occurred in the patients in whom the artery was not detected.

▶ In this study, when the artery of Adamkiewicz was identified by MR angiography, only the intercostal or lumbar artery from which it originated was reimplanted into the graft. The surgical technique also used femoral-femoral bypass and selective cannulation of visceral vessels. Spinal cord drainage was not mentioned. The mix of patients and the small number of patients precludes any definite conclusions, but when it comes to paraplegia, 0% is a very good number!

G. L. Moneta, MD

Descending Thoracic Aortic Aneurysm Repair: 12-Year Experience Using Distal Aortic Perfusion and Cerebrospinal Fluid Drainage
Estrera AL, Miller CC III, Chen EP, et al (Univ of Texas, Houston)
Ann Thorac Surg 80:1290-1296, 2005   8–5

Background.—The benefit of distal aortic perfusion and cerebrospinal fluid drainage over the "clamp and sew" technique during repairs of the descending thoracic aorta is still being debated. The purpose of this report is to analyze our experience with regard to neurologic deficit (paraplegia and paraparesis) and mortality using the adjuncts of distal aortic perfusion and cerebrospinal fluid drainage.

Methods.—Between February 1991 and September 2004, we repaired 355 descending thoracic aortic aneurysms. Excluded from analysis were 29 patients who required profound hypothermic circulatory arrest as a result of transverse arch involvement and 26 patients with aortic rupture, leaving a group of 300 patients for which outcomes were analyzed. Mean patient age was 67 years, and 102 (34%) of the patients were women. The adjunct group of distal aortic perfusion and cerebrospinal fluid drainage used in 238 (79.3%) patients was compared with a group of 62 patients who underwent simple cross-clamp with or without the addition of a single adjunct. Multivariable data were analyzed by Cox regression.

Results.—The incidence of neurologic deficit after all repairs was 2.3% (7 of 300 patients). The incidence of neurologic deficit (immediate and delayed) in the adjunct group was 1.3% (3 of 238 patients), and in the nonadjunct group was 6.5% (4 of 62 patients; $p < 0.02$). One case of delayed paraplegia occurred in each group. All neurologic deficits occurred in patients with aneurysmal involvement of the entire descending thoracic aorta (extent C; $p < 0.02$). Statistically significant predictors for neurologic deficit were the use of the adjunct (odds ratio [OR], 0.19; $p = 0.02$), previous repaired abdominal aortic aneurysm (OR, 7.0; $p = 0.005$), type C aneurysm (OR, 13.73; $p = 0.02$), and cerebrovascular disease history (OR, 4.7; $p < 0.03$). Thirty-day mortality was 8% (24 of 300 patients). Significant multivariate predictors of 30-day mortality were preoperative renal dysfunction (OR, 4.6; $p < 001$) and female sex (OR, 2.9; $p < 0.03$).

Conclusions.—Repairs of the descending thoracic aorta using the adjunct of distal aortic perfusion and cerebrospinal fluid drainage can be performed with a low incidence of neurologic deficit and an acceptable mortality. The use of the adjuncts should be considered during elective repairs of the descending thoracic aorta.

▶ This article from Safi's group in Houston indicates what is possible to achieve with open thoracic aneurysm repair. I doubt this volume of patients and this level of expertise is present in many institutions. Because of this, this article cannot really be used to justify or not justify endovascular techniques of thoracic aneurysm repair. However, with the data presented, it would seem silly not to provide, when possible, cerebrospinal fluid drainage and distal aortic perfusion in patients undergoing open descending thoracic aortic aneurysm repair.

G. L. Moneta, MD

Traumatic rupture of the thoracic aorta: Ten years of delayed management

Pacini D, Angeli E, Fattori R, et al (Univ of Bologna, Italy)
J Thorac Cardiovasc Surg 129:880-884, 2005

8–6

Objective.—Traumatic rupture of the thoracic aorta is a highly fatal condition in which patient outcome is strongly conditioned by other associated injuries. Delayed aortic treatment has been proposed to improve results.

Methods.—The charts of 69 patients with traumatic rupture of the thoracic aorta observed between 1980 and 2003 were reviewed. Patients were

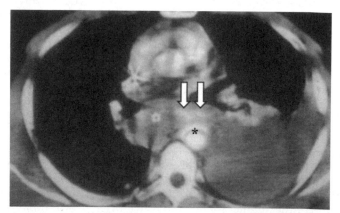

FIGURE 1.—Chest CT scan shows isthmic aortic rupture (*asterisk*) with massive left hemothorax and contrast media extravasation (*arrows*). (Reprinted from Pacini D, Angeli E, Fattori R, et al: Traumatic rupture of the thoracic aorta: Ten years of delayed management. *J Thorac Cardiovasc Surg* 129:880-884, 2005. Copyright 2005 with permission from The American Association for Thoracic Surgery.)

grouped according the timing of repair: group I, immediate repair (21 patients); and group II, delayed repair (48 patients). In group II, 45 patients were treated surgically or by endovascular procedure.

Results.—In-hospital mortalities were 4 of 21 patients (19%) in group I and 2 of 48 patients (4.2%) in group II. There were 3 cases of paraplegia in group I and none in group II.

Conclusion.—Improvement of patient outcome with traumatic rupture of the thoracic aorta can be achieved by delaying surgical repair until after management of major associated injuries if there are no signs of impending rupture. Endovascular treatment is feasible and safe and may represent a valid alternative to open surgery in selected cases (Fig 1).

▶ Most patients with thoracic aortic injuries are dead before the paramedics arrive. Those who survive are demonstrating they have a different sort of injury. It is therefore not surprising they can, in many cases, be managed conservatively for a while. With the availability of endoluminal thoracic grafts, it may be that the period of conservative management can be considerably shortened without an increase in mortality rates related to the thoracic aortic repair.

G. L. Moneta, MD

Open repair of chronic post-traumatic aneurysms of the aortic isthmus: The value of direct aortoaortic anastomosis
Kieffer E, Leschi J-P, Chiche L (Pitié-Salpêtrière Univ, Paris)
J Vasc Surg 41:931-935, 2005   8–7

Purpose.—This report presents our experience with open repair of post-traumatic aneurysms of the aortic isthmus using recent surgical techniques, including distal aortic perfusion and the preferential use of direct aortoaortic anastomosis without interposition of prosthetic material.

Methods.—From 1990 to 2004, the senior author's (EK) patients (21 men; mean age, 40.3 years) who presented with post-traumatic aneurysms of the aortic isthmus were treated operatively, either with (20 patients) or without (3 patients) distal aortic perfusion, or endovascularly with a stent graft (3 patients). In 15 (75 %) of the 20 patients treated with distal aortic perfusion, the technique consisted of resection followed by direct aortoaortic anastomosis. Eight patients, including the three patients treated with simple clamping, had prosthetic replacement.

Results.—No postoperative deaths or permanent spinal cord complications occurred. One patient required reoperation to control hemorrhage. Aortography or computed tomography angiography was performed on 12 of the 15 patients treated by direct aortoaortic anastomosis, with a mean follow-up of 58.7 ± 8.9 months. No morphologic abnormality was found.

Conclusion.—This study shows that low-risk patients with a chronic post-traumatic aneurysm of the aortic isthmus can be successfully treated with excellent long-term results by resection and direct aortoaortic anastomosis without prosthetic interposition. In our opinion, endovascular repair

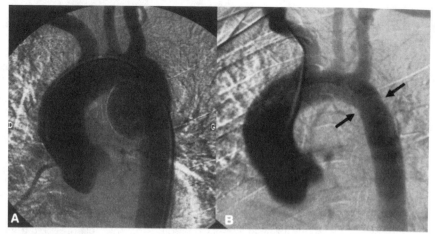

FIGURE 2.—A, Preoperative and (B) postoperative angiogram of a patient treated with direct suture, without prosthetic interposition, for a chronic post-traumatic aneurysm of the aortic isthmus. (Reprinted by permission of the publisher from Kieffer E, Leschi J-P, Chiche L: Open repair of chronic post-traumatic aneurysms of the aortic isthmus: The value of direct aortoaortic anastomosis. *J Vasc Surg* 41:931-935, 2005. Copyright 2005 by Elsevier.)

should only be used in patients who present with absolute contraindications for open surgical repair (Fig 2).

▶ Professor Kieffer's excellent results make a very good argument for direct repair of chronic thoracic aortic injuries without the use of interposition prosthetic material. The technique does require extensive mobilization of the aortic arch and the arch vessels and therefore is really not suitable for a "clamp and sew" mentality. The patients are also still at risk for recurrent nerve injury, and a thoracotomy is morbid even in a young patient. My guess is, despite Dr Kieffer's excellent results, this infrequent lesion will most often be treated with a thoracic stent graft in the very near future.

G. L. Moneta, MD

Long-Term Integrity of Teflon Felt-Supported Suture Lines in Aortic Surgery

Strauch JT, Spielvogel D, Lansman SL, et al (New York Univ)
Ann Thorac Surg 79:796-800, 2005

8–8

Background.—Although the ultimate success of aortic operations depends upon the integrity of graft-to-aorta anastomoses, little is known about different techniques used to assure their longevity. We report the incidence of reoperation for suture line disruptions arising from anastomoses using reinforcement with Teflon felt.

Methods.—Since 1987, 1475 patients underwent 2281 anastomoses in the thoracic aorta (mean 1.55/anastomoses per patient). All patients were followed with at least yearly computed tomographic scans, for a total

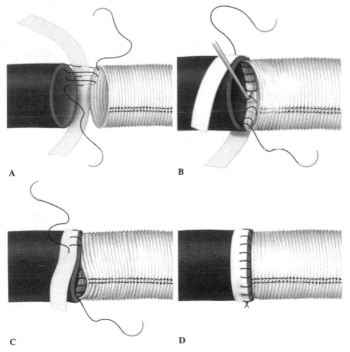

FIGURE 1.—(A) The back wall of the anastomosis is performed open, with the sutures passing from the Dacron graft to the Teflon felt and then to the wall of the aorta. The first stitch is taken inside the graft. (B) The Teflon felt strip is then carefully positioned outside the aorta; the graft is invaginated within the aorta, and the back suture line is tightened with a nerve hook. (C) The second needle, on the other suture end, is passed through the aorta and the Teflon felt, and the suture line is continued in either an open or closed fashion along the front wall. Care is taken to place the graft within the aorta and to position the Teflon felt carefully on the outside. (D) The completed anastomosis. The most important aspect of the anastomosis is that the suture does not pull directly on aortic tissue. In essence, the end of the aorta is clamped between the graft and the external Teflon felt by the running sutures. This not only reduces needle hole bleeding at the time of the anastomosis, but also prevents progressive erosion of the suture through the aortic wall as stress is applied to the suture line by the pulsating aortic pressure. The snugly fitted Teflon felt also heals securely to the aorta, as does the graft on the inside, and it is possible that the cuff of Teflon felt buffers the transition between the relatively noncompliant vascular graft and the variably compliant aorta. (Courtesy of Strauch JT, Spielvogel D, Lansman SL, et al: Long-term integrity of Teflon felt-supported suture lines in aortic surgery. *Ann Thorac Surg* 79:796-800, 2005. Reprinted with permission from the Society of Thoracic Surgeons.)

follow-up of 6483.8 patient-years. Those requiring reoperation were reviewed retrospectively for evidence of suture line disruption.

Results.—Only 34 patients, with a mean age of 55.1 years old (range 26–85 years old) underwent reoperation for suture-line disruptions following vascular graft-to-aorta anastomosis using Teflon felt. The previous operation was a Bentall procedure in 15 (44%); ascending aorta replacement in 9 (26%); total arch replacement in 6 (18%); descending aorta replacement in 2 (6%); thoracoabdominal repair in 1 (3%); and sinus of Valsalva repair in 1 (3%). The incidence of suture line disruption was 0.0052 per patient-year, and 0.0034 per anastomosis-year. The mean interval between operations was 55.9 months (range 4–180 months). In 21%, the pseudoaneurysm originated from the proximal anastomosis; in 71% from the distal anastomosis;

in 3% from both; in 3% from the innominate artery; and in 3% from a sinus of Valsalva repair. In only 1 patient was there evidence of infection. Reoperation involved ascending aorta replacement in 11 patients, and total arch replacement in 13 patients. Adverse outcome, such as hospital death or permanent stroke, occurred in 8% (3 patients).

Conclusions.—Use of Teflon felt to support aortic suture lines yields a very low incidence of suture line disruptions: 1 per 191 patient-years, or 1 per 296 anastomosis-years. Teflon felt reinforcement provides a secure, long-lasting graft-to-aorta anastomosis with minimal risk of infection (Fig 1).

▶ We have all faced abdominal aortic back walls where it seemed poor judgment to mobilize the back wall and best to include the spinal ligaments in the anastomosis as sort of an "autogenous Teflon." Nevertheless, this technique deserves consideration for thoracic aortic repairs where mobilization of the aortic back wall is easier than in selected abdominal aortic anastomoses. How much difference the Teflon really makes is unknown. There are no controls in this series.

G. L. Moneta, MD

Fate of the Visceral Aortic Patch After Thoracoabdominal Aortic Repair
Tshomba Y, Melissano G, Civilini E, et al (Vita-Salute Univ, Milan, Italy)
Eur J Vasc Endovasc Surg 29:383-389, 2005   8–9

Objective.—To analyse the fate of a visceral aortic patch (VAP) in patients that underwent thoracoabdominal aortic aneurysm (TAAA) repair.

Methods.—We reviewed 204 consecutive patients (158 M, 46 F) treated for TAAA between 1988 and 2004. We performed VAP in 182 cases. Among the 149 survivors at 6 months, we followed 138 cases, mean follow-up 7 years (range 0.6–16 years). The mean graft diameter we used was 29mm (range 24–34mm) from 1988 to 1999 (83 patients), and 21.7mm (range 16–24mm) from 2000 to 2003 (55 patients). In 23% of cases we performed a separate bypass to the left renal artery.

Results.—We observed 16 (12%) VAP dilatations (<5cm), 6 (4%) VAP aneurysms (>5cm) and one VAP pseudoaneurysm, at a mean time of 6 years after atherosclerotic TAAA was atherosclerotic repair. There were no VAP dilatations/aneurysms in the group of patients with separate left renal revascularization. Five VAP aneurysms were treated electively. In four cases the operation was performed with thoracophrenolaparotomy, in one case with a bilateral subcostal laparotomy. In all cases the visceral aorta was re-grafted. Reimplantation of a single undersized VAP was performed in one case, separate revascularization of visceral arteries was performed in the other four cases. Selective intraoperative hypothermic perfusion of visceral and renal arteries was used in all the patients. There was 1 perioperative death; 2 patients with preoperative renal failure required dialysis. The last VAP aneurysm has remained asymptomatic and stable at annual CT surveil-

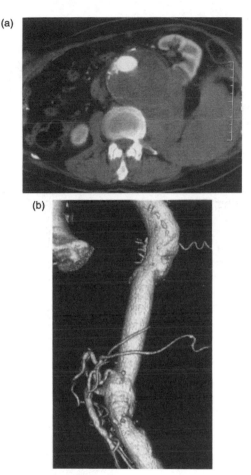

FIGURE 3.—(a) Emergent CT taken in patient (6 referred to our ER after hemorrhagic shock. The scan reveals the VAP pseudo-aneurysm and a retroperitoneal haematoma dislodging the left kidney. (b) 3-D spiral CT showing successful repair of the VAP pseudo-aneurysm. (Reprinted from Tshomba Y, Melissano G, Civillini E, et al: Fate of the visceral aortic patch after thoracoabdominal aortic repair. *Eur J Vasc Endovasc Surg* 29:383-389, 2005, by permission of the publisher.)

lance. The VAP pseudoaneurysm was successfully treated with an emergency thoracophrenolaparotomy and refashioning the left side suture line.

Conclusions.—Aneurysm of VAP is not uncommon in the patients operated on using larger grafts with a single VAP that includes the LRA (7.4%, 5/67 cases). Its treatment carries significant morbidity and mortality (Fig 3).

▶ We don't do all that much thoracoabdominal aortic surgery in Oregon (there are only 3.6 million people in the whole state). But I have never liked including the left renal artery in the visceral patch. It makes the patch seem too large and, on the basis of these data, that impression appears to be correct. If a separate side branch graft is attached to the main body of the aortic graft before the graft is implanted, the added ischemic time to the left kidney is only the time required to do the left renal artery anastomosis.

G. L. Moneta, MD

Endovascular repair of thoracic aortic lesions with the Zenith TX1 and TX2 thoracic grafts: Intermediate-term results
Greenberg RK, O'Neill S, Walker E, et al (Cleveland Clinic Found, Ohio)
J Vasc Surg 41:589-596, 2005   8–10

Purpose.—This prospective study was designed to assess the technical success and outcome after patients with thoracic aortic pathology at high risk for conventional therapy were treated with the Zenith TX1 and TX2 endovascular graft.

Methods.—Between 2001 and 2004, patients at high risk for conventional surgical therapy presenting with chronic aortic dissections, thoracic aneurysms, or aortobronchial or aortoesophageal fistulas were treated with a single- or multiple-piece endovascular grafts. Surgical modification of proximal or distal fixation sites was performed when necessary to establish adequate regions for device landing zones. Follow-up studies included radiographic evaluation before discharge and at 1, 6, 12, and 24 months. Aortic morphologic characteristics were determined by using three-dimensional imaging studies and centerline of flow measurements. Statistical analyses were performed with Kaplan Meier analysis to assess survival, factors predictive of poor outcome, and morphologic changes, including sac shrinkage.

Results.—A total of 100 patients (42% women) were treated, including 81 aneurysms, 15 aortic dissections (with aneurysms), 2 patients with fistulous connections (1 aortobronchial and 1 aortoesophageal), 1 subclavian artery aneurysm, and 1 aortic rupture. Mean follow-up and aneurysm size were 14 months and 62 mm, respectively. Most patients (55%) had undergone prior aortic aneurysm repair. Surgical modifications were required to create adequate implantation sites in 29% patients, including 14 elephant trunk/arch reconstructions, 18 carotid-subclavian bypasses, and 4 visceral vessel bypasses. Iliac conduits were required in 19 patients. Overall mortality was 17%, and aneurysm-related mortality was 14% at 1 year. Sac regression (>5 mm maximum diameter decrease) was observed in 52% and 56% at 12 and 24 months. Growth was noted in one patient (1.6%) at 12 months. Endoleaks were detected in eight patients (8.5%) at 30 days and three patients (6%) at 12 months Secondary interventions were required in 15 patients. Migration (>10 mm) of the proximal or distal stent was noted in three patients (6%) (two proximal and one distal), none of which required treatment or resulted in an adverse event.

Conclusions.—Acceptable intermediate-term outcomes have been achieved in the treatment of high-risk patients in the setting of both favorable and challenging anatomic situations with these devices. The complexity of the patient population, in contrast to endovascular infrarenal repair, attests to the differences in the pathophysiology aortic disease in the anatomic beds.

▶ Over a period of 40 months, approximately 125 thoracic aortic stent grafts were used at the Cleveland Clinic Foundation. This report includes 100 Zenith grafts in 100 patients considered at high risk for open surgery (authors do not elaborate on criteria to define "high-risk" for open surgery). A technical success rate of 87.6% was achieved with a mortality rate of 17% and neurologic event rate of 9% (spinal 6%, central nervous system 3%). Endoleaks were observed in 14.5%. Despite the intended seal zone of 30 mm used during this study, the authors report a migration (>10 mm) rate of 6% at a mean follow-up of only 14 months. The authors postulate that this "low migration" rate results from the use of barbs to achieve graft fixation. In my opinion, most thoracic grafts should be able to achieve better than a 6% migration rate with a 30-mm seal zone. Migration will be most often noted in the presence of short conical necks with significant angulation.

K. Kasirajan, MD

Changes in False Lumen After Transluminal Stent-Graft Placement in Aortic Dissections: Six Years' Experience

Kusagawa H, Shimono T, Ishida M, et al (Mie Univ, Tsu, Japan; Matsuzaka Chu-o Gen Hosp, Japan)
Circulation 111:2951-2957, 2005   8–11

Background.—Transluminal stent-graft placements (TSGPs) are a new, less invasive procedure now recognized as the choice for aortic disease repair. Treatment of aortic dissections with TSGPs has resulted in good early results, but the long-term results and changes in the false lumen have not been elucidated in detail.

Method and Results.—TSGPs were performed in 49 patients with primary tears in their descending aortas, and the follow-up period ranged from 4 months to 6 years. The patients were divided into 32 acute-onset and 17 chronic dissections; of the acute-onset cases, there were 15 Stanford type A retrograde dissections. Periodic enhanced spiral CT was conducted after TSGP. The false lumen in the ascending aorta in 14 (93%) of the Stanford type A cases was obliterated completely within 3 months. The CT study was continued for >2 years for 17 acute-onset dissection and 11 chronic dissection patients. The average false lumen diameters of the proximal, middle, and distal descending aorta before treatment were 15.9, 16.2, and 15.6 mm in the acute-onset dissection group and 28.1, 25.2, and 21.0 mm in the chronic dissection group, respectively. The false lumen diameters 2 years after treatment were 3.0, 3.7, and 3.1 mm in the acute-onset dissection group and 10.6, 105, and 11.9 mm in the chronic dissection group, respectively. Two years after TSGPs, the false lumen of the thoracic aorta totally disappeared in 76% of the acute-onset dissection group and 36% of the chronic dissection group. No cases showed rupture after TSGP.

Conclusions.—Complete obliteration of the false lumen is more likely in acute-onset cases than in chronic cases.

▶ The study suggests a move toward more catheter-based treatment of acute thoracic dissection. Certainly, the success of obliterating the retrograde dissection into the aortic arch from a descending primary tear suggests that acute treatment of type B dissections will be considered and performed at additional institutions. Medical management of type B dissection is highly effective (see Abstract 8–3) But the fact that chronic dissections have more difficulty in late obliteration of the false lumen after treatment with stent grafts suggests that it may be prudent to eventually treat type B dissections acutely with stent graft placement.

G. L. Moneta, MD

Endovascular stent-graft repair of pararenal and type IV thoracoabdominal aortic aneurysms with adjunctive visceral reconstruction

Fulton JJ, Farber MA, Marston WA, et al (Univ of North Carolina, Chapel Hill)
J Vasc Surg 41:191-198, 2005   8–12

Objective.—Pararenal and type IV thoracoabdominal aortic aneurysms (TAAA) are not currently considered as indications for endovascular repair given unfavorable neck anatomy or aneurysm involvement of the visceral vessels. Open repair of these aneurysms is associated with significant morbidity and mortality, particularly postoperative renal dysfunction. In selective high-risk patients, debranching of the visceral aorta to improve the proximal neck region can be used to facilitate endovascular exclusion of the aneurysm.

Methods.—Between October 2000 and July 2003, 10 patients were treated with open visceral revascularization and endovascular repair of pararenal and type IV TAAAs at a single institution. Patient demographics and procedural characteristics were obtained from medical records.

Results.—Overall 13 visceral bypasses were performed in 10 patients: 6 patients with a single iliorenal bypass, 3 with a hepatorenal bypass, and 1 patient with complete visceral revascularization. Juxtarenal aneurysms occurred in 5 patients (50%), suprarenal aneurysms in 3 patients (30%), and type IV TAAAs in 2 patients (20%). All patients had successful endovascular aneurysm exclusion. Mean follow-up was 8.7 months. There were no perioperative deaths, neurologic deficits coagulopathies, or renal dysfunction. Follow-up spiral computed tomography scans demonstrated patency of all bypass grafts with only one patient requiring a secondary intervention for late type I leak which was sealed with placement of a proximal cuff.

Conclusion.—These initial results suggest that are similar to infrarenal AAA endovascular repair. This combined approach to repair of pararenal and type IV TAAAs reduces the morbidity and mortality of open repair, and represents an attractive option in high-risk patients while endoluminal technology continues to evolve (Fig 3).

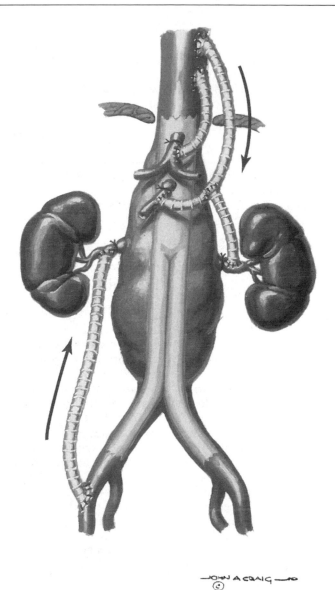

JOHN A CRAIG

FIGURE 3.—Complete revascularization and stent graft. (Reprinted by permission of the publisher from Fulton JJ, Farber MA, Marston WA, et al: Endovascular stent-graft repair of pararenal and type IV thoraco-abdominal aortic aneurysms with adjunctive visceral reconstruction. *J Vasc Surg* 41:191-196, 2006. Copyright 2006 by Elsevier.)

▶ The authors describe a novel means to improve the seal zone in patients who are not suited for a standard endovascular repair. The title may have been better labeled as "Renal bypass to facilitate aortic stent graft repair of aneurysms" because all but one patient required only renal bypass to allow the use of the perirenal aortic segment as the seal zone. A single patient required a total visceral debranching. This single patient had a thoracoabdominal exposure and a separate right retroperitoneal exposure. Total visceral debranching may be better performed from an iliac inflow site, eliminating a thoracotomy and an aortic cross-clamp. I have also noted better patient outcomes when total visceral debranching is staged than when it is combined with the aortic stent-graft implant. A lower incidence of renal dysfunction and paraplegia may be noted in staged procedures.

K. Kasirajan, MD

Repair of thoracoabdominal aortic aneurysms with fenestrated and branched endovascular stent grafts

Anderson JL, Adam DJ, Berce M, et al (Ashford Community Hosp, South Australia; Birmingham Heartlands Hosp, England; Royal Adelaide Hosp, South Australia; et al)

J Vasc Surg 42:600-607, 2005   8–13

Objective.—To report the repair of thoracoabdominal aortic aneurysms (TAAAs) with fenestrated and branched endovascular stent grafts (EVSGs).

Methods.—Four patients with asymptomatic TAAAs were treated with custom-designed Zenith fenestrated and branched EVSGs. Three patients had undergone previous open aortic aneurysm repair. Thirteen visceral vessels in four patients were targeted for incorporation by graft fenestrations and branches.

Results.—The fenestration/orifice interface was secured with balloon-expandable Genesis stents or Jostent stent grafts in 9 of 13 target vessels. Completion angiography demonstrated antegrade perfusion in 12 of 13 target vessels. One renal artery occluded because of graft rotation during deployment. There were no endoleaks. Three patients required additional surgical procedures related to access vessels. One patient required reoperation for bleeding from an extra-anatomic bypass graft and subsequently died from multisystem organ failure. Three patients made an uncomplicated recovery. No patient developed spinal cord ischemia. Computed tomography at 12 months in the 3 survivors demonstrated complete aneurysm exclusion with antegrade perfusion in all 10 target vessels.

Conclusions.—TAAA repair with fenestrated and branched EVSGs is feasible and provides an acceptable and promising alternative to conventional surgical repair in selected patients.

▶ This technology, although in its infancy, will be gladly welcomed by patients and physicians encountering TAAAs. The current need for custom design limits its use to only highly selected centers. This is partly responsible for the slow progress in this field.

K. Kasirajan, MD

Feasibility of the Inoue single-branched stent-graft implantation for thoracic aortic aneurysm or dissection involving the left subclavian artery: Short- to medium-term results in 17 patients
Saito N, Kimura T, Odashiro K, et al (Kyoto Univ, Japan; Kokura Mem Hosp, Japan; Takeda Hosp, Japan)
J Vasc Surg 41:206-212, 2005   8–14

Objective.—This study assessed the short- to medium-term clinical results of the Inoue single-branched stent graft for repair of thoracic aortic aneurysms or dissections involving the left subclavian artery.

Methods.—A retrospective review of experiences at two institutions was performed. We analyzed the data of consecutive 17 patients with thoracic aortic aneurysms or dissections who underwent endovascular repairs with the Inoue single-branched stent graft between July 1999 and April 2004. Complete baseline and follow-up data were available on all patients. The mean age was 71 ± 9 years, and 13 of the patients (76%) were men. Eight patients (47%) were considered unfit for open surgery because of advanced age or the presence of comorbid diseases.

Results.—The stent grafts were successfully delivered and deployed in all 17 patients. Periprocedural major complications, defined as those that caused any persistent disorder, occurred in one patient who developed spinal

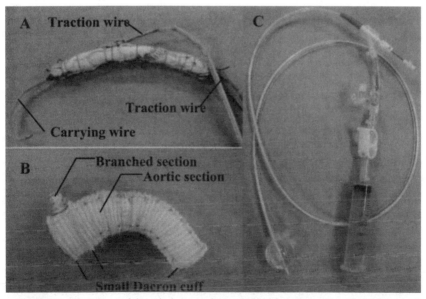

FIGURE 1.—The Inoue single branched stent-graft (*A* and *B*) and the balloon (*C*). A. The folded state. the carrying wire is attached to the proximal end of the aneurysm. Each traction wire is attached to the branched section and the aortic section. B. The unfolded state. The stent-graft consists of the aortic section and the branched section. (Reprinted by permission of the publisher from Saito N, Kimura T, Odashiro K, et al: Feasibility of the Inoue single-branched stent-graft implantation for thoracic aortic aneurysm or dissection involving the left subclavian artery: Short- to medium-term results on 17 patients. *J Vasc Surg* 41:206 212, 2005. Copyright 2005 by Elsevier.)

ischemia. A postoperative computed tomographic scan revealed three attachment site endoleaks; two endoleaks were from the proximal attachment sites and one endoleak was from the distal attachment site. The mean follow-up period was 26 months (range, 7 to 65 months). Two deaths occurred in the follow-up period from cerebral bleeding and pneumonia, both considered unrelated to the stent grafting. Two patients with attachment site endoleaks needed secondary stent-grafting; one patient required the implantation of a straight stent-graft in the distal attachment site and the other, the implantation of a double-branched stent-graft. Another patient with attachment site endoleak was considered very high-risk for open surgery or secondary stent grafting and did not undergo secondary intervention. The aneurysmal sac size of the patient has been stable for 28 months. The branched section of the stent graft was patent in all patients in the follow-up period.

Conclusion.—The results demonstrate the feasibility of the Inoue single-branched stent graft for thoracic aortic aneurysms or dissections involving the left subclavian artery (Fig 1).

▶ The authors describe the use of an innovative custom graft for preserving flow of the left subclavian artery during thoracic stent graft placement. This technique, however, may be more useful for thoracic aneurysms that require coverage of the left common carotid artery or the innominate artery. Very rarely is covering the left subclavian itself a major concern. The technique involves transbrachial snares. Total operative time is approximately 4 hours and an average of 250 mL of contrast medium is used. It appears therefore unlikely this technique will be used when subclavian coverage is required. A carotid-subclavian bypass is our revascularization technique of choice in the few patients who require this. Such patients include those with a left intermal mammary artery bypass, aberrant origin of the left vertebral artery, an innominate or right subclavian artery stenosis, or patients with an atreic or stenosed right vertebral artery.

K. Kasirajan, MD

Spinal cord ischemia after elective stent-graft repair of the thoracic aorta
Chiesa R, Melissano G, Marrocco-Trischitta MM, et al ("Vita-Salute" Univ, Milan, Italy)
J Vasc Surg 42:11-17, 2005   8–15

Objectives.—Neurologic deficit after endovascular treatment of the thoracic aorta is a complication reported with variable frequency that may be associated with severe morbidity and mortality. The mechanism of spinal cord ischemia appears to be multifactorial and remains ill-defined. We reviewed our experience to investigate the determinants of paraplegia after stent-graft repair of the thoracic aorta, identify patients at risk, and assess the effectiveness of ancillary techniques.

Methods.—Over a 5-year period (June 1999 to December 2004), 103 patients underwent elective endovascular repair of the thoracic aorta at a university referral center. Indications for treatment were atherosclerotic aneurysms in 88 patients, chronic type B dissection in 10 patients, and penetrating aortic ulcer in 5 patients. Four of the 103 patients affected with thoracoabdominal aortic aneurysms had hybrid procedures and were excluded from the cumulative analysis. Twelve patients with zone 0 and zone 1 aortic arch aneurysms were operated on with synchronous or staged surgical aortic debranching. Preoperative cerebrospinal fluid (CSF) drainage was instituted in seven selected patients. Neurologic deficits were assessed by an independent neurologist and classified as immediate or delayed. Patient demographics and perioperative factors related to the endovascular procedure were evaluated by using univariate statistical analyses.

Results.—A primary technical success was achieved in 94 patients (94.9%). At a mean follow-up of 34 ± 14 months, a midterm clinical success was obtained in 90 patients (90.9%). Four patients (4.04%) had delayed neurologic deficit that completely resolved after the institution of CSF drainage, steroids administration, and arterial pressure pharmacologic adjustment. None of the four patients who underwent hybrid procedures for thoracoabdominal aortic aneurysms had paraplegia or paraparesis. Univariate analyses identified only a perioperative lowest mean arterial pressure (MAP) of <70 mm Hg as a significant risk factor ($P < .0001$).

Conclusion.—Perioperative hypotension (MAP <70 mm Hg) was found to be a significant predictor of spinal cord ischemia; hence, careful monitoring and prompt correction of arterial pressure may prevent the development of paraplegia. When the latter occurred, reduction of the CSF pressure by drainage was useful. Patients with a previous or synchronous abdominal aortic repair may also benefit from CSF drainage as a perioperative adjunct.

▶ Four patients with transient paraplegia after thoracic stent graft are described. All 4 patients had significant postoperative hypotension and 2 patients had an infrarenal abdominal aortic aneurysm (AAA). The immediate correction of hypotension and the use of a CSF drain and steroids reversed the neurologic event in all patients. Also of interest, all 4 events developed after 48 hours; hence, the use of techniques such as motor-sensory evoked potentials intraoperatively may not be beneficial. In our center we routinely use CSF drains in patients with an AAA, prior AAA repair, or aortobifemoral bypass. Also patients with known internal iliac occlusions receive a CSF drain. We also routinely use motor-sensory evoked potentials in high-risk patients. Any change is immediately treated with induced hypertension and further CSF drainage. CSF drains are not removed for 48 hours.

K. Kasirajan, MD

Strategies to Manage Paraplegia Risk After Endovascular Stent Repair of Descending Thoracic Aortic Aneurysms

Cheung AT, Pochettino A, McGarvey ML, et al (Univ of Pennsylvania, Philadelphia)
Ann Thorac Surg 80:1280-1289, 2005
8–16

Background.—Paraplegia is a recognized complication after endovascular stent repair of descending thoracic aortic aneurysms. A management algorithm employing neurologic assessment, somatosensory evoked potential monitoring, arterial pressure augmentation, and cerebrospinal fluid drainage evolved to decrease the risk of postoperative paraplegia.

Methods.—Patients in thoracic aortic aneurysm stent trials from 1999 to 2004 were analyzed for paraplegic complications. Lower extremity strength was assessed after anesthesia and in the intensive care unit. A loss of lower extremity somatosensory evoked potential or lower extremity strength was treated emergently to maintain a mean arterial pressure 90 mmHg or greater and a cerebrospinal fluid pressure 10 mm Hg or less.

Results.—Seventy-five patients (male = 49, female = 26, age = 75 ± 7.4 years) had descending thoracic aortic aneurysms repaired with endovascular stenting. Lumbar cerebrospinal fluid drainage (n = 23) and somatosensory evoked potential monitoring (n = 15) were performed selectively in patients with significant aneurysm extent or with prior abdominal aortic aneurysm repair (n = 17). Spinal cord ischemia occurred in 5 patients (6.6%); two had lower extremity somatosensory evoked potential loss after stent deployment and 4 developed delayed-onset paraplegia. Two had full recovery in response to arterial pressure augmentation alone. Two had full recovery and one had near-complete recovery in response to arterial pressure augmentation and cerebrospinal fluid drainage. Spinal cord ischemia was associated with retroperitoneal bleed (n = 1), prior abdominal aortic aneurysm repair (n = 2), iliac artery injury (n = 1), and atheroembolism (n = 1).

Conclusions.—Early detection and intervention to augment spinal cord perfusion pressure was effective for decreasing the magnitude of injury or preventing permanent paraplegia from spinal cord ischemia after endovascular stent repair of descending thoracic aortic aneurysm. Routine somatosensory evoked potential monitoring, serial neurologic assessment, arterial pressure augmentation, and cerebrospinal fluid drainage may benefit patients at risk for paraplegia (Fig 2).

▶ Despite the use of adjunctive measures, the authors continued to have a paraplegia incidence of 6.6%. Similar to the article by Chiesa et al (Abstract 8–15), most patients recovered from the neurologic events. The avoidance of hypotension and placement of CSF drains in patients with AAA or prior infrarenal repair appear to be the most reliable means to minimize this dreaded complication.

K. Kasirajan, MD

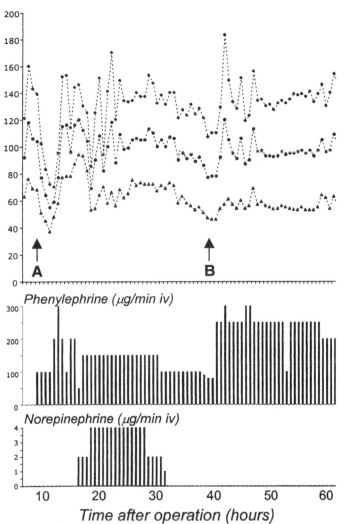

FIGURE 2.—Relation between arterial pressure and two separate episodes of delayed onset paraparesis after endovascular stent repair. A decrease in blood pressure preceded the onset of paraparesis at 9 hours (event A) and 39 hours after operation (event B). Full recovery of neurologic function coincided with increased arterial pressure. (*iv = intravenous.*) (Courtesty of Cheung AT, Pochettino A, McGarvey ML, et al: Strategies to manage paraplegia risk after endovascular stent repair of descending thoracic aortic aneurysms. *Ann Thorac Surg* 80:1280-1289, 2005. Reprinted with permission from the Society of Thoracic Surgeons.)

9 Leg Ischemia and Aortoiliac Disease

Relationship between objective measures of peripheral arterial disease severity to self-reported quality of life in older adults with intermittent claudication
Izquierdo-Porrerra AM, Gardner AW, Bradham DD, et al (Univ of Maryland, Baltimore; Univ of Oklahoma, Norman)
J Vasc Surg 41:625-630, 2005   9–1

Objectives.—The aim of this study was to determine the relation between functional measures of peripheral arterial disease (PAD) severity with both disease-specific and generic self-reported health-related quality-of-life (HR-QOL) measures, as well as the relation between the two types of HR-QOL measures.

Methods.—This was a cross-sectional observation of participants from the community and primary care or vascular surgery clinics in an academic Veterans Administration medical center. Eighty patients with symptomatic Fontaine stage II PAD provided physiologic measures and self-response questionnaires. Objective measures included the ankle-brachial index (ABI), time to maximum claudication pain on a graded exercise test, and a 6-minute floor-walking distance. Self-reports included the Walking Impairment Questionnaire (WIQ), a disease-specific HR-QOL measure and the Medical Outcomes Study (MOS) Short-Form 36 (SF-36), a generic HR-QOL measure.

Results.—Patients (mean age 70 ± 8 [± SD] and 85% men) exhibited moderate-to-severe PAD by objective measures of ABI (0.65 ± 0.19) and time in minutes to maximal claudication on a graded exercise test (7:54 ± 4:58). Significant correlations were found between these measures and the WIQ distance, MOS-Physical Function, and MOS-Role Limitations due to physical dysfunction. The SF-36 and the WIQ subscales were significantly correlated.

Conclusion.—In older PAD patients with intermittent claudication, objective measures of disease severity are correlated with a self-reported, disease-specific and generic HR-QOL.

▶ It is obvious from the following series of abstracts that assessment of the impact of peripheral arterial disease on quality of life and functional status is now an area of intense interest. This study correlates questionnaire data concerning quality of life with functional data. Most patients will not be willing or able to fill out all the forms or do all the tests outlined in this article. The data here, however, suggest that we may be able to get just as much information from fewer examinations or questions. There are other opinions (see Abstract 9–2).

G. L. Moneta, MD

Assessment of disease impact in patients with intermittent claudication: Discrepancy between health status and quality of life
Breek JC, de Vries J, van Heck GL, et al (Martini Hosp, Groningen, The Netherlands; Tilburg Univ, The Netherlands; St Elisabeth Hosp, Tilburg, The Netherlands; et al)
J Vasc Surg 41:443-450, 2005   9–2

Objective.—To describe similarities and differences between health status and quality of life in patients with intermittent claudication.

Methods.—This was an observational study in the vascular outpatient department of a teaching hospital; it concerned 200 consecutive patients with intermittent claudication. Health status was assessed with the RAND-36, and quality of life was assessed with a reduced version of the World Health Organization Quality of Life assessment instrument-100. Scores were compared with those of sex- and age-matched healthy controls. Mann-Whitney U tests were used to detect statistically significant differences ($P < .01$) between patients and healthy controls. Pearson correlations were calculated between health status and quality-of-life scores. Differences between correlations were examined by using Fisher z statistics. The upper and lower 10% of quality-of-life scores were compared with the response quartiles of the health status scores.

Results.—Health status was significantly impaired in all domains. Quality of life was significantly worse with respect to aspects of physical health and level of independence and one global evaluative facets overall quality of life and general health. Quality-of-life assessment with the World Health Organization Quality of Life instrument disclosed patient-reported problems that had not been identified in health status. Conversely, patients did not regard all objective functional impairments as a problem. Pearson correlations ranged from 0.20 to 0.74. There were patients with excellent and very poor quality-of-life scores in nearly all the quartiles of the corresponding health status domains.

Conclusions.—Health status and quality of life represent different outcomes in patients with intermittent claudication. In addition to functional restrictions as measured in health status, quality of life also permits a personal evaluation of these restrictions. Objective functioning and subjective appraisal of functioning are complementary and not identical. Combining these measures should direct treatment in a way that meets patients' needs.

► This and the preceding abstract reach different conclusions. It is not surprising patients do not regard the same level of functional impairment as affecting their quality of life equally. Perception is reality and perceptions vary. Questions on quality of life must somehow reflect the patient's subjective opinions. Perception of health and perception of quality of life are not going to always be the same.

G. L. Moneta, MD

D-Dimer and Inflammatory Markers as Predictors of Functional Decline in Men and Women with and without Peripheral Arterial Disease
McDermott MM, Ferrucci L, Liu K, et al (Northwestern Univ, Chicago; NIH, Baltimore, Md; Univ of California at San Diego; et al)
J Am Geriatr Soc 53:1688-1696, 2005   9–3

Objectives.—To determine whether higher circulating levels of inflammatory and thrombotic markers are associated with greater decline in lower extremity performance.

Design.—Prospective cohort.

Setting.—Academic medical center.

Participants.—Three hundred thirty-seven men and women with lower extremity peripheral arterial disease (PAD) and 215 without PAD.

Measurements.—Objective measures of leg function, including the 6-minute walk and Short Physical Performance Battery (SPPB), were obtained at baseline and annually for 3 years. D-dimer, high-sensitivity C-reactive protein, serum amyloid A, and fibrinogen levels were measured at baseline. Participants were categorized into one of three groups, ranging from low to high levels of inflammation, depending on the number of individual blood factors in the lowest and highest tertiles for each corresponding blood factor.

Results.—Adjusting for age, sex, race, ankle brachial index, comorbidities, and other confounders, greater inflammation was associated with greater decline in the SPPB ($P=.008$). Results were similar when repeated in participants with and without PAD separately (P for trend$=.04$ for participants with PAD and .07 for participants without PAD). In fully adjusted analyses, there were no significant associations between inflammation group and decline in 6-minute walk performance.

Conclusion.—Higher baseline levels of inflammatory markers and D-dimer were associated with greater decline in the SPPB at 3-year follow-up in persons with and without PAD.

► McDermott et al are finding more ways to assess functional status in patients with peripheral arterial disease than the number of fleas on a North Carolina dog in August (see Abstract 9–4). The impact of therapies on all these functional parameters needs to be assessed. We also need to know whether changes in functional status resulting from therapy actually matter to the patient (see Abstract 9–2).

G. L. Moneta, MD

Functional decline in lower-extremity peripheral arterial disease: Associations with comorbidity, gender, and race
McDermott MM, Guralnik JM, Ferrucci L, et al (Northwestern Univ, Chicago; Natl Inst on Aging, Bethesda, Md; Univ of California at San Diego)
J Vasc Surg 42:1131-1137, 2005   9–4

Purpose.—To identify comorbidities associated with increased rates of functional decline in persons with lower-extremity peripheral arterial disease (PAD). We also determined whether female sex and black race were associated with greater functional decline than male sex and white race, respectively, in PAD.

Methods.—Three-hundred ninety-seven men and women with PAD were followed prospectively for a median of 36 months. The presence of comorbid illnesses was determined with medical record review, patient report, medications, laboratory values, and a primary care physician questionnaire. Functional outcomes, measured annually, included the 6-minute walk, usual-paced and fast-paced 4-meter walking speed, and summary performance score. The summary performance score is a composite measure of lower-extremity functioning (score range, 0 to 12; 12 = best).

Results.—Adjusting for known and potential confounders, PAD patients with pulmonary disease had a significantly greater average annual decline in 6-minute walk performance of -34.02 ft/y (95% confidence interval [CI], -60.42 to -7.63; $P = .012$), rapid-paced 4-meter walk speed of -0.028 m/s/y (95% CI, -0.054 to -0.001; $P = .042$), and summary performance score of -0.460/y (95% CI, -0.762 to -0.157; $P = .003$) compared with those without pulmonary disease. PAD patients with spinal stenosis had a greater average annual decline in 6-minute walk performance of -77.4 ft/y (95% CI, -18.9 to -35.8; $P < .001$) and usual-paced 4-meter walking velocity of -0.045 m/s/y (95% CI, -0.081 to -0.009; $P = .014$) compared with participants without spinal stenosis.

Conclusion.—At 3-year follow-up, pulmonary disease and spinal stenosis were each associated with a significant decline in functioning among persons with PAD. In contrast, female sex and black race were not associated with functional decline among persons with PAD.

▶ The same comments apply here as to the previous abstract. At some time, investigators in this field need to evaluate whether all these functional tests are influenced by therapy and, if so, whether the changes actually matter to the patients. Again, patient perception is patient reality.

G. L. Moneta, MD

Upper- vs lower-limb aerobic exercise rehabilitation in patients with symptomatic peripheral arterial disease: A randomized controlled trial

Zwierska I, Walker RD, Choksy SA, et al (Sheffield Hallam Univ, England; Univ of Sheffield, England)
J Vasc Surg 42:1122-1130, 2005   9–5

Objectives.—To investigate the effects of a 24-week program of upper- and lower-limb aerobic exercise training on walking performance in patients with symptomatic peripheral arterial disease (PAD) and to study the mechanisms that could influence symptomatic improvement.

Methods.—After approval from the North Sheffield Local Research Ethics Committee, 104 patients (median age, 69 years; range, 50 to 85 years) with stable PAD were randomized into an upper- or lower-limb aerobic exercise training group (UL-Ex or LL-Ex), or to a nonexercise training control group. Training was performed twice weekly for 24 weeks at equivalent relative exercise intensities. An incremental arm- and leg-crank test (ACT and LCT) to maximum exercise tolerance was performed before and at 6, 12, 18, and 24 weeks of the intervention to determine peak oxygen consumption ($\dot{V}O_2$). Walking performance, defined as the claudicating distance (CD) and maximum walking distance (MWD) achieved before intolerable claudication pain, was assessed at the same time points by using a shuttle-walk protocol. Peak blood lactate concentration, Borg ratings of perceived exertion (RPE) and pain category ratio (CR-10) were recorded during all assessments.

Results.—CD and MWD increased over time ($P < .001$) in both training groups. At 24 weeks, CD had improved by 51% and 57%, and MWD had improved by 29% and 31% (all $P < .001$) in the UL-Ex and LL-Ex groups, respectively. An increase in peak heart rate at MWD in the UL-Ex group (109 ± 4 vs 115 ± 4 beats/min; $P < .01$) and LL-Ex group (107 ± 3 vs 118 ± 3 beats/min; $P = .01$) was accompanied by an increase in the amount of pain experienced in both groups ($P < .05$), suggesting that exercising patients could tolerate a higher level of cardiovascular stress and an increased intensity of claudication pain before test termination after training. Patients assigned to exercise training also showed an increase in LCT peak $\dot{V}O_2$ at the 24-week time point in relation to baseline ($P < .01$) and control patients ($P < .01$), whereas ACT peak $\dot{V}O_2$ was only improved in the UL-Ex group ($P < .05$).

Conclusions.—Our results suggest that a combination of physiologic adaptations and improved exercise pain tolerance account for the improvement in walking performance achieved through upper-limb aerobic exercise training in patients with PAD. Furthermore, that both arm- and leg-crank training could be useful exercise training modalities for improving cardiovascular function, walking performance, and exercise pain tolerance in patients with symptomatic PAD.

► The exact mechanisms by which exercise improves claudication is unknown. My former partner, Lloyd Taylor, liked to describe it as being essentially equivalent to "athletic training." Studies such as this indicate that there is a combination of psychologic, overall cardiovascular fitness, and lower extremity conditioning that combine to improve claudication distance with exercise training. It appears to maximize exercise-induced improvement in walking in patients with claudication; an exercise program that includes walking and other forms of exercise, perhaps swimming and biking, etc, will work best. How many claudicants can and will do all this is a different question.

G. L. Moneta, MD

The effect of exercise intensity on the response to exercise rehabilitation in patients with intermittent claudication
Gardner AW, Montgomery PS, Flinn WR, et al (Univ of Oklahoma, Oklahoma City; Univ of Maryland, Baltimore)
J Vasc Surg 42:702-709, 2005   9–6

Purpose.—The purpose of this randomized trial was to compare the efficacy of a low-intensity exercise rehabilitation program vs a high-intensity program in changing physical function, peripheral circulation, and health-related quality of life in peripheral arterial disease (PAD) patients limited by intermittent claudication.

Methods.—Thirty-one patients randomized to low-intensity exercise rehabilitation and 33 patients randomized to high-intensity exercise rehabilitation completed the study. The 6-month exercise rehabilitation programs consisted of intermittent treadmill walking to near maximal claudication pain 3 days per week at either 40% (low-intensity group) or 80% (high-intensity group) of maximal exercise capacity. Total work performed in the two training regimens was similar by having the patients in the low-intensity group exercise for a longer duration than patients in the high-intensity group. Measurements of physical function, peripheral circulation, and health-related quality of life were obtained on each patient before and after the rehabilitation programs.

Results.—After the exercise rehabilitation programs, patients in the two groups had similar improvements in these measures. Initial claudication distance increased by 109% in the low-intensity group ($P < .01$) and by 109% in the high-intensity group ($P < .01$), and absolute claudication distance increased by 61% ($P < 0.01$) and 63% ($P < .01$) in the low-intensity and high-intensity groups, respectively. Furthermore, both exercise programs elicited improvements ($P < .05$) in peak oxygen uptake, ischemic window, and health-related quality of life.

Conclusion.—The efficacy of low-intensity exercise rehabilitation is similar to high-intensity rehabilitation in improving markers of functional independence in PAD patients limited by intermittent claudication, provided that a few additional minutes of walking is accomplished to elicit a similar volume of exercise.

▶ Intensity of exercise does matter for some things. You will never run a marathon in 3 hours if all you do is stroll in the park. The overall level of exercise is relatively low here but, of course, the improvements derived may be very meaningful to the patients involved. The difference in the amount of time spent exercising in the low- versus high-intensity exercise groups is so small that, given equal results of high- versus low-intensity training, there seems to be no reason to use "high-intensity exercise" in patients with claudication.

G. L. Moneta, MD

Impaired health status and invasive treatment in peripheral arterial disease: A prospective 1-year follow-up study
Aquarius AE, Denollet J, Hamming JF, et al (Tilburg Univ, The Netherlands; Leiden Univ, The Netherlands; Martini Hosp, Groningen, The Netherlands)
J Vasc Surg 41:436-442, 2005   9–7

Objective.—It has been argued that health status and quality of life (QOL) should be taken into account in the treatment policy of patients with peripheral arterial disease (PAD). In cardiac patients, it has been shown that poor perceived health status is an independent predictor of mortality and hospitalization. We therefore examined (1) the role of health status, QOL, and clinical indices of disease severity as determinants of invasive treatment in patients with PAD and (2) the effect of invasive treatment on health status and QOL.

Methods.—At their first visit, patients completed the RAND 36-item Health Survey and World Health Organization Quality of Life assessment instrument questionnaires to assess health status and QOL, respectively. During the 1-year follow-up period, data concerning hospitalization were derived from the patients' medical files. Furthermore, patients completed the RAND 36 and the World Health Organization Quality of Life assessment instrument again at 1-year follow-up. The setting was a vascular outpatient clinic of a teaching hospital in Tilburg, The Netherlands; participants were 200 consecutive patients newly diagnosed with intermittent claudication, a common expression of PAD. Diagnosis was based on history, physical examination, treadmill walking distance, and ankle-brachial pressure indices. Main outcome measures were (1) invasive treatment of PAD that took place during the 1-year follow-up, derived from the patients' medical files, and (2) health status and QOL after 1 year of follow-up.

Results.—After 1 year of follow-up, 107 patients (53.5%) were event free, whereas 77 patients (38.5%) had been hospitalized for invasive treatment of PAD. Sixteen patients (8%) were hospitalized for other cardiovascular reasons. In a multivariate logistic regression model, age (odds ratio [OR], 0.95; 95% confidence interval [CI], 0.91-0.99; $P = .024$), pain-free walking distance (OR, 2.74; 95% CI, 1.05-7.17; $P = .04$), and physical functioning (OR, 4.46; 95% CI, 1.79-11.12; $P = .001$) were independent predictors of invasive treatment of intermittent claudication. After 1 year of follow-up, patients who were treated invasively experienced a significant improvement in their physical functioning ($P = .004$), role limitations due to emotional problems ($P = .018$), and bodily pain ($P = .026$).

Physical Functioning: □ High ■ Low

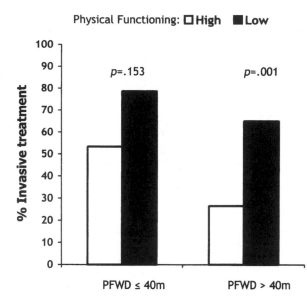

FIGURE 1.—Invasive treatment as a function of pain-free treadmill walking distance (*PFWD*) and RAND 36-item Health Survey subscale physical functioning at baseline. (Reprinted by permission of the publisher from Aquarius AE, Denollet J, Hamming JF, et al: Impaired health status and invasive treatment in peripheral arterial disease: A prospective 1-year follow-up study. *J Vasc Surg* 41:436-442, 2005. Copyright 2005 by Elsevier.)

Conclusions.—Patients with poor self-reported physical functioning, limited walking distance, and a younger age were likely to be treated invasively. The physician's clinical judgment about when to intervene adequately reflects the patient's own opinion about his or her health status. Invasive treatment led to a significant improvement in patients' health status. These findings indicate the effectiveness of the strategy to include patients' perceived physical functioning into the process of clinical decision-making (Fig 1).

▶ One cannot disagree with the statement that claudication patients perceive physical functioning as an important component of the decision-making process regarding therapy for claudication. However, follow-up was only 1 year in this study. That is too short to know whether the patient will regard intervention as having been helpful in the long run. A few emergency operations for failed grafts may change things!

G. L. Moneta, MD

Femorofemoral bypass with femoral popliteal vein

D'Addio V, Ali A, Timaran C, et al (Univ of Texas, Dallas; Univ of Arkansas, Little Rock)

J Vasc Surg 42:35-39, 2005   9–8

Background.—The femoropopliteal vein (FPV) has been used successfully for vascular reconstructions at multiple sites. To date, there have been no studies documenting patency of the FPV graft in the femorofemoral position. Our goal was to assess long-term patency of the FPV graft used for femorofemoral bypass (FFBP).

Methods.—Patients undergoing FFBP over a 10-year period were studied. Those in whom the FPV was used as a conduit were analyzed for runoff resistance score to assess how patients with poor runoff fared. *Poor runoff* was defined as a runoff resistance score of ≤7 (1 = normal runoff, 10 = total occlusion of all runoff vessels).

Results.—Fifty-four patients underwent FPV FFBP as a sole procedure (n = 16, 30%) or as a portion of an aortofemoral reconstruction with a FFBP component (n = 38, 70%). Mean (± SD) follow-up was 47 ± 33 months. The 1-, 3-, and 5-year primary patencies were 97%, 93%, and 76%. The 5-year assisted primary and secondary patency rates were 85% and 90%. Among 27 patients with poor runoff (runoff resistance score of ≤7), the cumulative 40 month patency rate was 90%. Among patients in whom FPV FFBP was performed as a primary procedure (no aortofemoral component), there were no graft failures.

Conclusions.—FFBP performed with FPV has excellent 1-, 3, and 5-year patency rates. FPV has sustained patency for FFBP in patients with poor runoff.

▶ I don't think prosthetic femorofemoral bypasses performed for occlusive disease work all that well. They occlude, and infectious complications are not infrequent. I am convinced a femorofemoral bypass performed with femoral popliteal vein is a more durable procedure. It is also a more extensive and more morbid procedure. We still do a few prosthetic femorofemoral bypasses when an endovascular reconstruction is not a reasonable option. However, if that graft fails, the next step, if the graft is still needed and a new femorofemoral bypass seems reasonable, should be consideration of a repeat femorofemoral bypass with femoropopliteal vein and not a new prosthetic graft or a simple thrombectomy.

G. L. Moneta. MD

Critical appraisal of femorofemoral crossover grafts

Pursell R, Sideso E, Magee TR, et al (Royal Berkshire Hosp, Reading, England)

Br J Surg 92:565-569, 2005   9–9

Background.—The aim of this study was to determine how often femorofemoral crossover grafting for critical ischaemia or intermittent claudication gives an ideal result. An ideal result is an uncomplicated operation with primary wound healing, relief of ischaemic symptoms without recurrence and no need for further intervention.

Methods.—All patients undergoing primary femorofemoral crossover grafting between January 1988 and December 2003 were studied.

Results.—Some 144 operations were analysed; 51 patients had critical ischaemia and 93 claudication. There was one postoperative death (0.7 per cent). Complications occurred within 30 days in 32 patients (22.2 per cent), including graft occlusion in three (2.1 per cent); six patients (4.2 per cent) required early reoperation. Primary patency for patients with critical ischaemia was 88, 82 and 74 per cent at 1, 3 and 5 years respectively. Respective figures for those who presented with claudication were 93, 92 and 90 per cent ($P = 0.034$). Late symptoms included graft occlusion (20 patients), disease progression (25), ongoing ulceration (six), graft infection (nine), false aneurysm formation (two) and late donor-site stenosis (two).

Conclusion.—When obtaining informed consent, simply describing patency and limb salvage rates does not provide an accurate picture of the outcome of femorofemoral grafting.

▶ The authors highlight problems with femorofemoral grafts other than just graft occlusion. This same analysis can be provided with respect to all arterial reconstructions. Not noted in the abstract, but mentioned in the article, was that freedom from symptoms in patients with femorofemoral grafts for critical limb ischemia was only 61% at 1 year and 54% at 3 years. Vascular surgery improves but in most cases does not cure critical limb ischemia when one looks at what matters to patients (ie, freedom from symptoms).

G. L. Moneta, MD

Endovascular management of iliac artery occlusions: extending treatment to TransAtlantic Inter-Society Consensus class C and D patients
Leville CD, Kashyap VS, Clair DG, et al (Cleveland Clinic Found, Ohio)
J Vasc Surg 43:32-39, 2006   9–10

Objective.—The preferential use of endovascular techniques to treat complex aortoiliac disease has increased in recent years. The purpose of this study was to review the outcomes and durability of recanalization, percuta-

---

FIGURE 1.—A, Transbrachial aortography documents a TransAtlantic Inter-Society Consensus class D iliac occlusion with right external iliac occlusion and complete occlusion of the left iliac system in a 46-year-old man with disabling claudication. B, Endovascular recanalization was performed with a hydrophilic guidewire and catheter, and femoral access was obtained with ultrasound guidance. Primary stenting with self-expanding nitinol stents with postdeployment balloon angioplasty restored normal pulsatile perfusion to both lower extremities, with palpable pedal pulses. Note that the right hypogastric circulation and other lumbar collateral arteries are preserved. (Reprinted by permission of the publisher from Leville CD, Kashyap VS, Clair DG, et al: Endovascular management of iliac artery occlusions: Extending treatment to TransAtlantic Inter-Society Consensus class C and D patients. *J Vasc Surg* 43:32-39, 2006. Copyright 2006 by Elsevier.)

FIGURE 1.

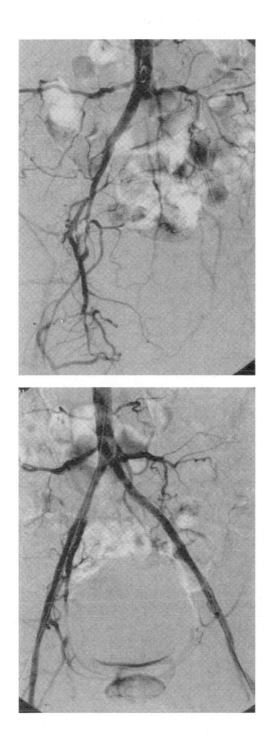

neous transluminal angioplasty, and stenting for iliac occlusions based on the patient's TransAtlantic Inter-Society Consensus (TASC) stratification.

Methods.—Between 1998 and 2004, more than 628 patients with a clinical diagnosis of aortoiliac atherosclerotic disease underwent arteriography. The endovascular treatment of 89 consecutive patients (mean age, 66 years; 58% male) with symptomatic iliac occlusions (TASC-B, -C, and -D) was the basis for this study. Original angiographic imaging was evaluated for lesion grade and runoff. Electronic and hard copy medical records were reviewed for demographic data, clinical variables, and noninvasive vascular laboratory testing. Kaplan-Meier estimators were used to determine patency rates according to Society for Vascular Surgery criteria. Univariate and multivariate analyses were performed. P values of <.05 were considered significant.

Results.—Recanalization and percutaneous transluminal angioplasty/stenting (total, 178 stents) of occluded iliac arteries was technically successful in 84 (91%) of 92 procedures. Patients in the TASC-C and -D groups often required multiple access sites (50%) and femoral artery endarterectomy/patch angioplasty for diffuse disease (24%). The mean ankle-brachial index increased from 0.45 to 0.83. Distal embolization led to major amputation and eventual death in one patient. Two other deaths occurred in the perioperative period secondary to cardiorespiratory causes. Three-year primary patency, secondary patency, and limb salvage rates were 76%, 90%, and 97%, respectively, and progression of infrainguinal disease led to late limb loss in two patients. Diabetes as a risk factor was significantly associated with decreased primary patency (57% vs 83%; $P = .049$). Critical ischemia at presentation was associated with decreased patency rates as well ($P = .002$), but TASC classification did not significantly alter patency rates.

Conclusions.—Complex long-segment and bilateral iliac occlusions can be safely treated via endovascular means with high rates of symptom resolution. Initial technical success, low morbidity, and mid-term durability are comparable to results with open reconstruction. A liberal posture to open femoral artery reconstruction extends the ability to treat diffuse TASC-C and -D lesions via endovascular means (Fig 1).

▶ These data will encourage more attempts at recanalization of occluded iliac arteries and will decrease the use of femorofemoral grafts (see Abstracts 9–8 and 9–9). It is, however, important to note these are surgeons very experienced and skilled in catheter-based interventions. It is not likely anyone will achieve the same results with their first few attempts at recanalizing an occluded iliac artery. The need for multiple access sites in 50% of the patients attests to the complexity of these procedures. Also note that procedures were performed in a setting where a concomitant open procedure was possible and, indeed, 24% of the time an open groin procedure was also performed.

G. L. Moneta, MD

Long-term Results of Above Knee Femoro-popliteal Bypass Depend on Indication for Surgery and Graft-material

Berglund J, for the SWEDVASC Femoro-popliteal Study Group (Univ Hosp of Linköping, Sweden; et al)
Eur J Vasc Endovasc Surg 29:412-418, 2005   9–11

Objective.—To determine the long-term results of above-knee femoro-popliteal bypass with autologous saphenous vein (SV) or expanded polytetrafluoroethylene (ePTFE) in routine surgical practice.

Methods.—Data from the Swedish vascular registry, Swedvasc, was reviewed retrospectively. Patients with bypass surgery in 1996 and 1997 were assessed 5–7 years later. Data were gathered from the case-records and from clinical follow-up. The composite endpoint of graft failure included death within 30 days, occlusion, major amputation, extension of the graft to below-knee position and removal of an infected graft. Kaplan-Meier curves and Cox proportional hazard ratios were calculated.

Results.—Four hundred and ninety-nine patients undergoing bypass for critical limb ischemia (CLI) (56%) or claudication (44%), SV (28%) or ePTFE (72%), were included. There were no significant differences in patient characteristics between patients with SV or ePTFE (Figs 3 and 4) CLI and ePTFE were risk factors for graft failure. For patients with both claudication and CLI SV grafts yielded better long-term results than ePTFE grafts

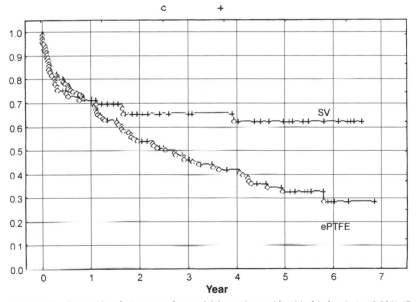

FIGURE 3.—Patency in relation to graft material for patients with critical ischemia ($p=0.031$). (Reprinted from Berglund J, for the SWEDVASC Femoro-popliteal Study Group: Long-term results of above knee femoro-popliteal bypass depend on indication for surgery and graft-material. *Eur J Vasc Endovasc Surg* 29:412-418, 2005, by permission of the publisher.)

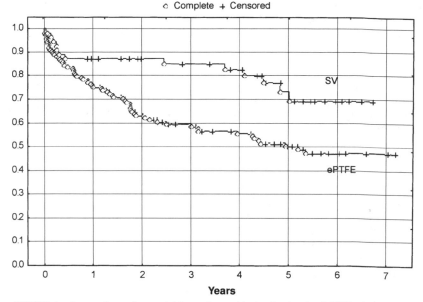

○ Complete + Censored

FIGURE 4.—Patency by graft material for patients with claudication ($p=0.0027$). (Reprinted from Berglund J, for the SWEDVASC Femoro-popliteal Study Group: Long-term results of above knee femoro-popliteal bypass depend on indication for surgery and graft-material. *Eur J Vasc Endovasc Surg* 29:412-418, 2005, by permission of the publisher.)

($p<0.03$) and ($p<0.003$), respectively. Symptom aggravation after graft occlusion was almost exclusively restricted to ePTFE grafts.

Conclusions.—Femoro-popliteal bypass above-knee with SV gives good long-term results, especially for claudication. ePTFE grafts cannot be recommended in claudicants, since occlusion occurs often and frequently leads to CLI.

▶ This study utilized a unique method in the evaluation of SV and PTFE grafts. A composite end point was utilized to include all graft-related events that may be considered procedural failures. The end point is unusual, but perhaps better reflects overall potential problems of infrainguinal bypass grafts than just usual patency end points. Based on the authors' data, it is difficult to argue with their conclusion that SV grafts should be utilized for femoropopliteal bypass whenever possible.

G. L. Moneta, MD

Sequential Femorodistal Composite Bypass with Second Generation Glutaraldehyde Stabilized Human Umbilical Vein (HUV)

Neufang A, Espinola-Klein C, Dorweiler B, et al (Johannes Gutenberg Univ, Mainz, Germany)

Eur J Vasc Endovasc Surg 30:176-183, 2005   9–12

Objective.—To evaluate the performance of sequential composite by-passes with second generation glutaraldehyde stabilized human umbilical vein (HUV) and autologous vein.

Design.—Retrospective study of consecutive patients, in a single centre.

Patients.—From January 1998 to December 2003, 54 femoro-distal HUV-autologous vein sequential composite bypasses were constructed in 52 patients with critical leg ischemia and absence of sufficient length of autologous vein (Fig 1).

Methods.—All infra-inguinal bypass operations were registered in a computerized database and prospectively followed. Bypasses using sequential HUV-composite technique were reviewed for graft patency, limb salvage and patient survival.

Results.—Primary patency and secondary patency rates at 1, 2, 3 and 4 years were 71, 61, 53 and 53% and 89, 80, 73 and 67%, respectively. Corresponding limb salvage rates were 96, 92, 88 and 88%. Patient survival was 56% at 4 years. After 30 days additional procedures to maintain graft patency were necessary in six bypasses. Asymptomatic occlusion of one sequential anastomosis was found in five patients.

Conclusion.—Graft patency and limb salvage rate support the use of the sequential composite technique with second generation HUV in femoro-distal bypass surgery, when autologous vein of sufficient length is not available.

▶ There still remains some interest in the use of HUV grafts. The authors' technique of using HUV grafts as the prosthetic component of a prosthetic/autologous sequential composite bypass has provided reasonable results in terms of both patency and limb salvage. The results differ little from what one would expect with similar procedures with polytetrafluorethylene grafts. Biodegeneration of the HUV grafts in this series of limb salvage patients appeared to be a nonissue. If a sequential composite prosthetic/autogenous graft is required, it appears to make little difference whether the prosthetic component is polytetrafluorethylene or HUV.

G. L. Moneta, MD

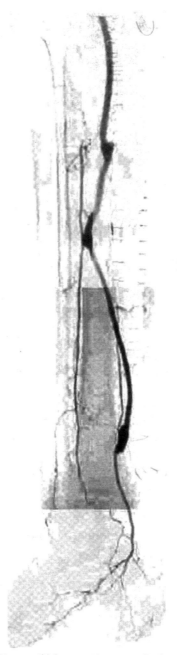

FIGURE 1.—Sequential HUV-compatible bypass with segment of ipsilateral greater saphenous vein. (Reprinted from Neufang A, Espinola-Klein C, Dorweiler B, et al: Sequential femorodistal composite bypass with second generation glutaraldehyde stabilized human umbilical vein (HUV). *Eur J Vasc Endovasc Surg* 30:176-183, 2005, by permission of the publisher.)

Effect of Warfarin Anticoagulation on Below-Knee Polytetrafluoroethylene Graft Patency

LeCroy CJ, Patterson MA, Taylor SM, et al (Univ of Alabama at Birmingham)
Ann Vasc Surg 19:192-198, 2005   9–13

When polytetrafluoroethylene (PTFE) must be used for below-knee bypass to achieve limb salvage, effective anticoagulation with warfarin may improve graft survival. We analyzed our practice of routinely using oral anticoagulation to improve graft patency rates for PTFE grafts to below-knee popliteal and crural vessels in limb salvage procedures. We reviewed our established vascular database from February 1999 through April 2003 to identify those patients who required below-knee and tibial artery bypass with PTFE for critical limb ischemia. All patients were initiated on warfarin anticoagulation postoperatively, with an international normalized ratio (INR) of 2.0-3.0 considered therapeutic. All patients were discharged in the therapeutic range. Life-table analysis and Kaplan-Meier estimates were used to compare primary patency rates with regard to INR and position of distal anastomosis (Fig 3). Cox proportional hazards analysis was performed to compare the patency rates for grafts with therapeutic versus subtherapeutic anticoagulation while correcting for variability in distal runoff. Between February 1999 and April 2003, 74 patients (mean age, 69.2 years; 58% men) had 77 below-knee PTFE bypasses. Indications for operation included rest pain (43), ischemic ulcer (27), and gangrene (7). Patients presenting with occluded grafts more often had a subtherapeutic INR. Patients with a subtherapeutic INR (≤1.9) had a median primary graft patency of 6.8 months and those with a therapeutic INR (≥2.0) had a median primary graft patency of 29.9 months (*p* = 0.0007). Analysis by Cox proportional hazards model demonstrated a significantly better graft patency rate in patients with a therapeutic INR regardless of outflow vessel. The patency rates of PTFE grafts to infrageniculate vessels may be improved by effective anticoagulation with warfarin. This improved patency rate may also result in improved limb salvage and further support the use of PTFE grafts for critical limb is-

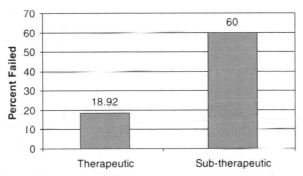

FIGURE 3.—Graft failure risk based on INR (therapeutic and subtherapeutic), *p* = 0.0002. (Courtesy of LeCroy CJ, Patterson MA, Taylor SM, et al: Effect of warfarin anticoagulation on below-knee polytetrafluoroethylene graft patency. *Ann Vasc Surg* 19:192-198, 2005.)

chemia when autogenous vein is not available. Predictably, the best results are seen with an INR therapeutic range of 2.0 to 3.0.

▶ There have been several randomized controlled trials designed to evaluate efficacy of anticoagulation in maintaining infrainguinal prosthetic bypass graft patency. Nevertheless, this remains an area of considerable debate. The investigators throw their hat into the ring on the side of anticoagulation, suggesting subtherapeutic anticoagulation leads to a 4-fold increase in graft failure. We agree with their bias, routinely anticoagulating good-risk patients. Not addressed in this study, however, is the substantial increase in wound and bleeding complications associated with this approach. This likely will offset some of the gains obtained in improved primary patency.

S. A. Berceli, MD, PhD

Infragenicular Polytetrafluoroethylene Bypass With Distal Vein Cuffs for Limb Salvage: A Contemporary Series

Lauterbach SR, Torres GA, Andros G, et al (St Joseph's Med Ctr, Burbank, Calif)

Arch Surg 140:487-494, 2005   9–14

Hypothesis.—Infragenicular polytetrafluoroethylene (PTFE)–venous cuff bypass grafting provides acceptable graft patency and limb salvage rates for limb salvage.

Design.—Retrospective clinical review of a consecutive series.

Setting.—Vascular surgical practice during the interval October 1, 2000, to September 1, 2004.

Patients.—Fifty-one male and 49 female patients whose mean age was 76.9 years were operated on for tissue loss (67%), chronic rest pain (28%), and severe claudication (6%). Fifty-two percent of patients were diabetic and 49% had undergone previous leg bypass surgery. All patients had absent or inadequate greater saphenous vein, and 84 patients had absent or inadequate arm vein.

Interventions.—One hundred five infragenicular PTFE bypasses were performed in these 100 patients. Distal targets were the infragenicular popliteal (40), posterior tibial (35), anterior tibial (16), and peroneal arteries (14). Sixty-eight venous cuffs were constructed from lesser saphenous vein.

Main Outcome Measures.—Graft patency, limb salvage, and patient survival were analyzed.

Results.—Twelve early graft failures resulted in 7 leg amputations. The mean ± SE 3-year primary patency and limb salvage rates were 64.4% ± 12.8% and 74.4% ± 11.9%, respectively. Perioperative mortality was 2.9% and 3-year survival was 38%. Graft follow-up ranged from 1 to 47 months with a mean of 13 months using life-table methods.

Conclusions.—For patients requiring arterial revascularization for limb salvage, in which autologous venous conduit is unavailable, distal venous cuff–PTFE bypass provides acceptable patency and limb salvage rates when viewed in the context of short life expectancy for these elderly patients.

▶ While not carefully studied, the addition of a venous cuff at the distal prosthetic graft anastomosis appears to confer some improvement in patency. The majority of patients were followed up for less than 18 months. This study, however, is in general agreement with previously published reports on this topic. Advancement in this area cries for a head-to-head comparison of cuffed-prosthetic versus cryopreserved venous grafts. The increasing use of endovascular tibial interventions, however, may soon make this a topic of historic interest only.

S. A. Berceli, MD, PhD

Risk of Major Haemorrhage in Patients after Infrainguinal Venous Bypass Surgery: Therapeutic Consequences? The Dutch BOA (Bypass Oral Anticoagulants or Aspirin) Study

Ariesen MJ, for the Dutch Bypass Oral Anticoagulants or Aspirin (BOA) Study Group (Univ Med Ctr Utrecht, The Netherlands; et al)
Eur J Vasc Endovasc Surg 30:154-159, 2005   9–15

Objectives.—The beneficial effect of oral anticoagulants after infrainguinal venous bypass surgery is compromised by bleeding complications. We developed a model to identify patients, treated with anticoagulation, at risk of major haemorrhage and estimated whether this complication could have been prevented if patients had received aspirin.

Design.—Randomised clinical trial.

Methods.—Data of patients who participated in the Dutch Bypass Oral Anticoagulation or Aspirin Study were reanalysed using Cox regression. After infrainguinal bypass surgery these patients were randomised to oral anticoagulants ($n = 1326$) or aspirin ($n = 1324$).

Results.—Predictors of major haemorrhage for patients on oral anticoagulants were increased systolic blood pressure (≥ 140 mm Hg, hazard ratio [HR] 1.62), age ≥ 75 years (HR 2.77) and diabetes mellitus (HR 1.60). If the 345 patients in the highest risk quartile had received aspirin, major haemorrhages would have been reduced from 46 to 22, with no major changes in ischemic events and graft occlusions. In the subgroup with venous bypasses major haemorrhages would have been reduced from 27 to 13, at the cost of seven more ischemic events (mostly fatal) and 17 more graft occlusions.

Conclusions.—Treating patients at highest risk of major haemorrhage with aspirin instead of oral anticoagulants would have resulted in a reduction of non-fatal haemorrhages, but for venous bypasses this reduction was outweighed by an increase in ischemic events and graft occlusions. We still recommend treatment with oral anticoagulants after peripheral venous bypass surgery.

▶ The BOA study is widely known and widely quoted, but thus far its findings have had little influence on the treatment of patients with vein bypass grafts. Part of the lack of acceptance of the BOA recommendations undoubtedly has to do with the increased hemorrhage rate with the use of anticoagulants. This analysis suggests that even with increased rates of hemorrhage, patients with vein bypasses still benefit from oral anticoagulants compared with aspirin. Although the authors' model is interesting, this type of retrospective analysis in itself is not going to convince many to utilize oral anticoagulants as routine prophylaxis against vein bypass graft occlusion.

G. L. Moneta, MD

Percutaneous angioplasty and stenting of the superficial femoral artery
Surowiec SM, Davies MG, Eberly SW, et al (Univ of Rochester, NY)
J Vasc Surg 41:269-278, 2005   9–16

Objectives.—The objectives of this study were to examine factors predictive of success or failure after percutaneous angioplasty (PTA) and stenting (S) of the superficial femoral artery (SFA) and to compare the results of PTA/S with a contemporary group of patients treated with femoropopliteal bypass.

Methods.—A database of patients undergoing PTA and/or S of the SFA between 1986 and 2004 was maintained. Intention-to-treat analysis was performed. Patients underwent duplex scanning follow-up at 1, 3, and every 6 months after the intervention. Angiograms were reviewed in all cases to assess lesion characteristics and preprocedure and postprocedure runoff. Results were standardized to current TransAtlantic Inter-Society Consensus (TASC) and Society for Vascular Surgery (SVS) criteria. Kaplan-Meier survival analyses were performed to assess time-dependent outcomes Cox proportional hazard analyses were performed to assess factors associated with patient survival and treatment efficacy.

Results.—Three hundred eighty total limbs underwent PTA/S in 329 patients (67% male, 33% female; average age, 65 years). Mean follow-up was 1.8 years from the date of initial intervention. Indications for intervention were claudication in 66%, rest pain in 16%, and tissue loss in 18%. Runoff at the tibial level was 2.1 0.8 patent vessels. Mean SVS ischemia grade was 3.1 (range, 1 to 5). TASC lesion grades were A (48%), B (18%), C (22%), and D (12%). Angioplasty alone was used in 63% of cases. Primary treatment failure (inability to cross lesion) was seen in 7% of patients. There was one periprocedural death. Primary patency rates were 86% at 3 months, 80% at 6 months, 75% at 12 months, 66% at 24 months, 60% at 36 months, 58% at 48 months, and 52% at 60 months. Assisted primary patency rates were slightly higher (P = not significant). By Cox proportional hazards analysis, patency of PTA/S was associated with higher preoperative ankle/brachial index ($P = .016$) and the performance of angioplasty only ($P = .011$). Failed or occluded PTA/S was associated with TASC C ($P < .0001$) and TASC D lesions ($P < .0001$). Patient death was associated with the presence of congestive heart failure ($P = .003$). Subgroup analysis revealed that primary patency rates are highly dependent on lesion type (A > B > C > D, $P < .0001$). PTA/S patency for TASC A and B lesions compared favorably to prosthetic and venous femoropopliteal bypass (Figs 1 and 2). Surgical bypass was superior to PTA/S for TASC C and D lesions.

Conclusions.—PTA and stenting of the SFA can be performed safely with excellent procedural success rates. Improved patency of these interventions was seen with increased ankle/brachial index and the performance of angioplasty only. Worse patency was seen with TASC C and TASC D lesions. Patency rates were strongly dependent on lesion type, and the results of angioplasty and stenting compared favorably with surgical bypass for TASC A and B lesions.

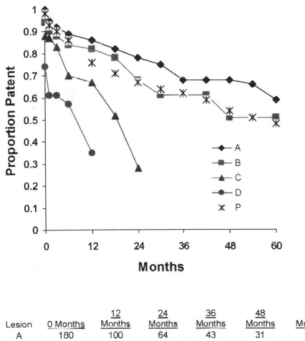

Lesion	0 Months	12 Months	24 Months	36 Months	48 Months	60 Months
A	180	100	64	43	31	17
B	83	26	10	7	5	5
C	69	16	2	1	0	
D	42	3	0			
P	350	180	129	97	70	50

FIGURE 1.—Primary patency of SFA PTA/S (broken down by lesion type) compared with femoropopliteal bypass with prosthetic (*asterisks within boxes*). Error bars omitted for clarity. All standard errors <10% for data shown. The number of patients at risk at each time interval is shown *below* the figure. *A*, TASC A lesion; *B*, TASC B lesion; *C*, TASC C lesion; *D*, TASC D lesion; *P*, prosthetic femoropopliteal bypass (polytetrafluoroethylene, Dacron). (Reprinted by permission of the publisher from Surowiec SM, Davies MG, Eberly SW, et al: Percutaneous angioplasty and stenting of the superficial femoral artery. *J Vasc Surg* 41:269-278, 2005. Copyright 2005 by Elsevier.)

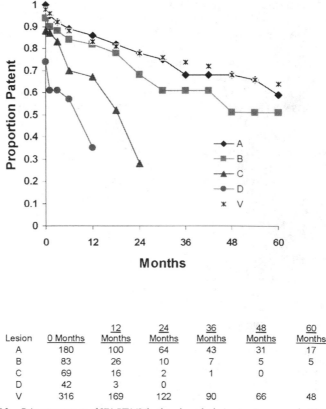

Lesion	0 Months	12 Months	24 Months	36 Months	48 Months	60 Months
A	180	100	64	43	31	17
B	83	26	10	7	5	5
C	69	16	2	1	0	
D	42	3	0			
V	316	169	122	90	66	48

FIGURE 2.—Primary patency of SFA PTA/S (broken down by lesion type) compared with femoropopliteal bypass with vein (*asterisks within boxes*). Error bars omitted for clarity. All standard errors <10% for data shown. The number of patients at risk at each time interval is shown *below* the figure. A, TASC A lesion; B, TASC B lesion; C, TASC C lesion; D, TASC D lesion; P, prosthetic femoropopliteal bypass (polytetrafluoroethylene, Dacron). (Reprinted by permission of the publisher from Surowiec SM, Davies MG, Eberly SW, et al: Percutaneous angioplasty and stenting of the superficial femoral artery. *J Vasc Surg* 41:269-278, 2005. Copyright 2005 by Elsevier.)

▶ Once again, we see percutaneous angioplasty of diffuse SFA disease or long-segment occlusions, with or without the use of adjunct stenting, yields poor primary patency rates. Despite increasing application of these techniques, useful data guiding their use are lacking. While retrospective analysis using our traditional end points of patency and limb salvage is easily accomplished, it provides overall limited insights. Only through prospective data collection, in well-characterized patient populations using a range of functional end points, can a true risk-benefit analysis be performed.

S. A. Berceli, MD, PhD

Efficacy of Hemobahn® in the Treatment of Superficial Femoral Artery Lesions in Patients with Acute or Critical Ischemia: A Comparative Study with Claudicants

Hartung O, Otero A, Dubuc M, et al (Hôpital Nord, Marseille, France)

Eur J Vasc Endovasc Surg 30:300-306, 2005   9–17

Purpose.—To assess the results of covered stents in the treatment of superficial femoral artery (SFA) occlusive disease.

Method.—From July 2000 till June 2003, 32 patients (34 limbs) were scheduled for procedures including Hemobahn® deployment in the SFA. Indication for treatment was claudication (group I, $N=15$ patients and 16 limbs, 31.2% occlusions) or critical and acute ischemia (group II, $N=17$ patients and 18 limbs, 61.1% occlusions). TASC D SFA lesions were excluded. No limb artery was patent pre-operatively in 19% and 89% of limbs in groups I and II, respectively ($p=0.00001$).

Results.—Outflow procedures were performed simultaneously in one limb in group I and 12 in group II ($p=0.0003$). The technical, hemodynamic and clinical success rates were 100, 100 and 94.1%, respectively. Mean follow-up was 18.1 months. Primary patency rates at 12 months were 81.310.6% in group I and 88.6±9.0% in group II ($p=0.547$). At 12 months, the secondary patency and limb salvage rates were, respectively, 87.5±8.9 and 100% in group I and 87.5±8.93 and 94.45±6.71% in group II.

Conclusion.—Treatment of SFA occlusive lesions (excluding TASC D lesions) with the Hemobahn covered stent yielded good results for both claudicants with good outflow and patients with critical or acute ischemia with bad outflow, if concomitant outflow-improving procedures were performed.

▶ Suggesting primary patency greater than 80% at 12 months, this report stands among the best performances of percutaneous endovascular SFA stent grafting reported in the literature to date. While the underlying reasons for this improved efficacy are not delineated, the small sample size of 32 patients may be contributing to the optimistic outlook. Larger retrospective series have suggested primary patency in the range of 60% at 12 months, and I suspect those data are more consistent with reality. With patency rates similar to angioplasty or uncovered stenting, the benefits of SFA stent grafting remain poorly defined.

S. A. Berceli, MD, PhD

Endovascular brachytherapy prevents restenosis after femoropopliteal angioplasty: results of the Vienna-3 randomised multicenter study
Pokrajac B, Pötter R, Wolfram RM, et al (Med Univ of Vienna; Lainz Hosp, Vienna)
Radiother Oncol 74:3-9, 2005   9–18

Background and Purpose.—The aim of the trial was to investigate the effect of Iridium-192 gamma endovascular brachytherapy on reduction of restenosis after femoropopliteal angioplasty.

Patients and Methods.—Between Oct, 1998 and Jul, 2001 a total of 134 patients have been randomized after successful angioplasty to brachytherapy or sham irradiation in a prospective, randomized, multicenter, double blind controlled trial. Patients with de novo lesion of at least 5 cm or recurrent lesion of any length after prior angioplasty have been enrolled. Brachytherapy was performed with 7F centering catheter. Mean lesion length was 9.1cm (1.5–25 cm) and mean intervention length 13.6 cm (4–27.5 cm) in brachytherapy cohort.

Results.—In placebo cohort mean lesion length was 10.3 cm (2–25 cm) and mean intervention length 14.1 cm (2–29 cm). A dose of 18 Gy was prescribed 2 mm from the surface of centering balloons. Analyzed (based on angiography) on intention to treat basis the binary restenosis rate at 12 months was 41.7% (28/67) in brachytherapy cohort and 67.1% (45/67) in placebo cohort (χ^2 test, $P<0.05$). Corresponding data for as treated analysis (A total of 38 patients was excluded from analysis due to lack of follow-up, early recurrence within 30 days and >30% residual stenosis after angioplasty) have been 23.4% in the brachytherapy and 53.3% in the placebo group ($P<0.05$), respectively. The cumulative patency rates after 24 months on intention to treat analysis were 54% in the brachytherapy and 27% in the placebo group ($P<0.005$). Corresponding data for as treated analysis were 77% in the brachytherapy and 39% in the placebo group ($P<0.001$) Late thrombosis was not seen.

Conclusions.—Significant reduction of restenosis rate was obtained with endovascular gamma brachytherapy after femoropopliteal angioplasty.

▶ Although efficacy in the coronary circulation has been demonstrated, the frequent occlusions and extensive lesion lengths in peripheral arteries provide a more formidable challenge for brachytherapy as an adjunct to percutaneous interventions. Despite the impressive results reported here, application will be limited by the inability to handle these high-intensity gamma emitters outside radiation oncology facilities. The investigators are to be commended for a well-designed study. This is, however, little more than proof-in-concept data. In the dizzying array of adjuncts to percutaneous revascularization, it is unlikely radiation therapy will ever become more than a fringe participant.

S. A. Berceli, MD, PhD

Endovascular Brachytherapy: Restenosis in de Novo versus Recurrent Lesions of Femoropopliteal Artery—The Vienna Experience

Wolfram RM, Budinsky AC, Pokrajac B, et al (Med Univ of Vienna)
Radiology 236:338-342, 2005   9–19

Purpose.—To determine the effectiveness of endovascular brachytherapy in the prevention of restenosis in recurrent versus de novo femoropopliteal lesions.

Materials and Methods.—Ethics committee approval and patient informed consent were obtained. After they had undergone femoropopliteal angioplasty, 199 patients (mean age, 71.9 years ± 9.6; 115 men, 84 women) were treated with either percutaneous transluminal angioplasty (PTA) and brachytherapy ($n = 100$) or PTA alone ($n = 99$). The patients were part of prospective randomized trials, the Vienna 2 and 3 trials, and were evaluated according to the stratification criterion of de novo or recurrent disease. Sixty-six of 134 patients with a de novo lesion and 34 of 65 patients with a recurrent lesion were randomly assigned to the PTA and brachytherapy arm; the remaining patients were treated with PTA alone. Outcomes were compared between the groups. The Student t test or one-way analysis of variance was used to compare continuous variables, and the χ^2 test or Fisher exact test was used to assess dichotomous variables. Kaplan-Meier curves were calculated, and the log-rank test was performed to determine freedom from recurrence at 12 months in both groups. A multivariate Cox proportional hazard

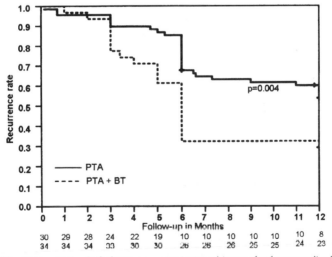

FIGURE 2.—Kaplan-Meier graph shows recurrence (restenosis) rates after femoropopliteal PTA in patients with recurrent lesions according to treatment group. Numbers below x-axis are numbers of patients who underwent PTA alone (top row) or PTA and brachytherapy (*BT*) (bottom row) and were at risk for recurrence. The difference in recurrence rates between the two treatment groups was significant ($P = .004$, log-rank test). (Courtesy of Wolfram RM, Budinsky AC, Pokrajac B, et al: Endovascular brachytherapy: Restenosis in de novo versus recurrent lesions of femoropopliteal artery—the Vienna experience. *Radiology* 236:338-342, 2005, Radiological Society of North America)

regression analysis was performed to evaluate the multivariate predictors of recurrence at 12-month follow-up.

Results.—For patients with de novo lesions, the frequency of recurrence at 12 months was not significantly different between those who underwent brachytherapy and PTA and those who underwent PTA alone (24 [36%] of 66 patients vs 30 [44%] of 68 patients, $P = 32$). For patients with recurrent lesions, however, the 12-month recurrence rate was significantly lower in those who received brachytherapy than in those who did not (nine [26%] of 34 patients vs 22 [71%] of 31 patients, $P = .004$) (Fig 2).

Conclusion.—Endovascular brachytherapy with gamma radiation significantly reduces the restenosis rate after femoropopliteal angioplasty of recurrent but not de novo lesions.

▶ The study suggests that different strategies may be required to reduce restenosis after PTA of original versus recurrent stenotic lesions. Brachytherapy continues to be evaluated as a means of reducing restenosis after PTA. Given the relatively cumbersome techniques involved and logistic difficulties administering gamma radiation, investigations in this field have been somewhat limited. Nevertheless, there appear to be some patient and lesion combinations that may benefit from brachytherapy. Continued investigation is warranted. Larger multicenter trials will be required to prove the utility of this technique as an adjunct to catheter-based arterial stenosis.

G. L. Moneta, MD

Prevalence and Clinical Impact of Stent Fractures After Femoropopliteal Stenting

Scheinert D, Scheinert S, Sax J, et al (Univ of Leipzig, Germany)
J Am Coll Cardiol 45:312-315, 2005   9–20

Objectives.—The aim of this study was to investigate the occurrence and the clinical impact of stent fractures after femoropopliteal stenting.

Background.—The development of femoral stent fractures has recently been described; however, there are no data about the frequency and the clinical relevance.

Methods.—A systematic X-ray screening for stent fractures was performed in 93 patients. In total, 121 legs treated by implantation of self-expanding nitinol stents were investigated after a mean follow-up time of 10.7 months. The mean length of the stented segment was 15.7 cm.

Results.—Overall, stent fractures were detected in 45 of 121 treated legs (37.2%). In a stent-based analysis, 64 of 261 stents (24.5%) showed fractures, which were classified as minor (single strut fracture) in 31 cases (48.4%), moderate (fracture of >1 strut) in 17 cases (26.6%), and severe (complete separation of stent segments) in 16 cases (25.0%). Fracture rates were 13.2% for stented length ≤8 cm, 42.4% for stented length >8 to 16 cm, and 52.0% for stented length >16 cm. In 21 cases (32.8%) there was a restenosis of >50% diameter reduction at the site of stent fracture (Fig 1). In 22

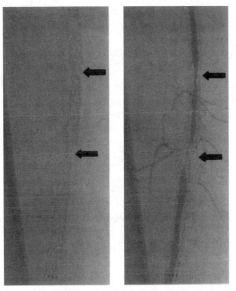

FIGURE 1.—Self-expanding nitinol stent nine months after implantation showing a severe stent fracture in the distal and a moderate stent fracture in the proximal part of the stent. Angiographically, both lesions were associated with a restenosis >50% diameter reduction. (Courtesy of Scheinert D, Scheinert S, Sax J, et al: Prevalence and clinical impact of stent fractures after femoropopliteal stenting. *J Am Coll Cardiol* 45:312-315, 2005. Reprinted with permission of the American College of Cardiology.)

cases (34.4%) with stent fracture there was a total stent reocclusion. According to Kaplan-Meier estimates, the primary patency rate at 12 months was significantly lower for patients with stent fractures (41.1% vs. 84.3%, p < 0.0001).

Conclusions.—There is a considerable risk of stent fractures after long segment femoral artery stenting, which is associated with a higher in-stent restenosis and reocclusion rate.

► There has been some thought that nitinol stents may improve the results of femoropopliteal artery stenting. Data such as this suggest this will not be the case, but other trials are ongoing. This is another in a long line of reports documenting the poor results of stenting of femoropopliteal arteries.

G. L. Moneta, MD

Balloon angioplasty of popliteal and crural arteries in elderly with critical chronic limb ischemia

Atar E, Siegel Y, Avrahami R, et al (Rabin Med Ctr, Petah Tikva, Israel; Univ of Tel Aviv, Israel; Hillel-Yoffe Med Ctr, Hadra, Israel)
Eur J Radiol 53:287-292, 2005   9–21

Objective.—Elderly patients with extensive infrainguinal peripheral vascular disease and critical chronic limb ischemia (CCLI) are poor surgical candidates. Our purpose was to evaluate angiographic and clinical results of popliteal, infrapopliteal, and multi-level disease percutaneous transluminal angioplasty (PTA) in such patients.

Design.—Retrospective study of angiographic and clinical files in selected group.

Materials and Methods.—Between 1996 and 2002, 38 elderly patients aged 80–94 years old (mean age 83.3) with critical leg ischemia were treated with PTA. All patients were at high surgical risk. 31/38 (81.5%) patients had chronic non-healing wounds, and 14/38 (37%) had multi-level disease of superficial femoral, popliteal and crural arteries. One hundred and two lesions were treated by angioplasty. Immediate angiographic and 1 year clinical results were retrospectively analyzed.

Results.—The overall procedural success rate was 32/38 (84.2%). There were three major complications (7.9%), but no deaths, and three technical failures, all were of infrapopliteal lesions. After 1 year, 27 patients could be followed, five patients died during the first year of unrelated causes. Twenty-three patients (85.2%), were clinically re-occluded within 1 year, but complete and partial wound healing was achieved in 80% (16/20) and rest pain improvement in 57% (4/7), so that overall limb salvage was 74% (20/27).

Conclusions.—Elderly patients with multi-level CCLI have a short patency term following angioplasty of 14.8% after 1 year. Nevertheless, this temporary vascular patency enables wound healing or improvement in 74% of these patients, thus such endovascular interventions are recommended in this age group.

▶ There is always a discrepancy between anatomic patency of arterial reconstructions for critical limb ischemia and limb salvage. However, the discrepancy is such that limb salvage is usually about 20% to 30% greater than reconstruction patency. The discrepancy between a limb salvage rate of 74% in this study and a clinical patency rate of 14% seems excessive when compared with surgical series. The implication is that some of these patients may have healed or resolved their rest pain without any intervention other than medical management and local wound care. An interesting bit of data lacking in all angioplasty and surgical series for critical limb ischemia is how many patients developed recurrent critical limb ischemia in the treated limb after an initial episode of critical limb ischemia resolved?

G. L. Moneta, MD

Bypass versus angioplasty in severe ischaemia of the leg (BASIL): multi-centre, randomised controlled trial
Bradbury AW, for the BASIL Trial Participants (Univ of Birmingham, England; et al)
Lancet 366:1925-1934, 2005

9–22

Background.—The treatment of rest pain, ulceration, and gangrene of the leg (severe limb ischaemia) remains controversial. We instigated the BASIL trial to compare the outcome of bypass surgery and balloon angioplasty in such patients.

Methods.—We randomly assigned 452 patients, who presented to 27 UK hospitals with severe limb ischaemia due to infra-inguinal disease, to receive a surgery-first (n=228) or an angioplasty-first (n=224) strategy. The primary endpoint was amputation (of trial leg) free survival. Analysis was by intention to treat. The BASIL trial is registered with the National Research Register (NRR) and as an International Standard Randomised Controlled Trial, number ISRCTN45398889.

Findings.—The trial ran for 5.5 years, and follow-up finished when patients reached an endpoint (amputation of trial leg above the ankle or death). Seven individuals were lost to follow-up after randomisation (three assigned angioplasty, two surgery); of these, three were lost (one angioplasty, two surgery) during the first year of follow-up. 195 (86%) of 228 patients assigned to bypass surgery and 216 (96%) of 224 to balloon angioplasty underwent an attempt at their allocated intervention at a median (IQR) of 6 (3–16) and 6 (2–20) days after randomisation, respectively. At the end of follow-up, 248 (55%) patients were alive without amputation (of trial leg; Fig 2), 38 (8%) alive with amputation, 36 (8%) dead after amputation, and 130 (29%) dead without amputation. After 6 months, the two strategies did not differ significantly in amputation-free survival (48 *vs* 60 patients; unadjusted hazard ratio 1.07, 95% CI 0.72–16; adjusted hazard ratio 0.73, 0.49–1.07). We saw no difference in health-related quality of life between the two strategies, but

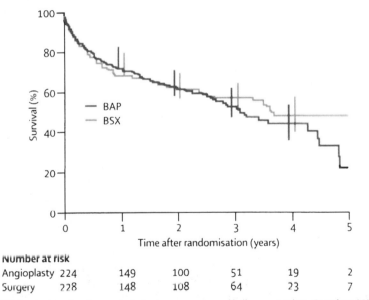

Number at risk						
Angioplasty	224	149	100	51	19	2
Surgery	228	148	108	64	23	7

FIGURE 2.—Amputation-free survival after bypass surgery and balloon angioplasty. Bars show 95% CIs for survival up to 1, 2, 3, and 4 years of follow-up, which were calculated from the cumulative hazards. (Reprinted by permission of the publisher from Bradbury AW, for the BASIL Trial Participants: Bypass versus angioplasty in severe ischaemia of the leg (BASIL): Multicentre, randomised controlled trial. *Lancet* 366:1925-1934, 2005. Copyright 2005 by Elsevier.)

for the first year the hospital costs associated with a surgery-first strategy were about one third higher than those with an angioplasty-first strategy.

Interpretation.—In patients presenting with severe limb ischaemia due to infra-inguinal disease and who are suitable for surgery and angioplasty, a bypass-surgery-first and a balloon-angioplasty-first strategy are associated with broadly similar outcomes in terms of amputation-free survival, and in the short-term, surgery is more expensive than angioplasty.

▶ This study raises a couple of interesting points. (1) It is very difficult to recruit for trials of critical limb ischemia. The audit data suggest less than 10% of the patients screened for the trial would be eligible for randomization. (2) In the short term, in patients who are suitable for both angioplasty or surgery, results are similar. Morbidity and expense are greater with surgery, but long-term, amputation-free survival may be improved by a surgery for strategy. Overall, the trial results would appear to be as expected. In the lower extremities there is a constant theme with respect to angioplasty and surgery. If short-term results are what matter, and the patient can be treated with either angioplasty or surgery, angioplasty is likely the preferred strategy. However, in patients with suitable anatomy and a reasonable life expectancy, surgery may be a better alternative, excepting more short-term morbidity as a price for greater long-term durability.

G. L. Moneta, MD

Midfoot Amputations Expand Limb Salvage Rates for Diabetic Foot Infections
Stone PA, Back MR, Armstrong PA, et al (Univ of South Florida, Tampa; Charleston Area Med Ctr, Charleston WV)
Ann Vasc Surg 19:805-811, 2005   9–23

The persistent high incidence of limb loss resulting from advanced forefoot tissue loss and infection in diabetic patients prompted an evaluation of transmetatarsal (TMA) and transtarsal/midfoot amputations in achieving foot salvage at our tertiary vascular practice. Over the last 8 years, 74 diabetic patients required 77 TMAs for tissue loss and/or infection. Twelve (16%) of the patients had a contralateral below-knee amputation (BKA) and 26% (*n* = 20) had dialysis-dependent renal failure. Thirty-five (45%) limbs had concomitant revascularization (bypass grafting or percutaneous transluminal angioplasty), 32 (42%) had arterial occlusive disease by noninvasive testing and/or arteriography but were not or could not be revascularized, and seven (13%) had normal hemodynamics. Patient factors, arterial testing, operative complications, operative mortality (<60 days), wound healing (at 90 days), limb salvage, functional status, and survival were evaluated during a mean follow-up of 20 months (range 3-48). Operative mortality was 5% (n = 4) after TMA and/or midfoot amputation. Although 32 TMAs initially healed (44%), six BKAs were required 5-38 months later. Of the 41 nonhealing TMAs (56%), progressive infection/tissue loss necessi-

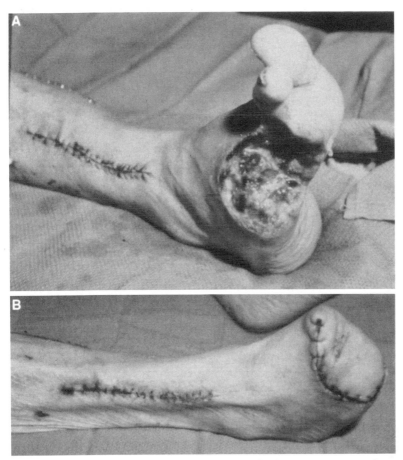

FIGURE 1.—A Open lateral TMA. **B** Use of medial-based skin flap for coverage. (Courtesy of Stone PA, Back MR, Armstrong PA, et al: Midfoot amputations expand limb salvage rates for diabetic foot infections. *Ann Vasc Surg* 19:805-811, 2005.)

tated major amputation of nine limbs. Chopart (*n* = 22) or Lisfranc (n = 10) midfoot amputations were done in the remaining 32 nonhealing TMAs. Despite additional wound revisions in 14 patients (44%), major amputation was needed in six limbs. However, functional ambulation was achieved in 23 of 25 (92%) limbs with healed midfoot amputations, and foot salvage was possible in 61% (25/41) of nonhealing TMAs. Overall limb salvage for TMA/midfoot procedures was estimated from Kaplan-Meier life tables to be 73%, 68%, and 62% at 1, 3, and 5 years, respectively, with only 50% of dialysis patients avoiding major amputation. Ankle pressure >100 mm Hg and a biphasic pedal waveform had a positive predictive value (PPV) of 79%, and toe pressure >50 mm Hg had a PPV of 91% for determining healing of TMA/midfoot amputations. One- and 3-year survival rates were only 72% and 69% for the entire cohort from life table estimates. Aggressive attempts at foot salvage are justified in diabetic patients with advanced forefoot tissue loss/infection after assuring adequate arterial perfusion. Transtarsal amputations salvaged over half of nonhealing TMAs with excellent functional results (Fig 1).

▶ Uncomplicated healing of forefoot amputations in the diabetic patient is infrequent, and despite successful healing recurrence rate is high. This study convincingly documents that a relatively high proportion of these failures may be salvaged with a midfoot amputation. The report, however, falls short in that there is limited documentation of the ambulatory status of these amputees. The real issue is whether patients are more functional with a below-knee prosthesis or a midfoot amputation. So far, there is no answer to this question.

S. A. Berceli, MD, PhD

Preoperative clinical factors predict postoperative functional outcomes after major lower limb amputation: An analysis of 553 consecutive patients

Taylor SM, Kalbaugh CA, Blackhurst DW, et al (Greenville Hosp System, SC; Clemson Univ, SC)

J Vasc Surg 42:227-235, 2005   9–24

Background.—Despite being a major determinant of functional independence, ambulation after major limb amputation has not been well studied.

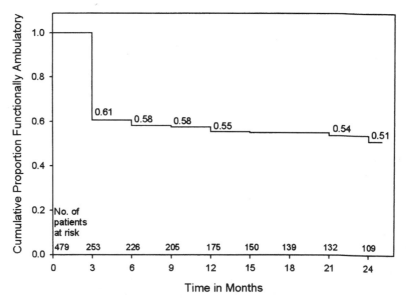

FIGURE 2.—Kaplan-Meier life tables showing overall maintenance of ambulation in a cohort of 533 consecutive lower limb amputees. (Reprinted by permission of the publisher from Taylor SM, Kalbaugh CA, Blackhurst DW, et al: Preoperative clinical factors predict postoperative functional outcomes after major lower limb amputation: An analysis of 553 consecutive patients. *J Vasc Surg* 42:227-235, 2005. Copyright 2005 by Elsevier.)

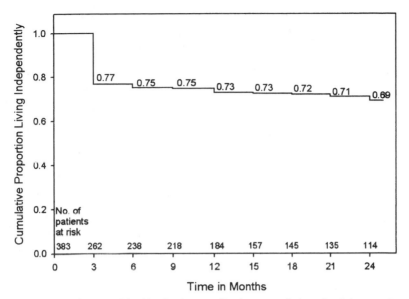

FIGURE 3.—Kaplan-Meier life tables showing overall maintenance of independent living status in a cohort of 533 consecutive lower limb amputees. (Reprinted by permission of the publisher from Taylor SM, Kalbaugh CA, Blackhurst DW, et al: Preoperative clinical factors predict postoperative functional outcomes after major lower limb amputation: An analysis of 553 consecutive patients *J Vasc Surg* 42:227-235, 2005. Copyright 2005 by Elsevier.)

The purpose, therefore, of this study was to investigate the relationship between a variety of preoperative clinical characteristics and postoperative functional outcomes in order to formulate treatment recommendations for patients requiring major lower limb amputation.

Methods.—From January 1998 through December 2003, 627 major limb amputations (37.6% below knee amputations, 4.3% through knee amputations, 34.5% above knee amputations, and 23.6% bilateral amputations) were performed on 553 patients. Their mean age was 63.7 years; 55% were men, 70.2% had diabetes mellitus, and 91.5% had peripheral vascular disease. A retrospective review was performed correlating various preoperative presenting factors such as age at presentation, race, medical comorbidities, preoperative ambulatory status, and preoperative independent living status, with postoperative functional endpoints of prosthetic usage, survival, maintenance of ambulation, and maintenance of independent living status. Kaplan-Meier survival curves were constructed and compared by using the log-rank test. Odds ratios (OR) and hazard ratios (HR) with 95% confidence intervals were constructed by using multiple logistic regressions and Cox proportional hazards models.

Results.—Statistically significant preoperative factors independently associated with not wearing a prosthesis in order of greatest to least risk were nonambulatory before amputation (OR, 9.5), above knee amputation (OR, 4.4), age >60 years (OR, 2.7), homebound but ambulatory status (OR, 3.0), presence of dementia (OR, 2.4), end-stage renal disease (OR, 2.3), and coronary artery disease (OR, 2.0). Statistically significant preoperative factors independently associated with death in decreasing order of influence included age ≥70 years (HR, 3.1), age 60 to 69 (HR, 2.5), and the presence of coronary artery disease (HR, 1.5). Statistically significant preoperative factors independently associated with failure of ambulation in decreasing order of influence included age ≥70 years (HR, 2.3), age 60 to 69 (HR, 1.6), bilateral amputation (HR, 1.8), and end-stage renal disease (HR, 1.4) (Fig 2). Statistically significant preoperative factors independently associated with failure to maintain independent living status in decreasing order of influence included age ≥70 years (HR, 4.0), age 60 to 69 (HR, 2.7), level of amputation (HR, 1.8), homebound ambulatory status (HR, 1.6), and the presence of dementia (HR, 1.6) (Fig 3).

Conclusions.—Patients with limited preoperative ambulatory ability, age ≥70, dementia, end-stage renal disease, and advanced coronary artery disease perform poorly and should probably be grouped with bedridden patients, who traditionally have been best served with a palliative above knee amputation. Conversely, younger healthy patients with below knee amputations achieved functional outcomes similar to what might be expected after successful lower extremity revascularization. Amputation in these instances should probably not be considered a failure of therapy but another treatment option capable of extending functionality and independent living.

▶ In support of our bias, this study demonstrates that a subset of patients facing major amputation are best served by primary above-knee amputation. In addition to the clearly bedridden individual, homebound patients with extensive renal or cardiac comorbidities were unlikely to ambulate with a prosthesis. While these concepts are not particularly new, the size of the dataset and the quantitative tools used for analysis provide significant insight. Elevating this study above the morass of published retrospective reports is the generation of an initial hypothesis and the prospective collection of data. The authors are to be commended.

S. A. Berceli, MD, PhD

The Impact of Immunological Parameters on the Development of Phantom Pain after Major Amputation
Stremmel C, Horn C, Eder S, et al (Friedrich Alexander Universität Erlangen-Nürnberg, Germany; Univ of Erlangen-Nürnberg, Erlangen, Germany)
Eur J Vasc Endovasc Surg 30:79-82, 2005   9–25

Objectives.—To investigate the relationship between local and systemic inflammatory markers and phantom limb pain.

Methods.—In 39 consecutive patients undergoing major amputations nerve biopsies, serum and clinical data was collected. Patients were followed up for 12 months to report on the incidence and severity of phantom limb pain.

Results.—After 12 months, 78% of the surviving patients had phantom pain, the symptom usually commencing within 14 days of operation. The severity of macrophage infiltration within the nerve biopsy was negatively correlated to the inception of phantom pain ($P = 0.026$). While serum TNF-alpha concentration was positively correlated to mortality ($P = 0.021$).

Conclusions.—The immune status existing before the amputation and the local immunological milieu influence the onset of phantom pain.

▶ With limited data and the absence of an underlying mechanistic hypothesis, it is difficult to draw any useful conclusions from this study. Treatment of phantom pain as a binary variable is oversimplistic, and the concept that leukocyte infiltration into the resected nerve affects phantom pain is suspect. Similarly, the usefulness of a single preoperative serum sample in providing insight into long-term survival after major amputation is limited. Overlying these issues is the fact that 16 statistical tests were performed, with 2 being significant just below the 0.05 level. In the absence of any correction for multiple testing, even these limited conclusions are dubious.

S. A. Berceli, MD, PhD

Popliteal Aneurysms: Distortion and Size Related to Symptoms
Galland RB, Magee TR (Royal Berkshire Hosp, Reading, England)
Eur J Vasc Endovasc Surg 30:534-538, 2005   9–26

Objectives.—To examine size and distortion of popliteal aneurysms (PA) in relation to symptoms produced at presentation.

Methods.—A prospective study of all PA presenting to a single unit 1988–1994. Wherever possible patients underwent angiography, duplex scanning and measurement of both PA diameter and the most proximal angle of distortion. Symptoms and measurements were noted at the time of first presentation (Fig 1).

Results.—Seventy-three patients presented with 116 PA. At initial diagnosis 44 PA (38%) were asymptomatic and 39 (34%) produced acute ischaemia. As the PA increased in diameter so did the degree of distortion ($p<0.0001$). Size and distortion were greater in PA producing acute ischaemia or acute thrombosis than in asymptomatic PA ($p<0.01$). Degree of distortion differentiated symptomatic from asymptomatic PA ($p=0.0066$). Size was not significantly different between these two groups. For PA 3 cm or larger in diameter with greater than 45° distortion sensitivity, specificity and positive and negative predictive values for thrombosis were 90, 89, 83 and 94%, respectively.

Conclusion.—Distortion and size can differentiate between PA producing different symptoms. Combining the two provides a reliable method of differentiating PA which should be managed by early elective repair.

▶ Not surprisingly, popliteal artery aneurysm diameter and proximal neck angle are closely correlated. In the absence of any multivariate analysis dem-

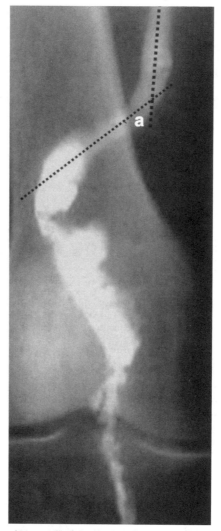

FIGURE 1.—Thrombosed PA partially cleared by thrombolysis. Distortion is shown. The most proximal angle of distortion (*a*) was measured. (Reprinted from Galland RB, Magee TR: Popliteal aneurysms: Distortion and size related to symptoms. *Eur J Vasc Endovasc Surg* 30:534-538, 2005, by permission of the publisher.)

onstrating neck distortion to be independently associated with the development of symptoms, conclusions from this report are limited. Couple this with the retrospective nature of the study, and it essentially eliminates any support for neck angle as a useful parameter in the clinical management of these patients. In the absence of prospective validation, this concept remains little more than curiosity.

S. A. Berceli, MD, PhD

Endovascular treatment of popliteal artery aneurysms: Results of a prospective cohort study
Tielliu IFJ, Verhoeven ELG, Zeebregts CJ, et al (Univ Med Ctr Groningen, The Netherlands)
J Vasc Surg 41:561-567, 2005   9–27

Objective.—Popliteal artery aneurysms can be treated endovascularly with less perioperative morbidity compared with open repair. To evaluate suitability of the endovascular technique and the clinical results of this treatment, we analyzed a prospective cohort of consecutive popliteal aneurysms referred to a tertiary university vascular center.

Methods.—All popliteal artery aneurysms between June 1998 and June 2004 that measured >20 mm in diameter were analyzed for endovascular repair. Anatomic suitability was based largely on quality of the proximal and distal landing zone as determined by angiography. Endovascular treatment was performed by using a nitinol-supported expanded polytetrafluoroethylene lined stent graft introduced through the common femoral artery.

Results.—We analyzed 67 aneurysms in 57 patients. Ten aneurysms (15%) were excluded from endovascular repair, or from any repair at all, for various reasons. The remaining 57 (85%) were treated endovascularly, of which 5 were treated emergently for acute ischemia. During a mean 24-month follow-up, 12 stent grafts (21%) occluded. Primary and secondary

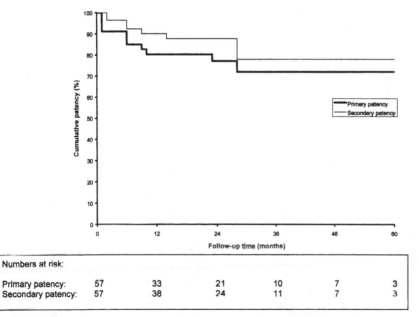

Numbers at risk:						
Primary patency:	57	33	21	10	7	3
Secondary patency:	57	38	24	11	7	3

FIGURE 1.—Cumulative primary and secondary patency rates. Standard errors ranged from 1.7% to 7.7% and from 1.8% to 7.8% for primary and secondary patency, respectively. (Reprinted by permission of the publisher from Tielliu IFJ, Verhoeven ELG, Zeebregts CJ, et al: Endovascular treatment of popliteal artery aneurysms: Results of a prospective cohort study. *J Vasc Surg* 41:561-567, 2005. Copyright 2005 by Elsevier.)

patency rates were 80% and 90% at 1 year, and 77% and 87% at 2 years of follow-up (Fig 1). Postoperative treatment with clopidogrel proved to be the only significant predictor for success.

Conclusions.—Endovascular repair of a popliteal artery aneurysm is feasible. Changes in the material used and the addition of clopidogrel may improve patency rates.

▶ This single study provides the largest experience detailing endovascular treatment of popliteal aneurysms. The investigators were aggressive. Over a 6-year period, 85% of the popliteal aneurysms undergoing repair were treated by stent grafting. Although limited essentially to 24-month follow-up, they demonstrate primary and secondary patency rates of 77% and 87%, respectively. Even though patency is less than can be expected from open repair, endograft performance is sufficiently durable to make it a reasonable treatment option in high-risk or limited-conduit patients. Subset analysis of these patients suggested clopidogrel to be an independent predictor for a successful long-term outcome.

S. A. Berceli, MD, PhD

Open repair versus endovascular treatment for asymptomatic popliteal artery aneurysm: Results of a prospective randomized study
Antonello M, Frigatti P, Battocchio P, et al (Univ of Padua, Italy)
J Vasc Surg 42:185-193, 2005   9–28

Purpose.—The aim of this prospective randomized study was to evaluate the relative risks and advantages of using the Hemobahn graft for popliteal artery aneurysm (PAA) treatment compared with open repair (OR). The primary end point was patency rate; secondary end points were hospital stay and length of surgical procedure.

Methods.—The study was a prospective, randomized clinical trial carried out at a single center from January 1999 to December 2003. Inclusion criteria were an aneurysmal lesion in the popliteal artery with a diameter ≥2 cm at the angio-computed tomography (CT) scan, and proximal and distal neck of the aneurysm with a length of >1 cm to offer a secure site of fixation of the stent graft. Exclusion criteria were age <50 years old, poor distal runoff, contraindication to antiplatelet, anticoagulant, or thrombolytic therapy, and symptoms of nerve and vein compression. The enrolled patients were thereafter prospectively randomized in a 1-to-1 ratio between OR (group A) or endovascular therapy (ET) (group B). The follow-up protocol consisted of duplex ultrasound scan and ankle-brachial index (ABI) measured during a force leg flexion at 1, 3, and 6 months. Group B patients underwent an angio-CT scan and plain radiography of the knee with leg flexion (>120°) at 6 and 12 months, and then yearly.

Results.—Between January 1999 and December 2003, 30 PAAs were performed: 15 OR (group A) and 15 ET (group B). Bypass and exclusion of the PAA was the preferred method of OR; no perioperative graft failure was ob-

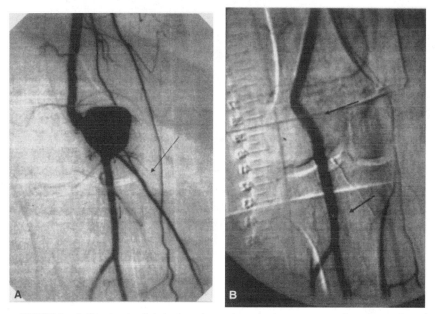

FIGURE 1.—A. Preoperative digital subtraction angiography demonstrates a collateral artery (*arrow*) originating from the aneurismal sack of the popliteal aortic aneurysm. **B.** Digital subtraction angiography after coil-embolization of the collateral vessel and endograft deployment (*arrows* point to endograft location). (Reprinted by permission of the publisher from Antonello M, Frigatti P, Battocchio P, et al: Open repair versus endovascular treatment for asymptomatic popliteal artery aneurysm: Results of a prospective randomized study. *J Vasc Surg* 42:185-193, 2005. Copyright 2005 by Elsevier.)

served. Twenty stent grafts were placed in 15 PAAs. Endograft thrombosis occurred in one patient (6.7%) in the postoperative period. The mean follow-up period was 46.1 months (range, 12 to 72 months) for group A and 45.9 months (range, 12 to 65 months) for group B Kaplan-Meier analysis showed a primary patency rate of 100% at 12 months for OR and 86.7% at 12 months with a secondary patency rate of 100% at 12 and 36 months for ET. No statistical differences were observed at the log-rank test. The mean operation time (OR, 155.3 minutes; ET, 75.4 minutes) and hospital stay (OR, 7.7 days; ET, 4.3 days) were statistically longer for OR compared with ET ($P < .01$).

Conclusion.—We can conclude, with the power limitation of the study, that PAA treatment can be safely performed by using either OR or ET. ET has several advantages, such as quicker recovery and shorter hospital stay (Fig 1).

▶ Initial reports detailing the early experience of endovascular popliteal aneurysm repair were mixed, calling for prospective evaluation of this issue. Although modest in enrollment, the current study nicely fills this void. Thirty patients with appropriate proximal and distal fixation sites and reasonable distal runoff were randomized between open and endovascular popliteal aneurysm repair. Results demonstrate primary patency rates of 86.7% and 100% at 36 months in the endovascular and open groups, respectively. While underpowered to show equivalency (approximately 300 patients would be required to power the study at the 0.80 level), this study firmly establishes endograft repair as a viable alternative for some patients.

S. A. Berceli, MD, PhD

The value of duplex surveillance after open and endovascular popliteal aneurysm repair
Stone PA, Armstrong PA, Bandyk DF, et al (Univ of South Florida, Tampa)
J Vasc Surg 41:936-941, 2005   9–29

Objective.—The objective of this study was to determine the clinical value of vascular laboratory surveillance after open or endovascular repair of popliteal aneurysm by analysis of the frequency and nature of secondary interventions performed.

Methods.—Over an 8-year period, 55 popliteal artery aneurysms were repaired in 46 men (mean age, 72 years) by aneurysm ligation and bypass grafting (vein, 37; prosthetic, 7), endoaneurysmorrhaphy and interposition grafting (prosthetic, 3; vein, 1), or endograft exclusion (n = 7). Indications for intervention included aneurysm thrombosis with critical limb ischemia (n = 8), symptomatic (n = 10) or asymptomatic (n = 37), >1.75 cm popliteal aneurysm with mural thrombus. Catheter-directed thrombolysis was used in three limbs to restore aneurysm and tibial artery patency before open repair. Duplex ultrasound surveillance was performed after repair to identify residual and acquired lesions. Life-table analysis was used to estimate repair site intervention-free (primary) and assisted-primary patency.

Results.—During a mean 20-month follow-up interval, 20 secondary procedures were performed in 18 (31%) limbs to repair duplex-detected graft stenosis (n = 10), repair site thrombosis (n = 5), vein graft aneurysm (n = 3), graft entrapment (n = 1), or type 1 endoleak (n = 1). Primary patency was 76% and 68% at 1 and 3 years, and was uninfluenced by tibial artery runoff status or type of bypass conduit. Open (n = 12) or endovascular (n = 8) secondary procedures were performed on 15 (12 vein, 3 prosthetic) bypass grafts, 2 endografts, and 1 interposition graft. Mean time to repair graft stenosis (11 months) was shorter than to repair of vein graft aneurysm (37 months). Assisted-primary patency was 93% and 88% at 1 and 3 years; redo bypass grafting was required and successful in five limbs. Limb salvage was 100%.

Conclusions.—One third of popliteal artery aneurysms repaired by open or endovascular procedures required a secondary intervention within 2 years of repair. Repair-site surveillance using duplex ultrasound was able to identify lesions that threaten patency, which resulted in excellent assisted patency and limb preservation rates when corrected.

▶ Trying to provide statistical validity to a retrospective study, the investigators present the outcomes for a mixed group of popliteal aneurysms repaired by open and endovascular techniques. Primary patency for this group was 68% at 3 years, somewhat below other contemporary series, but a significant number of potential failures were identified with duplex scanning prior to actual failure, yielding an assisted primary patency of 88% at 3 years. An important role for routine surveillance after popliteal aneurysm repair was therefore suggested. Useful conclusions from this study are limited. The authors appear to be creating a controversy where none exists. Few would argue that routine surveillance for vein graft pathology or aneurysm exclusion after endografting is justifiable. This study does little to support or challenge this approach.

S. A. Berceli, MD, PhD

10 Upper Extremity Ischemia

Selective use of ultrasonographic vascular mapping in the assessment of patients before haemodialysis access surgery
Wells AC, Fernando B, Butler A, et al (Addenbrooke's Hosp, Cambridge, England)
Br J Surg 92:1439-1443, 2005   10–1

Background.—Use of routine preoperative ultrasonography to determine the optimum site for haemodialysis access surgery increases the number of distal arteriovenous fistulas formed and improves overall patency rates. Nevertheless its use in all patients is time consuming and costly. This study examined whether clinical parameters could be used to determine the requirement for preoperative ultrasonography.

Methods.—Between March 2002 and October 2003, 145 consecutive patients were reviewed in the vascular access clinic. Patients were first assessed clinically, a site for vascular access surgery was proposed, and the need for radiological mapping studies recorded. A second, blinded, clinician determined the site for vascular access surgery using ultrasonography. The correlation between clinical and ultrasonographic findings was then examined.

Results.—Ultrasonography was considered unnecessary using clinical criteria in 106 patients. Subsequent ultrasonographic mapping altered the management of only one patient. In contrast, the management of 18 of the 39 patients in whom ultrasonography was thought necessary was influenced by radiological imaging. A 1-year primary patency rate of 77.0 per cent was achieved following vascular access surgery on the study population.

Conclusion.—Clinical parameters could be used to determine the need for preoperative vascular ultrasonographic mapping; imaging was not required in the majority of patients.

▶ All but 20 of the patients in this study had construction of either a radiocephalic or brachiocephalic fistula. The data suggest that when the cephalic vein is adequate clinically for construction of an autogenous fistula, preoperative US studies are unnecessary. Studies from the United States have suggested that preoperative US mapping can alter planned dialysis access surgery in up to 53% of patients.[1,2] Perhaps the demographics of the US population with the higher proportion of diabetic, obese, and black patients contribute to a greater reliance on preoperative imaging studies.

G. L. Moneta, MD

References

1. Silva MB Jr, Hobson RW II, Pappas PJ, et al: A strategy for increasing use of autogenous hemodialysis access procedures: Impact of noninvasive evaluation. *J Vasc Surg* 27:302-307, 1998.
2. Robbin ML, Gallichio MH, Deierhoi MH, et al: US vascular mapping before hemodialysis access placement. *Radiology* 217:83-88, 2000.

Vascular Access Stenosis: Comparison of Arteriovenous Grafts and Fistulas

Maya ID, Oser R, Saddekni S, et al (Univ of Alabama at Birmingham; Statistical Consulting of Montana, Bozeman)

Am J Kidney Dis 44:859-865, 2004   10–2

Background.—Vascular access stenosis is a frequent problem in hemodialysis patients. There is little published literature comparing the features of stenosis between arteriovenous fistulas and grafts, relative outcomes of elective angioplasty, and clinical factors predictive of access patency after angioplasty.

Methods.—Prospective data were collected for all patients referred for a fistulogram during a 2-year period because of suspected access stenosis. Angioplasty was performed if there was greater than 50% stenosis. For each procedure, we recorded the number and location of stenotic lesions, degree of stenosis (on a scale of 1 to 4), and ratio of access to systemic systolic pressure. All subsequent access procedures were tracked prospectively to calculate intervention-free access survival. Multivariable analysis was used to evaluate clinical factors affecting access patency after angioplasty.

Results.—Five hundred forty-three fistulograms were obtained: 358 in grafts and 185 in fistulas. The likelihood of finding a significant stenosis was substantially lower in fistulas than grafts (39.4% versus 68.7%; $P < 0.001$). Among patients with a significant stenosis, those with fistulas were less likely to have 2 or more stenotic lesions (12.5% versus 33.1%; $P < 0.001$). After angioplasty, degree of stenosis (1.35 ± 0.70 versus 1.23 ± 0.52) and access to systemic pressure ratio (0.34 ± 0.15 versus 0.32 ± 0.14) were similar between fistulas and grafts. Intervention-free survival was similar for fistulas and grafts (median survival, 7.5 versus 6.2 months; $P = 0.36$). Using multivariable stepwise proportional hazard regression analysis, only female sex, residual access stenosis, and postangioplasty access pressure ratio greater than 0.4 significantly predicted access survival ($P = 0.0006$).

Conclusion.—The positive predictive value of clinical evaluation for access stenosis is substantially lower for fistulas than grafts. The technical success of angioplasty and subsequent primary patency are similar for fistulas and grafts. Finally, female sex, residual stenosis, and high postprocedure ac-

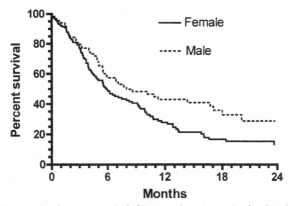

FIGURE 2.—Intervention-free access survival after angioplasty, comparing female (solid lines) with male patients (broken line). Analysis was restricted to the first angioplasty for each patient. $P = 0.02$ by log-rank test for the comparison between the 2 survival curves. (Courtesy of Maya ID, Oser R, Saddekni S, et al: Vascular access stenosis: Comparison of arteriovenous grafts and fistulas. *Am J Kidney Dis* 44:859-865, 2004. Copyright National Kidney Foundation.)

cess pressure ratio are each predictive of shorter access patency after elective angioplasty (Fig 2).

▶ Fistulas require fewer interventions than grafts to maintain patency. The current data, however, suggest that, once angioplasty is required, subsequent patency is no better for fistulas than for grafts. Once stenosis develops in a dialysis access, the prognosis for intervention-free access survival is poor, regardless if the access is synthetic or native.

G. L. Moneta, MD

Frequency of critical stenosis in primary arteriovenous fistulae before hemodialysis access: Should duplex ultrasound surveillance be the standard of care?
Grogan J, Castilla M, Lozanski L, et al (Univ of Chicago)
J Vasc Surg 41:1000-1006, 2005   10–3

Objective.—Increasing use of primary arteriovenous fistulae (pAVFs) is a desired goal in hemodialysis patients (National Kidney Foundation/Dialysis Outcome Quality Initiative guidelines). However, in many instances, pAVFs fail to adequately mature due to ill-defined mechanisms. We therefore investigated pAVFs with color duplex ultrasound (CDU) surveillance 4 to 12 weeks postoperatively to identify hemodynamically significant abnormalities that may contribute to pAVF failure.

Methods.—From March 2001 to October 2003, 54 upper extremity pAVFs were subjected to CDU assessment before access. A peak systolic velocity ratio (SVR) of ≥2:1 was used to detect ≥50% stenosis involving arterial inflow and venous outflow, whereas an SVR of ≥3:1 was used to detect

≥50% anastomotic stenosis. CDU findings were compared with preoperative vein mapping and postoperative fistulography when available.

Results.—Of 54 pAVFs, there were 23 brachiocephalic, 14 radiocephalic, and 17 basilic vein transpositions. By CDU surveillance, 11 (20%) were occluded and 14 (26%) were negative. Twenty-nine (54%) pAVFs had 38 hemodynamically significant CDU abnormalities. These included 16 (42%) venous outflow, 13 (34%) anastomotic, and 2 (5%) inflow stenoses. In seven (18%), branch steal with reduced flow was found. In 35 of 54 (65%) pAVFs, preoperative vein mapping was available and demonstrated adequate vein size (≥3 mm) and outflow in 86% of cases. Twenty-one fistulograms (38%) were available for verifying the CDU abnormalities. In each fistulogram, the arterial inflow, anastomosis, and venous outflow were compared with the CDU findings (63 segments). The sensitivity, specificity, and accuracy of CDU in detecting pAVF stenoses ≥50% were 93%, 94%, was 97%, respectively.

Conclusions.—Before initiation of hemodialysis, an unexpectedly high prevalence of critical stenoses was found in patent pAVFs using CDU surveillance. These de novo stenoses appear to develop rapidly after arterialization of the upper extremity superficial veins and can be reliably detected by CDU surveillance. Turbulent flow conditions in pAVFs may play a role in inducing progressive vein wall and valve leaflet intimal thickening, although stenoses may be due to venous abnormalities that predate AVF placement. Routine CDU surveillance of pAVFs should be considered to identify and correct flow-limiting stenoses that may compromise pAVF long-term patency and use.

▶ It is remarkable that three quarters of the native fistulas created in this study had a significant duplex detected "abnormality" or had occluded by 3 months postoperatively. Only 1 of 17 basilic vein transpositions did not have an "abnormality." Given the high prevalence of abnormalities detected in this study, and the assumption that the authors have a fistula maturation rate greater than 25%, one has to wonder if the author's criteria for "abnormalities" are too stringent. This, combined with the retrospective study design, incomplete use of fistulograms, and varying surgeons' approach to identified "abnormalities," along with incomplete use of preoperative vein mapping, make it difficult to derive any useful information from this article.

G. L. Moneta, MD

The timely construction of arteriovenous fistulae: a key to reducing morbidity and mortality and to improving cost management
Ortega T, Ortega F, Diaz-Corte C, et al (Hosp Universitario Central de Asturias, Oviedo, Spain; Inst Reina Sofia, Oviedo, Asturias, Spain)
Nephrol Dial Transplant 20:598-603, 2005   10–4

Background.—Some investigators have shown that the initial placement of a catheter or graft, instead of the timely construction of an arteriovenous fistula (AVF), late referral to nephrology services and unplanned dialysis increase morbidity and mortality in chronic haemodialysis (CHD) patients. Furthermore, a delay in providing an adequate AVF entails significant increases in treatment-related costs. This study was limited to the analysis of the effects of the lack of an adequate vascular access for CHD on morbidity and mortality.

Methods.—According to the vascular access they had in the first 3 months of CHD treatment 96 patients were divided into three groups (VA group): Group 1 (G1), having an adequate AVF in the first 3 months; Group 2 (G2), starting with a catheter but finishing with an AVF; and Group 3 (G3) starting and finishing with a catheter. Time-dependent Cox regression analysis was performed to identify variables associated with survival, and the standardized mortality index (SMI) was calculated. Finally, we studied cost-effectiveness.

Results.—Time-dependent Cox regression and logistic regression analyses showed the statistically significant variable to be the VA group. To ensure that mortality was comparable between VA groups, eliminating age bias, the findings were adjusted applying SMI. G1 patients appear to have a lesser risk of death (relative risk, 0.39) than G2 and G3 patients, as do G2 relative to G3 patients. Also, after adjustment with SMI, patients over 65 years, presumably at greater risk of death, have a lower mortality than the ≥ 65 age group. Patients with an adequate and functioning AVF lived longer than the others, and the cost of each 'death prevented' was lower (€3318/patient).

Conclusions.—The lack of an adequate AVF at the start of haemodialysis decreases survival significantly—even if patients are not diabetic, are referred to a nephrologist early and planned haemodialysis is initiated. It also increases the cost of each prevented death.

▶ It would be nice to blame the morbidity of dialysis access management on only the timing of creation of an AVF. Although starting dialysis with an AVF, intuitively, seems better than starting with a venous dialysis catheter, there are many variables that likely confound these data. These include coexisting vascular disease, varying blood flow rates, and other comorbidities that delay or limit creation of an AVF.

G. L. Moneta, MD

Autogenous radial-cephalic or prosthetic brachial-antecubital forearm loop AVF in patients with compromised vessels? A randomized, multicenter study of the patency of primary hemodialysis access
Rooijens PPGM, Burgmans JPJ, Yo TI, et al (Med Ctr Rijnmond Zuid, The Netherlands; Diakonessenhuis, The Netherlands; Erasmus Med Ctr, The Netherlands; et al)
J Vasc Surg 42:481-487, 2005   10–5

Background.—A properly functioning vascular access is vital for the survival of patients with end-stage renal disease in need of chronic intermittent

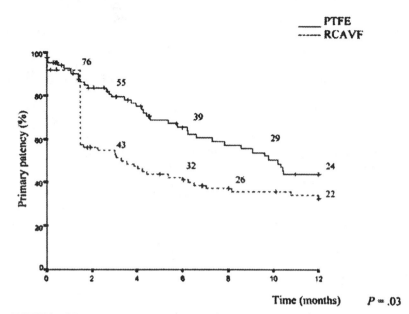

FIGURE 2.—Primary patency rates. Patency rate is shown in percentages and time in months. Number of patients is presented in the graph. *P* values calculated with the log-rank test. (Reprinted by permission of the publisher from Rooijens PPGM, Burgmans JPJ, Yo TI, et al: Autogenous radial-cephalic or prosthetic brachial-antecubital forearm loop AVF in patients with compromised vessels? A randomized, multicenter study of the patency of primary hemodialysis access. *J Vasc Surg* 42:481-487, 2005. Copyright 2005 by Elsevier.)

hemodialysis. The Kidney Dialysis Outcomes Quality Initiative and European guidelines for vascular access have proposed the construction of an autogenous radial-cephalic direct wrist arteriovenous fistula (RCAVF) as the primary and best option for these patients. However, studies have found that 10% to 24% of RCAVFs thrombose directly after operation or do not function adequately because of failure of maturation.

The outcomes for RCAVFs may be worse in patients with poor arterial or poor venous vessels, and in these patients an alternative vascular access is probably indicated. A prosthetic graft implant may be the second-best option. A multicenter study comparing RCAVF with polytetrafluoroethylene graft (a prosthetic graft) implantation for patients with poor vessels was presented.

Methods.—A randomized multicenter study was conducted among 383 consecutive new patients needing primary vascular access. Preoperative duplex scanning was used to allocate 140 patients to primary placement of an RCAVF and 61 patients to primary prosthetic graft implantation. The remaining 182 patients were randomly assigned to receive either an RCAVF (92 patients) or prosthetic graft implant (90 patient). The patency rate was defined as the percentage of arteriovenous fistulas (AVFs) that functioned well after implantation.

Results.—The primary and assisted primary 1-year patency rates were 33% ± 5.3% versus 44% ± 6.2% and 48% ± 5.5% versus 79% ± 5.1% for

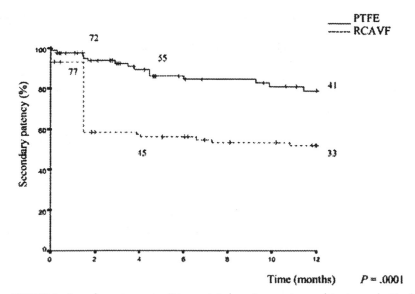

FIGURE 4.—Secondary patency rates. Patency rate is shown in percentages and time in months. Number of patients is presented in the graph. *P* values calculated with the log-rank test. (Reprinted by permission of the publisher from Rooijens PPGM, Burgmans JPJ, Yo TI, et al: Autogenous radial-cephalic or prosthetic brachial-antecubital forearm loop AVF in patients with compromised vessels? A randomized, multicenter study of the patency of primary hemodialysis access. *J Vasc Surg* 42:481-487, 2005. Copyright 2005 by Elsevier.)

the RCAVF and prosthetic AVF, respectively (Fig 2). Secondary patency rates were 52% ± 5.5% versus 79% ± 5.1% for the RCAVF and prosthetic AVF, respectively (Fig 4). Patients with RCAVFs had a total of 102 complications versus 122 complications for patients with prosthetic AVFs. A total of 43 interventions in the RCAVF group and 79 interventions in the prosthetic graft group were needed for access salvage.

Conclusions.—More interventions were required for patients in the prosthetic implant group, yet it appeared that patients with poor forearm vessels do derive some benefit from implantation of a prosthetic graft for vascular access.

▶ I always say that with respect to lower extremity arterial reconstruction, good vein is better than prosthetic but that prosthetic is better than bad vein. The same apparently holds true for construction of dialysis access.

G. L. Moneta, MD

Experience with Autogenous Arteriovenous Access for Hemodialysis in Children and Adolescents

Gradman WS, Lerner G, Mentser M, et al (Cedars-Sinai Med Ctr, Los Angeles; Children's Hosp, Los Angeles)

Ann Vasc Surg 19:609-612, 2005

10–6

The National Kidney Foundation's DOQI-NKF recommendation to construct an autogenous arteriovenous access (AAVA) for chronic hemodialysis whenever possible can be a challenge in the pediatric population. This report reviews recent surgical experience in this patient subgroup. From March 1999 to April 2004, 47 consecutive children requiring permanent vascular access had construction of AAVA. There were 16 girls and 31 boys, with a mean age of 14.6 years (range 5-20). The surgeon preoperatively mapped veins with ultrasound in all patients. Access sites were radial-cephalic ($n = 16$), upper arm brachial-cephalic ($n = 15$), transposed upper arm brachial-basilic ($n = 7$), and transposed femoral vein ($n = 9$). An operating microscope was used to construct three radial-cephalic accesses in individuals with small arteries. Three forearm cephalic veins were transposed (one at the original surgical procedure and two postoperatively). Five upper arm cephalic veins were transposed (three at the original surgical procedure and two postoperatively). Femoral vein accesses were constructed for either exhausted access in the upper extremities ($n = 7$) or patient preference ($n = 2$). Primary patency at 1 and 2 years was 100% and 96%, respectively. Secondary patency at 1 and 2 years was 100%. One individual with a radial-cephalic AAVA and severe radial artery calcification required an inflow procedure. Thirty-five accesses are currently in use (functionally patent), eight are in individuals with successful renal transplants, and two are maturing; one individual declines using the access. Two accesses are secondarily patent (thrombosed and repaired 12 and 29 months after construction, respectively), and one access thrombosed after 27 months (abandoned). Construction of an AAVA is possible in virtually all pediatric age individuals if attention is given to preoperative vein mapping, selective use of an operating microscope, and creation of a transposed femoral vein when upper extremity access is neither possible nor desired.

▶ Clearly, autogenous access in the pediatric population can be performed with outstanding results. Although vessels are smaller in children, it appears with proper surgical technique and planning and a willingness to transpose veins as necessary, durable long-term autogenous dialysis access can be provided in the pediatric population.

G. L. Moneta, MD

Femoral vein transposition for arteriovenous hemodialysis access: Improved patient selection and intraoperative measures reduce postoperative ischemia

Gradman WS, Laub J, Cohen W (Cedars Sinai Med Ctr, Los Angeles)
J Vasc Surg 41:279-284, 2005   10–7

Purpose.—Construction of prosthetic arteriovenous access for hemodialysis in the thigh results in a high incidence of graft failure and infection. Autogenous femoral artery-common femoral thigh transposition (transposed femoral vein [tFV]) arteriovenous accesses have superior patency, but our previous report documented a high incidence of ischemic events requiring secondary surgical intervention. Recent results of improved patient selection and intraoperative maneuvers to reduce ischemia are unknown.

Methods.—During a 6-year period eight children (mean age, 13.3 years) and 46 adults (mean age, 52.3 years; 27 female, 19 male) underwent construction of 55 tFV thigh accesses for hemodialysis access. Adult patients were divided into groups I and II on the basis of the introduction of specific

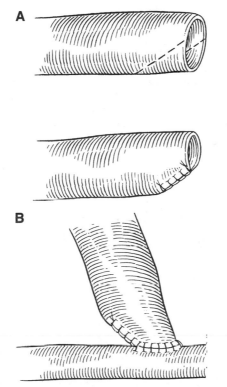

FIGURE 1.—In selected cases, the femoral vein is tapered to a 4.5- to 5.0- mm diameter (**A**) before implantation on the distal femoral artery (**B**). (Reprinted by permission of the publisher from Gradman WS, Laub J, Cohen W: Femoral vein transposition for arteriovenous hemodialysis access: Improved patient selection and intraoperative measures reduce postoperative ischemia. *J Vasc Surg* 41:279-284, 2005. Copyright 2005 by Elsevier.)

strategies to reduce the incidence of ischemic complications. In the cohort of children, steal prophylaxis included one banded femoral vein, three tapered femoral veins, two distal femoral artery pressure measurements taken before and after access construction (mean ratio, 0.70), and two closed anterior and superficial posterior compartment fasciotomies. Of the first 25 accesses in adults (group I, mean age, 55.9 years), 10 had access banding (six at the initial procedure and four in the immediate postoperative period to treat ischemia). Of the second 22 accesses (group II, mean age, 48.2 years), steal prophylaxis included 14 tapered femoral veins, 6 distal femoral artery pressure measurements (mean ratio, 0.76; range, 0.62 to 0.86), and 1 fasciotomy. Patients with significant distal occlusive disease were not offered a tFV access in the time frame of group II.

Results.—Eight accesses in children had 100% primary functional patency at 2 years, with no reoperations for ischemia. Nine group I adult patients underwent remedial procedures to correct distal ischemia. No adult patient in group II required a remedial procedure to correct ischemia. Groups I and II 2-year secondary functional access patency was 87% and 94%, respectively. There were no access infections in either group. Femoral vein tapering significantly reduced the need for remedial correction of ischemia ($P = .03$).

Conclusions.—Improved patient selection and selective intraoperative femoral vein tapering eliminated remedial procedures to correct ischemia in patients undergoing tFV access. Patency rates were excellent despite the liberal use of vein tapering. Transposed FV access should be considered for good risk individuals undergoing their first lower extremity access (Fig 1).

▶ By excluding patients with diminished ankle brachial indices and tapering the FV so the anastomosis to the artery was between 0.4 and 0.5 cm, the authors achieved excellent patency of tFV access without inducing arterial ischemia. Despite the increased magnitude of this procedure compared with that of a prosthetic lower-extremity access, the improved patency and lack of infectious complications make this a preferred access in properly selected patients. I would caution against using this type of access in obese patients. The length of the transposed vein available for cannulation will be too short unless a prosthetic component is added to lengthen the available vein to be brought to the surface.

G. L. Moneta, MD

Determinants of Failure of Brachiocephalic Elbow Fistulas for Haemodialysis

Zeebregts CJ, Tielliu IFJ, Hulsebos RG, et al (Univ Med Ctr Groningen, The Netherlands)

Eur J Vasc Endovasc Surg 30:209-214, 2005   10–8

Objectives.—The aim of this study was to analyse the results of brachiocephalic fistulas for haemodialysis and to determine possible predictors of failure.

Patients and Methods.—Between April 1999 and September 2004, a consecutive series of 100 autologous brachiocephalic fistulas were created in 96 patients. There were 57 men and 39 women with a mean (SD) age of 59.2 (15.6) years. Data were prospectively gathered.

Results.—The mean (SD) follow-up was 20.1 (16.4) months. The primary, primary assisted, and secondary patency rates after 6 months were 73.4, 83.2 and 86.4%, respectively. After 1 year, these figures were 54.7, 72.3 and 79.2%, and after 2 years 40.4, 59.2 and 67.5%, respectively. Predictors of failure with regard to primary patency, determined with Cox regression multivariate analysis, included diabetes mellitus (HR 2.81, p < 0.001) and a history of contralateral PTFE loop graft (HR 7.79, p = 0.007).

Conclusion.—Primary patency of brachiocephalic fistulas is comparable to that of radiocephalic fistulas. Primary assisted and secondary patency rates can, however, be brought to a much higher level, especially in patients without diabetes and a large-diameter venous outflow tract.

▶ Brachiocephalic fistulas provide excellent dialysis access. Articles such as this suggest meticulous follow-up of dialysis access, in particular, native fistulas, can result in significant increases in secondary patency. Aggressive monitoring and interventions for detected abnormalities are now widespread. In most but not all series, this results in improved overall patency of arteriovenous fistulas. (See also Abstracts 10–12 and 10–14.)

G. L. Moneta, MD

Hyperhomocysteinemia and Arteriovenous Fistula Thrombosis in Hemodialysis Patients

Mallamaci F, Bonanno G, Seminara G, et al (Instituto di Biomedicina, Epidemiologia Clinica e Fisiopatologia, Reggio Calabria, Italy; Univ of Cantania, Italy)

Am J Kidney Dis 45:702-707, 2005   10–9

Background.—To date, the relationship between vascular access (VA) failure and plasma total homocysteine level has been investigated only in mixed dialysis populations (ie, patients with a native arteriovenous [AV] fistula or arterial graft), whereas almost no data exist for hemodialysis patients with a native AV fistula.

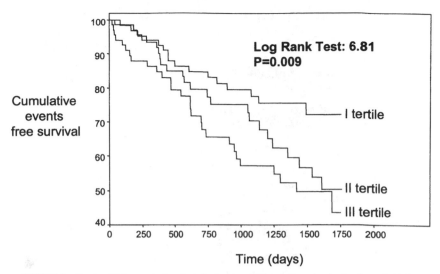

FIGURE 1.—Kaplan-Meier survival analysis for incident AV fistula thrombosis of patients divided into 3 tertiles according to individual levels of plasma total homocysteine. (Courtesy of Mallamaci F, Bonanno G, Seminara G, et al: Hyperhomocysteinemia and arteriovenous fistula thrombosis in hemodialysis patients. *Am J Kidney Dis* 45:702-707, 2005. Copyright National Kidney Foundation.)

Methods.—In this prospective cohort study, we examined the relationship between plasma total homocysteine level and the methylenetetrahydrofolate reductase (MTHFR) gene and VA-related incident morbidity in a cohort of 205 hemodialysis patients, all with a native AV fistula.

Results.—During follow-up, 78 patients experienced 1 or more VA thrombotic episodes. Patients with incident VA thrombosis had a significantly greater plasma total homocysteine level compared with patients without this event ($P = 0.046$). In Kaplan-Meier survival analysis, the hazard ratio for VA thrombosis increased in parallel with homocysteine level, such that patients in the third homocysteine level tertile had a relative risk for this outcome 1.72 times (95% CI, 1.21 to 2.24) greater than in those in the first tertile (log-rank test, 6.81; $P = 0.009$). In a multiple Cox regression model, plasma total homocysteine level was confirmed to be an independent predictor of AV fistula outcome. Plasma total homocysteine level was significantly greater ($P < 0.001$) in patients with the TT genotype of the MTHFR gene than in those with the CT or CC genotype.

Conclusion.—VA thrombosis in dialysis patients is associated with hyperhomocysteinemia. Intervention studies are needed to clarify whether decreasing plasma homocysteine concentrations may prevent VA failure in hemodialysis patients (Fig 1).

▶ There are many studies implicating increased homocysteine levels as a risk factor for atherothrombotic events, venous thrombosis, and now failure of native dialysis access. So far, however, intervention to lower homocysteine levels with folate and B12 supplementation has failed to decrease any vascular event associated with increased homocysteine levels. I doubt failure of dialysis access will be any different, but the study needs to be done. It certainly would be easy to give everyone a vitamin pill with their dialysis run.

G. L. Moneta, MD

Haemoglobin level and vascular access survival in haemodialysis patients

Garrancho JM, Kirchgessner J, Arranz M, et al (Fresenius Med Care Spain, Madrid; Fresenius Med Care Dentschland Gubh, Bad Homburg, Germany)
Nephrol Dial Transplant 20:2453-2457, 2005   10–10

Background.—A full correction of anaemia in haemodialysis (HD) patients may lead to an increased risk of vascular access (VA) failure. We studied the relationship between haemoglobin (Hb) level and VA survival.

Methods.—Incident patients between January 2000 and December 2002 with <1 month on HD were considered. The relative risk (RR) of access failure was evaluated in four different groups of patients divided according to their Hb level (<10, 10-12, 12-13 and >13 g/dl). Other factors possibly influencing VA survival were also considered: age, gender, diabetes, vascular disease, intact parathyroid hormone (iPTH) and treatment with an angiotensin-converting enzyme (ACE) inhibitor, angiotensin receptor blocker (ARB) or recombinant human erythropoietin therapy.

Results.—We studied 1254 patients (1057 with autologous fistulae, 75 grafts and 122 permanent catheters at admission). Based on Cox analysis, we found the next statistically significant RR of VA failure to be 2.3 times higher with grafts than with arterio-venous fistulae (AVFs) and 1.8 times higher in AVFs with Hb <10 g/dl than in AVFs of the next Hb group. There was no statistically significant difference in the RR of VA failure between patients with Hb 10-12 g/dl and those with Hb 12-13 g/dl or >13 g/dl. Diabetes (RR: 1.41, $P = 0.06$), age >65 years (RR: 1.32; $P = 0.11$) and iPTH (RR: 1.56; $P = 0.01$) were identified as predictive factors for VA failure; ACE inhibitors or ARB (RR: 0.69; $P = 0.03$) were found to be protective factors.

Conclusions.—In the studied population, the correction of Hb level to >12 g/dl was not associated with a higher incidence of VA thrombosis than in patients with Hb between 10 and 12 g/dl. ACE inhibitors or ARBs were found to be protective factors, and diabetes, age >65 years and iPTH >400 pg/ml were negative predictive factors for VA survival.

▶ This is an important study. Dialysis patients feel better with higher Hb levels. This study indicates preservation of dialysis access is no reason to keep Hb levels low. This may translate into nephrologists being willing to be more aggressive with erythropoietin therapy in patients with dialysis-dependent chronic renal failure. This should translate into better quality of life for the dialysis patient.

G. L. Moneta, MD

Colour Doppler ultrasound assessment of well-functioning arteriovenous fistulas for haemodialysis access

Pietura R, Janczarek M, Zaluska W, et al (Univ Med School of Lublin, Poland)
Eur J Radiol 55:113-119, 2005   10–11

Background.—A well-functioning mature arteriovenous fistula is essential for the maintenance of haemodialysis in patients with chronic renal failure. The Brescia-Cimino arteriovenous fistula has the best survival characteristics and low rate of complications. The most common reason of fistula failure is thrombosis caused by stenosis. Colour Doppler ultrasonography has proven to be effective in the assessment of anatomical vascular features. The majority of studies were done in patients with clinically presumed arteriovenous fistula complications. However, only limited data are available about the well-functioning mature arteriovenous fistulas. The purpose of the present study was to evaluate completely asymptomatic, mature arteriovenous fistulas with colour Doppler ultrasound.

Materials and Methods.—From July 2001 to April 2003, we examined 139 patients with the end-stage renal disease. They were in the range of 19-79 years of age (mean, 46.7 years). The study included only the patients who met the following criteria: (1) no difficulties with haemodialysis (as reported by nurses); (2) normal venous diastolic blood pressure (<150 mmHg) at monthly evaluation; (3) normal urea clearance × time/urea volume of distribution; (4) blood cells count, plasma electrolytes, and liver function at monthly evaluation. The mean fistula age was 26 months (S.D.=21.9). The mean time of dialysis therapy was 49 months. Thirty-eight percent patients had primary fistulas, 23%—secondary, 11%—third and 11%—fourth, 4%—fifth, 5%—sixth, and 8% patients had more than sixth.

Results.—There was no correlation between: (1) patient's age and fistula age; (2) patient's age and number of fistulas in one patient; (3) fistula age and number of fistulas in one patient; (4) localization of fistula and fistula age. There was a strong correlation between dialysis therapy period and number of fistulas in one patient. The mean flow volume was 1204.1 ml/min (S.D.=554). It was significantly higher in the fistulas with aneurysms, calcifications and tortuous vessels and lower in those with stenosis. There was no correlation between the flow volume or presence of stenosis and fistula age. Stenosis was detected in 64% fistulas. Fifty-seven percent of stenoses were located in the anastomotic region, 22% stenoses were in vein junction, 19% were at one or both ends of aneurysm, and 2% in the remaining region of the efferent vein. Perivascular colour artefacts were present at the 94% fistulas with stenosis. Chronic venous occlusion with collateral veins was detected in 6% of fistulas. The aneurysms were observed in 54% fistulas. The mean diameter of aneurysms was 12.4 mm. Ninety-six percent of aneurysms were located at puncture sites. Ten patients had a small thrombus in an aneurysm and at puncture sites.

Conclusions.—We conclude that there was a high level of abnormalities present in well-functioning mature arteriovenous fistulas. However, these

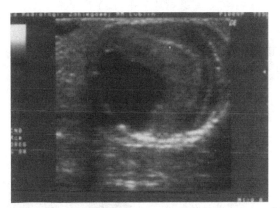

FIGURE 6.—Ultrasound images of thrombus in vein. (Reprinted by permission of the publisher from Pietura R, Janczarek M, Zaluska W, et al: Colour Doppler ultrasound assessment of well-functioning mature arteriovenous fistulas for haemodialysis access. *Eur J Radiol* 55:113-119, 2005. Copyright 2005 by Elsevier.)

abnormalities were not sufficient to affect the functioning of the dialysis fistula (Fig 6).

▶ If one looks for abnormalities, one can find them. Unfortunately, this study indicates one cannot determine those which are important; that is, which ones threaten the patency of the vascular access. Overall, dialysis access surveillance with color duplex is controversial for identifying lesions that threaten vascular access patency. This is another study adding to the controversy. (See also Abstracts 10–9 and 10–14.)

G. L. Moneta, MD

Stenosis detection in failing hemodialysis access fistulas and grafts: Comparison of color Doppler ultrasonography, contrast-enhanced magnetic resonance angiography, and digital subtraction angiography

Doelman C, Duijm LEM, Liem YS, et al (Catharina Hosp, Eindhoven, The Netherlands; Erasmus MC-Univ Med Ctr, Rotterdam, The Netherlands)
J Vasc Surg 42:739-746, 2005   10–12

Objective.—Several imaging modalities are available for the evaluation of dysfunctional hemodialysis shunts. Color Doppler ultrasonography (CDUS) and digital subtraction angiography (DSA) are most widely used for the detection of access stenoses, and contrast-enhanced magnetic resonance angiography (CE-MRA) of shunts has recently been introduced. To date, no study has compared the value of these three modalities for stenosis detection in dysfunctional shunts. We prospectively compared CDUS and CE-MRA with DSA for the detection of significant (≥50%) stenoses in failing dialysis accesses, and we determined whether the interventionalist would benefit from CDUS performed before DSA and endovascular intervention.

Methods.—CDUS, CE-MRA, and DSA were performed of 49 dysfunctional hemodialysis arteriovenous fistulas and 32 grafts. The vascular tree of

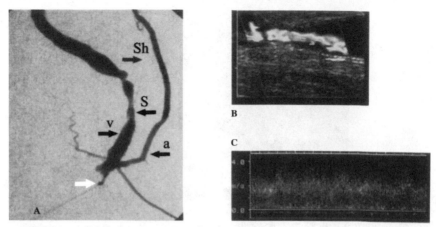

FIGURE 3.—A digital subtraction angiography (DSA) image (**A**) shows the introduction of a sheath (*Sh*) at the location of stenosis (*S*) in the venous outflow of an arteriovenous fistula. DSA was complicated by leakage of contrast (*white arrow*) through the puncture site of a previous hemodialysis. A color Doppler ultrasonography image at the area of narrowing shows a more than 50% diameter reduction of the fistula (**B**) in combination with spectral broadening due to turbulent flow and increased peak systolic velocity (**C**). *a,* Artery; *v,* vein. (Reprinted by permission of the publisher from Doelman C, Duijm LEM, Liem YS, et al: Stenosis detection in failing hemodialysis access fistulas and grafts: Comparison of color Doppler ultrasonography, contrast-enhanced magnetic resonance angiography, and digital subtraction angiography. *J Vasc Surg* 42:739-746, 2005. Copyright 2005 by Elsevier.)

the accesses was divided into three to eight segments depending on the access type (arteriovenous fistula or arteriovenous graft) and the length of venous outflow. CDUS was performed and assessed by a vascular technician, whereas CE-MRA and DSA were interpreted by two magnetic resonance radiologists and two interventional radiologists, respectively. All readers were blinded to information from each other and from other studies. DSA was used as reference standard for stenosis detection.

Results.—DSA detected 111 significant ($\geq$50%) stenoses in 433 vascular segments. Sensitivity and specificity of CDUS for the detection of significant stenosed vessel segments were 91% (95% CI, 84%-95%) and 97% (95% CI, 94%-98%), respectively. We found a positive predictive value of 91% (95% CI, 84%-95%) and a negative predictive value of 97% (95% CI, 94%-98%). The sensitivity, specificity, positive predictive value, and negative predictive value of MRA were 96% (95% CI, 90%-98%), 98% (95% CI, 96%-99%), 94% (95% CI, 88%-97%), and 98% (95% CI, 96%-99%), respectively. CDUS and CE-MRA depicted respectively three and four significant stenoses in six nondiagnostic DSA segments. The interventionalist would have chosen an alternative cannulation site in 38% of patients if the CDUS results had been available.

Conclusions.—We suggest that CDUS be used as initial imaging modality of dysfunctional shunts, but complete access should be depicted at DSA and angioplasty to detect all significant stenoses eligible for intervention. CE-MRA should be considered only if DSA is inconclusive (Fig 3).

▶ Bottom line: color duplex US alone is not sufficient to plan revision of failing access grafts, and angiography is required. MRA will be only rarely necessary. Color duplex US, however, may help plan the approach to a catheter-based revision of a failing access graft. The contrast study remains necessary to identify all lesions.

G. L. Moneta, MD

Monthly access flow monitoring with increased prophylactic angioplasty did not improve fistula patency
Shahin H, Reddy G, Sharafuddin M, et al (Univ of Iowa, Iowa City)
Kidney Int 68:2352-2361, 2005   10–13

Background.—Regular access monitoring is recommended to detect and treat access stenosis in order to prevent access thrombosis and failure.

Methods.—In 1999, we instituted monthly access blood flow monitoring using the ultrasound dilution technique (UDT). In a sequential observational trial, 222 patients were studied for the impact of UDT monitoring on patency of their first arteriovenous autogenous fistula. Group 1, the historic group (before 1999), had 146 arteriovenous fistulas (50.7% upper arm), followed for 259 access-years. Group 2, the UDT-monitored group, had 76 arteriovenous fistulas (60.5% upper arm), followed for 123 access-years. De-

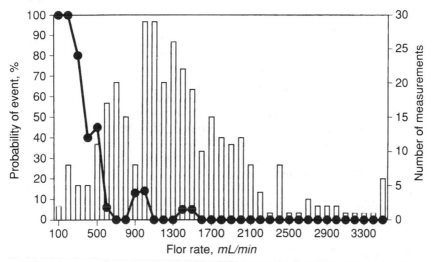

FIGURE 1.—Probability of an adverse access event within 1 month of the reported ultrasound dilution technique (UDT) measured flow rate. These data were collected during a 10-month prestudy observation period prior to January 1999, in which UDT flow monitoring was performed but the data were not provided to the dialysis physicians not used to direct access management. A total of 321 monthly flow measurements were obtained on 42 subjects (nine grafts and 33 fistulas). All access events (i.e., thrombosis, angioplasty, or surgery for stenosis) were recorded and linked to the preceding monthly flow measurement. The solid line shows the percent probability of an adverse event; the bars represent the number of measurements at each UDT measured flow. (Courtesy of Shahin H, Reddy G, Sharafuddin M, et al: Monthly access flow monitoring with increased prophylactic angioplasty did not improve fistula patency. *Kidney Int* 68:2352-2361, 2005. Reprinted by permission of Blackwell Publishing.)

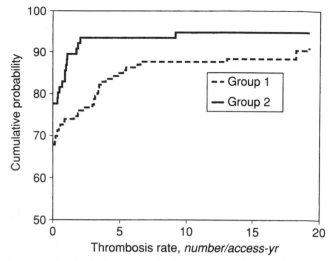

FIGURE 2.—Cumulative distribution function for thrombosis rate. The graph plots the cumulative probability of having a thrombosis rate at or below the rate shown on the horizontal access. The thrombosis rates are expressed as number of events per access-year per patient starting from the time of fistula placement until fistula failure, death, transplant, or transfer out of the unit or the end of the study. The thrombosis rates were higher in group 1 compared to group 2. However only 23% of group 2 and 33% of group 1 patients had any thrombosis over the life of their fistula. Note that the cumulative probability axis is truncated at 0.5 for thrombosis. (Courtesy of Shahin H, Reddy G, Sharafuddin M, et al: Monthly access flow monitoring with increased prophylactic angioplasty did not improve fistula patency. *Kidney Int* 68:2352-2361, 2005. Reprinted by permission of Blackwell Publishing.)

cision to refer for angiography was based on clinical criteria for group 1, and clinical criteria plus results of UDT flow monitoring in group 2.

Results.—Cumulative patency was longer ($P < 0.01$) and the thrombosis rate was lower ($P < 0.05$) in group 2. However, the improvement occurred prior to initiation of UDT flow monitoring. Comparing outcomes in group 2 patients whose fistula survived to start flow monitoring with group 1 patients whose fistula survived at least 160 days (the median time to starting UDT monitoring in group 2), there was a sevenfold increase in angioplasty procedures (0.67 vs. 0.09 per access-year) but no improvement in the thrombosis rate or cumulative fistula patency.

Conclusion.—UDT monitoring increased the rate of angioplasty procedures and thereby shortened primary unassisted patency, but did not decrease the thrombosis rate or improve cumulative fistula patency (Figs 1 and 2).

▶ This study and another recent study[1] do not justify sequentially monitoring of dialysis access fistulas or grafts, at least with the monitoring techniques used. Others are more optimistic. (See also Abstracts 10–9 and 10–12.) There is clearly no consensus on this topic.

G. L. Moneta, MD

Reference

1. Dember LM, Holmberg EF, Kaufman JS: Randomised controlled trial of prophylactic repair of hemodialysis arteriovenous graft stenosis. *Kidney Int* 66:390-398, 2004.

Central venous stenosis in haemodialysis patients without a previous history of catheter placement

Oguzkurt L, Tercan F, Yildirim S, et al (Baskent Univ, Adana, Turkey)
Eur J Radiol 55:237-242, 2005   10–14

Objective.—To evaluate dialysis history, imaging findings and outcome of endovascular treatment in six patients with central venous stenosis without a history of previous catheter placement.

Material and Methods.—Between April 2000 and June 2004, six (10%) of 57 haemodialysis patients had stenosis of a central vein without a previous central catheter placement. Venography findings and outcome of endovascular treatment in these six patients were retrospectively evaluated. Patients were three women (50%) and three men aged 32-60 years (mean age: 45 years) and all had massive arm swelling as the main complaint. The vas-

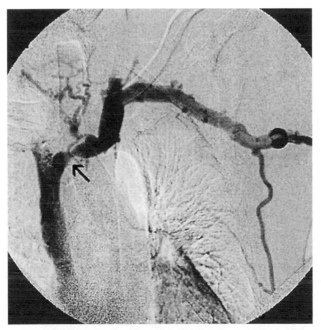

FIGURE 3.—60-year-old male with a brachiocephalic fistula. (A) Venography shows focal narrowing of the left brachiocephalic vein (arrow) with a few collaterals. (Reprinted by permission of the publisher from Oguzkurt L, Tercan F, Yildirim S, et al: Central venous stenosis in haemodialysis patients without a previous history of catheter placement. *Eur J Radiol* 55:237-242, 2005. Copyright 2005 by Elsevier.)

cular accesses were located at the elbow in five patients and at the wrist in one patient.

Results.—Three patients had stenosis of the left subclavian vein and three patients had stenosis of the left brachiocephalic vein. The mean duration of the vascular accesses from the time of creation was 25.1 months. Flow volumes of the vascular access were very high in four patients who had flow volume measurement. The mean flow volume was 2347 ml/min. One of three patients with brachiocephalic vein stenosis had compression of the vein by the brachiocephalic artery. All the lesions were first treated with balloon angioplasty and two patients required stent placement on long term. Number of interventions ranged from 1 to 4 (mean: 2.1). Symptoms resolved in five patients and improved in one patient who had a stent placed in the left BCV.

Conclusion.—Central venous stenosis in haemodialysis patients without a history of central venous catheterization tends to occur or be manifested in patients with a proximal permanent vascular access with high flow rates. Balloon angioplasty with or without stent placement offers good secondary patency rates in mid-term (Fig 3).

▶ All of the patients in this study were symptomatic with significant arm swelling. The abstract implies the central lesions are due to high flow rates secondary to the access. It is also possible that the central lesions were already there before the access was placed and only became manifest when the dialysis access flow rates increased over time. I still don't think visualization of central veins prior to placement of first-time access in a patient without previous central venous catheters should be routine. That approach is not likely to be cost effective.

G. L. Moneta, MD

Durability of percutaneous transluminal angioplasty for obstructive lesions of proximal subclavian artery: Long-term results

de Vries J-PPM, Jager LC, van den Berg JC, et al (St Antonius Hosp, Nieuwegein, The Netherlands)
J Vasc Surg 41:19-23, 2005   10–15

Purpose.—Percutaneous transluminal angioplasty (PTA) is one of the treatment options for localized obstruction of the subclavian artery. To document long-term durability of this kind of PTA we report a 10-year single-center experience in 110 patients.

Methods.—From January 1993 to July 2003, 110 patients (72 women; mean age, 62 ± 10 years) underwent PTA of symptomatic (>75%) stenosis (n = 90) or occlusion of the proximal subclavian artery (84 left-sided). Forty one patients (37%) had symptoms of vertebrobasilar insufficiency, 29 patients (26%) had disabling chronic arm ischemia, and 20 patients had both symptoms. Twenty patients with coronary artery disease underwent PTA in preparation for myocardial revascularization with the internal mammary artery. Duplex scans and arteriograms confirmed significant stenosis or oc-

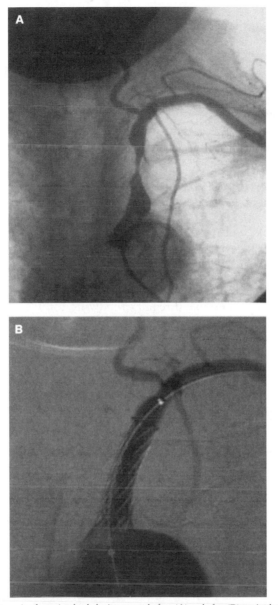

FIGURE 1.—Stenosis of proximal subclavian artery before (A) and after (B) angioplasty with additional stent placement via transfemoral route. (Reprinted by permission of the publisher from de Vries J-PPM, Jager LC, van den Berg JC, et al: Durability of percutaneous transluminal angioplasty for obstructive lesions of proximal subclavian artery: Long-term results. *J Vasc Surg* 41:19-23, 2005. Copyright 2005 by Elsevier.)

clusion. All PTA procedures were performed with the patient under local anesthesia, through the femoral artery (n = 89), brachial artery (n = 6), or combined route (n = 15). In 59 patients (58%) an additional stent was placed.

Results.—Angioplasty was initially technically and clinically successful in 102 patients (93%). Seven occlusions could not be recanalized, and 1 procedure had to be stopped because of ischemic stroke. Of the 102 patients in whom treatment was successful, 1 patient (1%) had a minor stroke in the contralateral hemisphere 2 hours post-PTA. Seven patients (7%) had minor problems, all without permanent sequelae. Follow-up with duplex scanning ranged from 3 months to 10 years (mean, 34 months). Primary clinical patency at 5 years was 89%, with a median recurrent obstruction-free period of 23 months. The local complication rate was 4.5%, and the combined stroke and death rate was 3.6%. Significant recurrent obstruction (>70%) developed in 8 patients with clinical symptoms. Four stenoses were successfully treated with repeat PTA (2 with additional stent placement); 4 occlusions required surgery.

Conclusions.—PTA of obstructive lesions of the proximal subclavian artery is not only an effective initial treatment, but is also successful over the long-term. Inasmuch as all clinical failures occurred within 26 months after initial therapy, we recommend regular follow-up for at least 2 years post-PTA. All clinically significant recurrent stenoses can be treated with repeat endovascular procedures. We could not prove positive or negative influence of additional placement of stents; however, the number of recurrent stenoses might be too small in this retrospective study to draw firm conclusions. Adverse events of any kind are certainly no greater than with invasive surgical procedures. Therefore PTA must be seriously considered in patients with localized obstruction of the proximal subclavian artery (Figs 1 and 2).

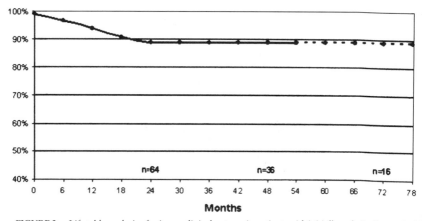

FIGURE 2.—Life table analysis of primary clinical patency in patients with initially technically successful percutaneous transluminal angioplasty of subclavian artery. (Reprinted by permission of the publisher from de Vries J-PPM, Jager LC, van den Berg JC, et al: Durability of percutaneous transluminal angioplasty for obstructive lesions of proximal subclavian artery: Long-term results. *J Vasc Surg* 41:19-23, 2005. Copyright 2005 by Elsevier.)

▶ The authors are treating a lot of subclavian lesions, probably too many. The main message is that PTA of a stenotic subclavian artery is a good technical procedure with good long-term durability. The idea of also trying to dilate occluded lesions because it may work (65% technical success) is a matter of philosophy. The authors dance around the issue of indications for their procedures and indicate in their discussion that half the patients they see with subclavian stenoses were treated. Perhaps this reflects referral patterns. But I doubt if even 10% of the patients I see with subclavian stenosis require any sort of procedure.

G. L. Moneta, MD

11 Carotid and Endovascular Disease

Association Between Carotid Plaque Characteristics and Subsequent Ischemic Cerebrovascular Events: A Prospective Assessment With MRI—Initial Results

Takaya N, Yuan C, Chu B, et al (Univ of Washington, Seattle; Juntendo Univ, Tokyo; Mountain-Whisper-Light Statistical Consulting, Seattle; et al)

Stroke 37:818-823, 2006   11–1

Background and Purpose.—MRI is able to quantify carotid plaque size and composition with good accuracy and reproducibility and provides an opportunity to prospectively examine the relationship between plaque features and subsequent cerebrovascular events. We tested the hypothesis that the characteristics of carotid plaque, as assessed by MRI, are possible predictors of future ipsilateral cerebrovascular events.

Methods.—A total of 154 consecutive subjects who initially had an asymptomatic 50% to 79% carotid stenosis by ultrasound with ≥12 months of follow-up were included in this study. Multicontrast-weighted carotid MRIs were performed at baseline, and participants were followed clinically every 3 months to identify symptoms of cerebrovascular events.

Results.—Over a mean follow-up period of 38.2 months, 12 carotid cerebrovascular events occurred ipsilateral to the index carotid artery. Cox regression analysis demonstrated a significant association between baseline MRI identification of the following plaque characteristics and subsequent symptoms during follow-up: presence of a thin or ruptured fibrous cap (hazard ratio, 17.0; $P \geq 0.001$), intraplaque hemorrhage (hazard ratio, 5.2; $P=0.005$), larger mean intraplaque hemorrhage area (hazard ratio for 10 mm2 increase, 2.6; $P=0.006$), larger maximum %lipid-rich/necrotic core (hazard ratio for 10% increase, 1.6; $P=0.004$), and larger maximum wall thickness (hazard ratio for a 1-mm increase, 1.6; $P=0.008$).

Conclusions.—Among patients who initially had an asymptomatic 50% to 79% carotid stenosis, arteries with thinned or ruptured fibrous caps, intraplaque hemorrhage, larger maximum %lipid-rich/necrotic cores, and larger maximum wall thickness by MRI were associated with the occurrence of subsequent cerebrovascular events. Findings from this prospective study provide a basis for larger multicenter studies to assess the risk of plaque features for subsequent ischemic events.

▶ This is the type of paper we need. Articles such as this one represent the second phase of determining which patients with asymptomatic carotid plaques will most likely benefit from prophylactic carotid interventions. Initial studies were all retrospective. Prospective studies are thankfully now appearing. The data here are extremely interesting and potentially highly clinically significant if larger multicenter studies can validate measurements of plaque characteristics as predictive of which asymptomatic carotid plaques truly place the patient at risk for an ipsilateral neurologic event.

G. L. Moneta, MD

Carotid Atherosclerotic Plaque Characteristics Are Associated With Microembolization During Carotid Endarterectomy and Procedural Outcome
Verhoeven BAN, de Vries JPPM, Pasterkamp G, et al (Univ Med Centre, Utrecht, The Netherlands; St Antonius Hosp, Nieuwegein, The Netherlands; Interuniv Cardiology Inst of the Netherlands, Utrecht)
Stroke 36:1735-1740, 2005   11–2

Background and Purpose.—During carotid endarterectomy (CEA), microemboli may occur, resulting in perioperative adverse cerebral events. The objective of the present study was to investigate the relation between atherosclerotic plaque characteristics and the occurrence of microemboli or adverse events during CEA.

Methods.—Patients (n=200, 205 procedures) eligible for CEA were monitored by perioperative transcranial Doppler. The following phases were discriminated during CEA: dissection, shunting, release of the clamp, and wound closure. Each carotid plaque was stained for collagen, macrophages, smooth muscle cells, hematoxylin, and elastin. Semiquantitative analyses were performed on all stainings. Plaques were categorized into 3 groups based on overall appearance (fibrous, fibroatheromatous, or atheromatous).

Results.—Fibrous plaques were associated with the occurrence of more microemboli during clamp release and wound closure compared with atheromatous plaques ($P=0.04$ and $P=0.02$, respectively). Transient ischemic attacks and minor stroke occurred in 5 of 205 (2.4%) and 6 of 205 (2.9%) patients, respectively. Adverse cerebral outcome was significantly related to the number of microembolic events during dissection ($P=0.003$) but not during shunting, clamp release, or wound closure. More cerebrovascular adverse events occurred in patients with atheromatous plaques (7/69) compared with patients with fibrous or fibroatheromatous plaques (4/138) ($P=0.04$).

Conclusions.—Intraoperatively, a higher number of microemboli were associated with the presence of a fibrous but not an atheromatous plaque.

However, atheromatous plaques were more prevalent in patients with subsequent immediate adverse events. In addition, specifically the number of microemboli detected during the dissection phase were related to immediate adverse events.

▶ "Vulnerable" plaque may be a better predictor of stroke risk than stenosis alone in patients treated medically, surgically, or endoluminally. This study confirms our suspicion of worse outcomes after CEA for atheromatous plaques. It also emphasizes that it is the dissection portion of the procedure, not shunting, clamp release, or wound closure, that is the time of greatest risk for adverse neurologic outcome.

M. K. Eskandari, MD

Soluble CD40L and cardiovascular risk in asymptomatic low-grade carotid stenosis
Novo S, Basili S, Tantillo R, et al (Univ of Palermo, Italy; Univ of Rome "La Sapienza"; Univ of Chieti, Italy)
Stroke 36:673-675, 2005   11–3

Background and Purpose.—We investigated whether soluble CD40L (sCD40L) may predict the risk of cardiovascular (CV) events in patients with asymptomatic carotid plaques.

Methods.—Forty-two patients with asymptomatic low-grade carotid stenosis (ALCS) and 21 controls without any carotid stenosis were enrolled. All subjects had at least a major cardiovascular risk factor (CRF). Plasma levels of C-reactive protein (CRP), IL-6, and sCD40L were measured. Subjects were reviewed every 12 months (median follow-up, 8 years).

Results.—ALCS patients had higher ($P<0.0001$) CRP, IL-6, and sCD40L than controls. Fourteen patients experienced a CV event. Cox regression analysis showed that only high sCD40L levels ($P=0.003$) independently predicted cardiovascular risk.

Conclusions.—High levels of sCD40L may predict the risk of CV events in ALCS.

▶ Thrombosis is the end point of atherosclerosis and inflammation is linked to the development of atherosclerosis. This study suggests that CD40-CD40L interactions may be one molecular mechanism linking the inflammation and the thrombosis associated with atherosclerosis.

G. L. Moneta, MD

Increased platelet count and leucocyte–platelet complex formation in acute symptomatic compared with asymptomatic severe carotid stenosis

McCabe DJH, Harrison P, Mackie IJ, et al (Univ College London; London School of Hygiene and Tropical Medicine; Churchill Hosp, Oxford, England)
J Neurol Neurosurg Psychiatry 76:1249-1254, 2005   11–4

Objective.—The risk of stroke in patients with recently symptomatic carotid stenosis is considerably higher than in patients with asymptomatic stenosis. In the present study it was hypothesised that excessive platelet activation might partly contribute to this difference.

Methods.—A full blood count was done and whole blood flow cytometry used to measure platelet surface expression of CD62P, CD63, and PAC1 binding and the percentage of leucocyte–platelet complexes in patients with acute (0-21 days, n = 19) and convalescent (79-365 days) symptomatic (n = 16) and asymptomatic (n = 16) severe ($\geq70\%$) carotid stenosis. Most patients were treated with aspirin (37.5-300 mg daily), although alternative antithrombotic regimens were more commonly used in the symptomatic group.

Results.—The mean platelet count was higher in patients with acute and convalescent symptomatic compared with asymptomatic carotid stenosis. There were no significant differences in the median percentage expression of CD62P and CD63, or PAC1 binding between the acute or convalescent symptomatic and asymptomatic patients. The median percentages of neutrophil–platelet ($p = 0.004$), monocyte-platelet ($p = 0.046$), and lymphocyte-platelet complexes ($p = 0.02$) were higher in acute symptomatic than in asymptomatic patients. In patients on aspirin monotherapy, the percentages of neutrophil-platelet and monocyte-platelet complexes ($p = 0.03$) were higher in acute symptomatic (n = 11) than asymptomatic patients (n = 14). In the convalescent phase, the median percentages of all leucocyte–platelet complexes in the symptomatic group dropped to levels similar to those found in the asymptomatic group.

Conclusion.—Increased platelet count and leucocyte–platelet complex formation may contribute to the early excess risk of stroke in patients with recently symptomatic carotid stenosis.

▶ Most patients with even severe carotid stenosis do not have strokes. Much research has focused on the plaque as a factor for risk of stroke in patients with carotid stenosis. This article is highly interesting in that it suggests the risk of stroke is going to be affected not only by stenosis and plaque composition but also by blood rheology. It makes sense to me.

G. L. Moneta, MD

Inflammatory markers, rather than conventional risk factors, are different between carotid and MCA atherosclerosis
Bang OY, Lee PH, Yoon SR, et al (Ajou Univ, Suwon, Republic of Korea; Shin Hosp, Suwon, Republic of Korea)
J Neurol Neurosurg Psychiatry 76:1128-1134, 2005   11–5

Background.—The apparent differences in risk factors for intra- and extracranial atherosclerosis are unclear and the mechanisms that underlie strokes in patients with intracranial atherosclerosis are not well known. We investigated the conventional vascular risk factors as well as other factors in stroke patients with large artery atherosclerosis.

Methods.—Using diffusion weighted imaging (DWI) and vascular and cardiologic studies, we selected patients with acute non-cardioembolic cerebral infarcts within the middle cerebral artery (MCA) territory. Patients were divided into two groups: those with atherosclerotic lesions on the carotid sinus (n = 112) and those with isolated lesions on the proximal MCA (n = 160). Clinical features, risk factors, and DWI patterns were compared between groups.

Results.—There were no differences in conventional risk factors, but markers for inflammation were significantly higher in patients with carotid atherosclerosis than in those with isolated MCA atherosclerosis (p < 0.01 for both). After adjustments for age/sex and the severity of stroke, an inverse correlation was observed between C-reactive protein levels and MCA atherosclerosis (odds ratio 0.57 per 1 mg/dl increase; 95% confidence interval 0.35 to 0.92; p = 0.02). Internal borderzone infarcts suggestive of haemodynamic causes were the most frequent DWI pattern in patients with MCA occlusion, whereas territorial infarcts suggesting plaque ruptures were most common in those with carotid occlusion.

Conclusions.—Our results indicate that inflammatory markers, rather than conventional risk factors, reveal clinical and radiological differences between patients with carotid and MCA atherosclerosis. Plaques associated with MCA atherosclerosis may be more stable than those associated with carotid atherosclerosis.

▶ Different patterns of atherosclerosis may be, in part, secondary to varying patterns of risk factors, both clinical and biochemical. Just as the presence of diabetes predisposes to infrageniculate disease, markers of inflammation may lead to more extracranial than intracranial atherosclerosis.

M. K. Eskandari, MD

Severity of Asymptomatic Carotid Stenosis and Risk of Ipsilateral Hemispheric Ischaemic Events: Results from the ACSRS Study

Nicolaides AN, for the Asymptomatic Carotid Stenosis and Risk of Stroke (ACSRS) Study Group (Cyprus Inst of Neurology and Genetics, Nicosia; et al)
Eur J Vasc Endovasc Surg 30:275-284, 2005   11–6

Objectives.—This study determines the risk of ipsilateral ischaemic neurological events in relation to the degree of asymptomatic carotid stenosis and other risk factors.

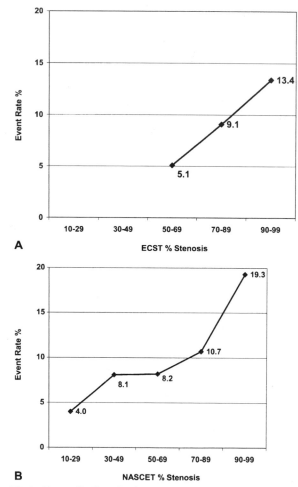

FIGURE 2.—The incidence of ipsilateral eschaemic hemispheric events (A) in relation to the ECST % stenosis of the internal carotid artery and (B) in relation to the NASCET % stenosis of the internal carotid artery. *Abbreviations: ECST*, European Carotid Surgery Trial; *NASCET*, North American Symptomatic Carotid Endarterectomy Trial. (Reprinted from Nicolaides AN, Kakkos SK, Griffin M, et al: Severity of asymptomatic carotid stenosis and risk of ipsilateral hemispheric ischaemic events: Results from the ACSRS Study. *Eur J Vasc Endovasc Surg* 30:275-284, 2005. Copyright 2005, by permission of Elsevier Ltd.)

Methods.—Patients ($n=1115$) with asymptomatic internal carotid artery (ICA) stenosis greater than 50% in relation to the bulb diameter were followed up for a period of 6–84 (mean 37.1) months. Stenosis was graded using duplex, and clinical and biochemical risk factors were recorded.

Results.—The relationship between ICA stenosis and event rate is linear when stenosis is expressed by the ECST method, but S-shaped if expressed by the NASCET method. In addition to the ECST grade of stenosis (RR 1.6; 95% CI 1.21–2.15), history of contralateral TIAs (RR 3.0; 95% CI 1.90–4.73) and creatinine in excess of 85 µmol/L (RR 2.1; 95% CI 1.23–3.65) were independent risk predictors. The combination of these three risk factors can identify a high-risk group (7.3% annual event rate and 4.3% annual stroke rate) and a low-risk group (2.3% annual event rate and 0.7% annual stroke rate).

Conclusions.—Linearity between ECST per cent stenosis and risk makes this method for grading stenosis more amenable to risk prediction without any transformation not only in clinical practice but also when multivariable analysis is to be used. Identification of additional risk factors provides a new approach to risk stratification and should help refine the indications for carotid endarterectomy (Fig 2).

▶ The interim analysis of the ACSRS study provided in this article shows there is more to stroke risk than severity of stenosis. A third of all neurologic events occurred among asymptomatic patients with less than 60% stenosis. This is a remarkable observation. It raises the question as to the efficacy of any interventions for asymptomatic carotid stenosis.

M. K. Eskandari, MD

Gender Differences in Outcome of Conservatively Treated Patients With Asymptomatic High Grade Carotid Stenosis

Dick P, Sherif C, Sabeti S, et al (Med Univ Vienna)
Stroke 36:1178-1183, 2005   11-7

Background and Purpose.—Gender differences are currently becoming increasingly recognized as an important prognostic factor in patients with atherosclerotic disease. We investigated gender-related differences in vascular outcome and mortality of asymptomatic patients with high-grade internal carotid artery (ICA) stenosis.

Methods.—We enrolled 525 consecutive patients (325 males with a median age of 72 years and 200 females with a median age of 75 years) from a single center registry who were initially treated conservatively with respect to a neurologically asymptomatic ≥70% ICA stenosis. Patients were followed-up for a median of 38 months (interquartile range, 18 to 65) for major adverse cardiovascular, cerebral, and peripheral vascular events (MACE: combined end point including myocardial infarction, stroke, [partial] limb amputation, and death), vascular mortality, and all-cause mortality.

Results.—Cumulative MACE-free survival rates in males and females at 1, 3, and 5 years were 83%, 65%, 48% versus 85%, 73%, and 67% ($P=0.004$), respectively. Adjusted hazard ratios for MACE, vascular mortality, and all-cause mortality for males were 1.96 ($P=0.016$), 2.48 ($P<0.001$), and 1.70 ($P=0.007$) as compared with females, irrespective of age, vascular risk factors, comorbidities, and the individual risk status estimated by the American Society of Anesthesiologists (ASA) score.

Conclusions.—Male patients with high-grade carotid artery stenosis are at a considerably higher risk for poor outcome than their female counterparts. In particular, the risk for fatal vascular events is substantially increased in males.

▶ The authors found male patients with asymptomatic high-grade carotid stenosis do poorly compared with female patients. The findings are irrespective of vascular risk factors, comorbidities, and age. Gender-related differences in outcomes of patients with asymptomatic high-grade carotid stenosis may have some implication for monitoring as well as strategies for interventions and prophylactic repair of asymptomatic high-grade carotid stenosis.

G. L. Moneta, MD

Population-based study of event-rate, incidence, case fatality, and mortality for all acute vascular events in all arterial territories (Oxford Vascular Study)

Rothwell PM, for the Oxford Vascular Study (Univ of Oxford, England; et al)
Lancet 366:1773-1783, 2005   11–8

Background.—Acute coronary, cerebrovascular, and peripheral vascular events have common underlying arterial pathology, risk factors, and preventive treatments, but they are rarely studied concurrently. In the Oxford Vascular Study, we determined the comparative epidemiology of different acute vascular syndromes, their current burdens, and the potential effect of the ageing population on future rates.

Methods.—We prospectively assessed all individuals presenting with an acute vascular event of any type in any arterial territory irrespective of age in a population of 91 106 in Oxfordshire, UK, in 2002-05.

Findings.—2024 acute vascular events occurred in 1657 individuals: 918 (45%) cerebrovascular (618 stroke, 300 transient ischaemic attacks [TIA]); 856 (42%) coronary vascular (159 ST-elevation myocardial infarction, 316 non-ST-elevation myocardial infarction, 218 unstable angina, 163 sudden cardiac death); 188 (9%) peripheral vascular (43 aortic, 53 embolic visceral or limb ischaemia, 92 critical limb ischaemia); and 62 unclassifiable deaths. Relative incidence of cerebrovascular events compared with coronary events was 1.19 (95% CI 1.06-1.33) overall; 1.40 (1.23-1.59) for non-fatal events; and 1.21 (1.04-1.41) if TIA and unstable angina were further excluded. Event and incidence rates rose steeply with age in all arterial territories, with 735 (80%) cerebrovascular, 623 (73%) coronary, and 147 (78%) peripheral

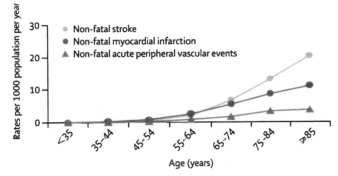

FIGURE 6.—Age-specific event rates for non-fatal stroke, non-fatal myocardial infarction, and non-fatal acute peripheral vascular events. (Courtesy of Rothwell PM, for the Oxford Vascular Study: Population-based study of event-rate, incidence, case fatality, and mortality for all acute vascular events in all arterial territories [Oxford Vascular Study]. *Lancet* 366:1773-1783. Copyright 2005 by Elsevier.)

vascular events in 12 886 (14%) individuals aged 65 years or older; and 503 (54%), 402 (47%), and 105 (56%), respectively, in the 5919 (6%) aged 75 years or older. Although case-fatality rates increased with age, 736 (47%) of 1561 non-fatal events occurred at age 75 years or older.

Interpretation.—The high rates of acute vascular events outside the coronary arterial territory and the steep rise in event rates with age in all territories have implications for prevention strategies, clinical trial design, and the targeting of funds for service provision and research (Fig 6).

▶ There is nothing particularly surprising in this study except that perhaps cerebral vascular events were more common than coronary events. It is also interesting that half of all events occurred in patients 75 years or older. The age distribution of vascular events suggests that trials designed to assess interventions for atherosclerotic vascular disease must include a large proportion of older patients. Limiting studies to patients younger than 80 years old, as is frequently done, will exclude that segment of the population with the largest number of events.

G. L. Moneta, MD

A simple score (ABCD) to identify individuals at high early risk of stroke after transient ischaemic attack
Rothwell PM, Giles MF, Flossmann E, et al (Univ of Oxford, England; Univ of Edinburgh, Scotland)
Lancet 366:29-36, 2005   11 9

Background.—Effective early management of patients with transient ischaemic attacks (TIA) is undermined by an inability to predict who is at highest early risk of stroke.

Methods.—We derived a score for 7-day risk of stroke in a population-based cohort of patients (n=209) with a probable or definite TIA (Oxfordshire Community Stroke Project; OCSP), and validated the score in a similar population-based cohort (Oxford Vascular Study; OXVASC, n=190). We assessed likely clinical usefulness to front-line health services by using the score to stratify all patients with suspected TIA referred to OXVASC (n=378, outcome: 7-day risk of stroke) and to a hospital-based weekly TIA clinic (n=210; outcome: risk of stroke before appointment).

Results.—A six-point score derived in the OCSP (age [≥60 years=1], blood pressure [systolic >140 mm Hg and/or diastolic ≥90 mm Hg=1], clinical features [unilateral weakness=2, speech disturbance without weakness=1, other=0], and duration of symptoms in min [≥60=2, 10-59=1, <10=0]; ABCD) was highly predictive of 7-day risk of stroke in OXVASC patients with probable or definite TIA (p<0.0001), in the OXVASC population-based cohort of all referrals with suspected TIA (p<0.0001), and in the hospital-based weekly TIA clinic-referred cohort (p=0.006). In the OXVASC suspected TIA cohort, 19 of 20 (95%) strokes occurred in 101 (27%) patients with a score of 5 or greater: 7-day risk was 0.4% (95% CI 0-1.1) in 274 (73%) patients with a score less than 5, 12.1% (4.2-20.0) in 66 (18%) with a score of 5, and 31.4% (16.0-46.8) in 35 (9%) with a score of 6. In the hospital-referred clinic cohort, 14 (7.5%) patients had a stroke before their scheduled appointment, all with a score of 4 or greater.

Conclusions.—Risk of stroke during the 7 days after TIA seems to be highly predictable. Although further validations and refinements are needed, the ABCD score can be used in routine clinical practice to identify high-risk individuals who need emergency investigation and treatment.

▶ The article underlies the fact that all transient ischemic attacks (TIAs) do not have the same clinical significance. The findings here make sense in that elderly patients with more severe risk factors and more marked TIAs are at higher risk of stroke. Especially remarkable is the very high 1-week risk of stroke in patients with a high Oxfordshire Community Stroke Project (OCSP) score. Patients with high OCSP scores after TIA should be subject to urgent evaluation and appropriate intervention.

G. L. Moneta, MD

Population-based study of delays in carotid imaging and surgery and the risk of recurrent stroke
Fairhead JF, Menta Z, Rothwell PM (Radcliffe Infirmary, Oxford, England)
Neurology 65:371-375, 2005   11–10

Background.—Benefit from carotid endarterectomy is greatest when performed within 2 weeks of a presenting TIA or stroke and decreases rapidly thereafter.

Objective.—To determine the delays to carotid imaging and endarterectomy in Oxfordshire, UK, and the consequences for the effectiveness of stroke prevention.

Methods.—All patients undergoing carotid imaging for ischemic retinal or cerebral TIA or stroke were identified in two populations: the population of Oxfordshire, UK (n = 680,772), from April 1, 2002, to March 31, 2003, and the Oxford Vascular Study (OXVASC) subpopulation (n = 92,000) from April 1, 2002, to March 31, 2004. The times from presenting event to referral, scanning, and endarterectomy (Oxfordshire population) and the risk of stroke prior to endarterectomy in patients with ≥50% symptomatic carotid stenosis (OXVASC population) were determined.

Results.—Among 853 patients who had carotid imaging in the Oxfordshire population, median (interquartile range) times from presenting event to referral, scanning, and endarterectomy were 9 (3 to 30), 33 (12 to 62), and 100 (59 to 137) days. Eighty-five patients were found to have 50 to 99% symptomatic stenosis, of whom 49 had endarterectomy. Only 3 (6%) had surgery within 2 weeks of their presenting event and only 21 (43%) within 12 weeks. The risk of stroke prior to endarterectomy in the OXVASC subpopulation with ≥50% stenosis was 21% (8 to 34%) at 2 weeks and 32% (17 to 47%) at 12 weeks, in half of which strokes were disabling or fatal.

Conclusion.—Delays to carotid imaging and endarterectomy after TIA or stroke in the United Kingdom are similar to those reported in several other countries and are associated with very high risks of otherwise preventable early recurrent stroke.

▶ Delays in treatment are not good when the problem is symptomatic carotid stenosis. Lack of expedient care can result in a higher incidence of what could have been a preventable stroke. Perhaps these results should also be published in the emergency medicine and primary care literature.

M. K. Eskandari, MD

The Role of Carotid Endarterectomy in the Endovascular Era
Chong PL, Salhiyyah K, Dodd PDF (Northern Gen Hosp, Sheffield, England)
Eur J Vasc Endovasc Surg 29:597-600, 2005   11–11

Objective.—Carotid artery angioplasty and stenting (CAS) has been proposed as an alternative to surgery for patients with high-grade symptomatic carotid disease. The purpose of this study was to determine the proportion of patients that were suitable for each type of intervention and to analyse the reasons that precluded stenting.

Materials and Methods.—This was a prospective observational study. All patients considered for intervention for carotid artery disease during an 18-month period were analysed. The management decision was recorded, as were the reasons for unsuitability for stenting.

Results.—Two hundred and sixty eight patients' data were analysed; 224 had complete records. Forty-seven patients did not require intervention and received best medical treatment alone. One hundred and seventy-seven patients required intervention; 113 were suitable for stenting and 64 were not. In 51 patients stenting was preferred. Sixty-two patients were suitable for either stent or surgery. Sixty-four patients were unsuitable for stenting. Carotid tortuosity and proximal disease accounted for 70% of this group.

Conclusions.—Current enthusiasm for carotid stenting might well be supported by the results of ongoing randomised-controlled clinical trials. However, this study highlights a significant proportion (64/177; 36%) of our patients is presently unsuitable for stenting. The common technical difficulties and limitations of stenting encountered in our unit are related predominantly to carotid anatomy.

▶ The article suggests enthusiasm for CAS has to be tempered with its limitations, the predominant one being unfavorable anatomy. Another limitation is the tendency to stretch the indication for carotid intervention with the availability of carotid stenting.

M. K. Eskandari, MD

Clinical and operative predictors of outcomes of carotid endarterectomy
Halm EA, Hannan EL, Rojas M, et al (Mount Sinai School of Medicine, New York; Univ of Albany, NY; New York Univ)
J Vasc Surg 42:420-428, 2005   11–12

Objective.—The net benefit for patients undergoing carotid endarterectomy is critically dependent on the risk of perioperative stroke and death. Information about risk factors can aid appropriate selection of patients and inform efforts to reduce complication rates. This study identifies the clinical, radiographic, surgical, and anesthesia variables that are independent predictors of deaths and stroke following carotid endarterectomy.

Methods.—A retrospective cohort study of patients undergoing carotid endarterectomy in 1997 and 1998 by 64 surgeons in 6 hospitals was performed (N = 1972). Detailed information on clinical, radiographic, surgical, anesthesia, and medical management variables and deaths or strokes within 30 days of surgery were abstracted from inpatient and outpatient records. Multivariate logistic regression models identified independent clinical characteristics and operative techniques associated with risk-adjusted rates of combined death and nonfatal stroke as well as all strokes.

Results.—Death or stroke occurred in 2.28% of patients without carotid symptoms, 2.93% of those with carotid transient ischemic attacks, and 7.11% of those with strokes ($P < .0001$). Three clinical factors increased the risk-adjusted odds of complications: stroke as the indication for surgery (odds ratio [OR], 2.84; 95% confidence interval [CI] = 1.55-5.20), presence of active coronary artery disease (OR, 3.58; 95% CI = 1.53-8.36), and contralateral carotid stenosis ≥50% (OR, 2.32; 95% CI = 1.33-4.02). Two surgical techniques reduced the risk-adjusted odds of death or stroke: use of local anesthesia (OR, 0.30; 95% CI = 0.16-0.58) and patch closure (OR, 0.43; 95% CI = 0.24-0.76).

Conclusions.—Information about these risk factors may help physicians weigh the risks and benefits of carotid endarterectomy in individual patients.

Two operative techniques (use of local anesthesia and patch closure) may lower the risk of death or stroke.

▶ The complication rate for carotid endarterectomy when the indication for operation was stroke seems a bit high here. Otherwise, there are no surprises. This is another article that implies benefit of local anesthesia for carotid endarterectomy. It is not true science, but it is a good series.

G. L. Moneta, MD

3-Hydroxy-3-methylglutaryl Coenzyme A Reductase Inhibitors Reduce the Risk of Perioperative Stroke and Mortality After Carotid Endarterectomy
McGirt MJ, Perler BA, Brooke BS, et al (Johns Hopkins Med Insts, Baltimore, Md)
J Vasc Surg 42:829-836, 2005   11–13

Objective.—There is increasing evidence that 3-hydroxy-3-methylglutaryl coenzyme A reductase inhibitors (statins) reduce cardiovascular and cerebrovascular events through anti-inflammatory, plaque stabilization, and neuroprotective effects independent of lipid lowering. This study was designed to investigate whether statin use reduces the incidence of perioperative stroke and mortality among patients undergoing carotid endarterectomy (CEA).

Methods.—All patients undergoing CEA from 1994 to 2004 at a large academic medical center were retrospectively reviewed. The independent as-

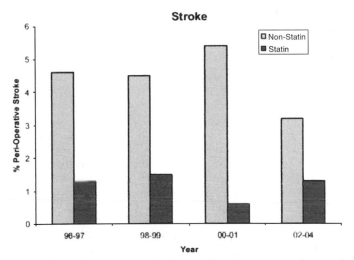

FIGURE 1.—Incidence of postoperative stroke after carotid endarterectomy as a function of statin vs no statin use over time. The postoperative stroke rate remained lower in patients receiving statins, regardless of the year of operation. (Reprinted by permission of the publisher from McGirt AJ, Perler BA, Brooke BS, et al: 3-Hydroxy-3-methylglutaryl coenzyme A reductase inhibitors reduce the risk of perioperative stroke and mortality after carotid endarterectomy. *J Vasc Surg* 42:829-836, 2005. Copyright 2005 by Elsevier.)

sociation of statin use and perioperative morbidity was assessed via multi-variate logistic regression analysis.

Results.—CEA was performed by 13 surgeons on 1566 patients (987 men and 579 women; mean age, 72 ± 10 years), including 1440 (92%) isolated and 126 (8%) combined CEA/coronary artery bypass grafting procedures. The indication for CEA was symptomatic disease in 660 (42%) cases. Six hundred fifty-seven (42%) patients received a statin medication for at least 1 week before surgery. Statin use was associated with a reduction in perioperative strokes (1.2% vs 4.5%; $P < 01$), transient ischemic attacks (1.5% vs 3.6%; $P < .01$), all-cause mortality (0.3% vs 2.1%; $P < .01$), and median (interquartile range) length of hospitalization (2 days [2-5 days] vs 3 days [2-7 days]; $P < .05$). Adjusting for all demographics and comorbidities in multivariate analysis, statin use independently reduced the odds of stroke threefold (odds ratio [95% confidence interval], 0.35 [0.15-0.85]; $P < .05$) and death fivefold (odds ratio [95% confidence interval], 0.20 [0.04-0.99]; $P < .05$) (Fig 1).

Conclusions.—These data suggest that perioperative statin use may reduce the incidence of cerebrovascular events and mortality among patients undergoing CEA.

▶ There seems to be no reason not to have vascular patients on statins. This article suggests that placing vascular patients on statins before surgery may be a good thing. The patients in this study on statins were on a statin for at least 1 week. However, the retrospective nature of this study does not allow determination of actually how long the patients should be on statins before surgery. Now that would be very useful information! See Abstract 11–14.

G. L. Moneta, MD

Statins are associated with better outcomes after carotid endarterectomy in symptomatic patients
Kennedy J, Quan H, Buchan AM, et al (Univ of Calgary, Alta, Canada; Univ of Oxford, England; Univ of Alberta, Edmonton, Canada)
Stroke 36:2072-2076, 2005   11–14

Background and Purpose.—Statins have been associated with a reduction in mortality from noncardiac surgery. This study aimed to determine whether statin use on admission to hospital for carotid endarterectomy was associated with a reduction of in-hospital adverse outcomes.

Methods.—Data describing patient characteristics, surgical indication, statin treatment, and in-hospital outcomes of death, ischemic stroke or death and cardiac outcomes were collected from a chart review of all patients (3360) undergoing carotid endarterectomy in Western Canada from January 2000 to December 2001. Outcomes of patients on statins versus those not on statins were compared using logistic regression to account for differences in patient characteristics, and propensity score methods to account for factors influencing patient allocation to statins.

Results.—Eight hundred and fifteen of 2031 symptomatic patients and 665 of 1252 asymptomatic patients were on a statin at the time of hospital admission. Statin use by symptomatic patients was associated with reduced in-hospital mortality and in-hospital ischemic stroke or death, but not in-hospital cardiac outcomes (adjusted odds ratio 0.25 [CI, 0.07 to 0.90], 0.55 [CI, 0.32 to 0.95], 0.87 [CI, 0.49 to 1.54], respectively). The improvement in outcomes was robust when tested using propensity score matching. This association was not seen in asymptomatic patients on statins (adjusted odds ratio, in-hospital mortality 0.54 [CI, 0.13 to 2.24]; in-hospital ischemic stroke or death 1.34 [CI, 0.61 to 2.93]; in-hospital cardiac outcomes 1.37 [CI, 0.73 to 2.58]).

Conclusions.—These findings are suggestive of a protective effect of statin therapy in symptomatic patients pre-treated at the time of carotid endarterectomy, though this needs confirmation in a randomized controlled trial.

▶ This study, like the previous abstract (see Abstract 11–13), adds to the growing impression that statins improve perioperative outcomes in patients undergoing vascular surgery. The lack of effect of statins in the asymptomatic patients undergoing carotid endarterectomy may be the result of an inability to detect the statin effect due to the low frequency of adverse events in the asymptomatic patients. Since this was not a randomized study, statins may be just serving as a marker of overall better perioperative care. The results of this observational study, and others like it, will need to be confirmed in large multicenter randomized trials specifically addressing the perioperative use of statins to improve operative outcomes.

G. L. Moneta, MD

Postcarotid Endarterectomy Hyperperfusion or Reperfusion Syndrome
Karapanayiotides T, Meuli R, Devuyst G, et al (Centre Hospitalier Universitaire Vaudois, Lausanne, Switzerland; CHUV, Lausanne, Switzerland)
Stroke 36:21-26, 2005   11–15

Background and Purpose.—Hyperperfusion syndrome (HS) after carotid endarterectomy (CEA) has been related to impaired cerebrovascular autoregulation in a chronically hypoperfused hemisphere. Our aim was to provide new insight into the pathophysiology of the HS using magnetic resonance imaging (MRI) studies with diffusion-weighted imaging (DWI) and perfusion weighted imaging (PWI).

Methods.—Five out of 388 consecutive patients presented 2 to 7 days after CEA, partial seizures (n=5), focal deficits (n=5), and intracerebral hemorrhage (n=3). In 4 patients, using sequential examinations, we identified vasogenic or cytotoxic edema by DWI; we assessed relative interhemispheric difference (RID) of cerebral blood flow (CBF) by PWI; and we measured middle cerebral artery mean flow velocities (MCA Vm) by transcranial Doppler (TCD).

Results.—None of the patients presented pathological DWI hyperintensities, consistent with the absence of acute ischemia or cytotoxic edema. In 2 patients, we found an MRI pattern of reversible vasogenic edema similar to that observed in the posterior leukoencephalopathy syndrome. Middle cerebral artery (MCA) mean flow velocities (Vm) were not abnormally increased at any time. PWI documented a 20% to 44% RID of CBF in favor of the ipsilateral to CEA hemisphere.

Conclusions.—HS can occur in the presence of moderate relative hyperperfusion of the ipsilateral hemisphere. MCA Vm values may not accurately reflect RID of CBF over the cortical convexity. We suggest that the hemodynamic pathogenetic mechanisms of the HS are more complicated than hitherto believed and that they may be more accurately described by the term "reperfusion syndrome."

▶ The classic definition of hyperperfusion syndrome after carotid endarterectomy is a 100% increase in cerebral blood flow compared to preoperative values.[1] The current study suggests that symptoms and pathology consistent with what is regarded as hyperperfusion syndrome after carotid endarterectomy can occur in the presence of relatively mild increased cerebral perfusion. Hemodynamic abnormalities leading to the clinical manifestations of hyperperfusion syndrome may be milder and more complicated than previously appreciated.

G. L. Moneta, MD

Reference

1. Ogasawara K, Yukawa H, Kobayashi M, et al: Prediction and monitoring of cerebral hyperperfusion after carotid endarterectomy by using single-photon emission computerized tomography scanning. *J Neurosurg* 99:504-510, 2003.

Safety and efficacy of reoperative carotid endarterectomy: A 14-year experience
Stoner MC, Cambria RP, Brewster DC, et al (Massachusetts Gen Hosp, Boston)
J Vasc Surg 41:942-949, 2005   11–16

Background.—Reoperative carotid endarterectomy (CEA) is an accepted treatment for recurrent carotid stenosis. With reports of a higher operative morbidity than primary CEA and the advent of carotid stenting, catheter-based therapy has been advocated as the primary treatment for this reportedly "high-risk" subgroup. This study reviews a contemporary experience with reoperative CEA to validate the high-risk categorization of these patients.

Methods.—From 1989 to 2002, 153 consecutive, isolated (excluding CEA/coronary artery bypass graft and carotid bypass operations) reoperative CEA procedures were reviewed. Clinical and demographic variables potentially associated with the end points of perioperative morbidity, long-term durability, and late survival were assessed with multivariate analysis.

Results.—There were 153 reoperative CEA procedures in 145 patients (56% men, 36% symptomatic) with an average age of 69 ± 1.3 years. The average time from primary CEA (68% primary closure, 23% prosthetic, 9% vein patch) to reoperative CEA was 6.1 ± 0.4 years (range, 0.3 to 20.4 years). At reoperation, patch reconstruction was undertaken in 93% of cases. The perioperative stroke rate was 1.9%, with no deaths or cardiac complications. Other complications included cranial nerve injury (1.3%) and hematoma (3.2%). Average follow-up after reoperative CEA was 4.4 ± 0.3 years (range, 0.1 to 12.7 years), with an overall total stroke-free rate of 96% and a restenosis rate (>50%) by carotid duplex of 9.2% (Fig 2). Among variables assessed for association with restenosis after reoperative CEA, only younger age was found to be significant (66 ± 2.5 years vs 70 ± 0.7 years, $P < .05$). The all-cause long-term mortality rate was 29%. Multivariate analysis of long-term survival identified diabetes mellitus as having a negative impact (hazard ratio, 3.4 ± 0.3, $P < .05$) and lipid-lowering agents as having a protective effect (hazard ratio, 0.42 ± 0.4, $P < .05$) on survival.

Conclusion.—Reoperative CEA is a safe and durable procedure, comparable to reported standards for primary CEA, for long-term protection from stroke. These data do not support the contention that patients who require

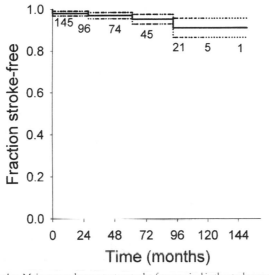

FIGURE 2.—Kaplan-Meier curve demonstrates stroke-free survival in the study population as measured from the date of reoperative carotid endarterectomy (*CEA*) (*broken arrow* shows standard error). (Reprinted by permission of the publisher from Stoner MC, Cambria RC, Brewster DC, et al: Safety and efficacy of reoperative carotid endarterectomy: a 14-year experience. *J Vasc Surg* 41:942-949, 2005. Copyright 2005 by Elsevier.)

reoperative CEA constitute a "high-risk" subgroup in whom reoperative therapy should be avoided.

▶ Redo CEA can be done with good results at centers of excellence. *When* to intervene in asymptomatic recurrent carotid stenotic lesions remains controversial, but the results of any intervention will have to be truly excellent to improve over the relatively benign natural history of recurrent carotid stenosis.

M. K. Eskandari, MD

High Rate of Early Restenosis After Carotid Eversion Endarterectomy in Homozygous Carriers of the Normal Mannose-Binding Lectin Genotype
Rugonfalvi-Kiss S, Dósa E, Madsen HO, et al (Semmelweis Univ, Budapest, Hungary; Rigshospitalet, Copenhagen; Szeged Univ, Hungary; et al)
Stroke 36:944-948, 2005   11–17

Background and Purpose.—Mannose-binding lectin (MBL) is thought to influence the pathophysiology of cardiovascular disease by decreasing the risk of advanced atherosclerosis and by contributing to enhanced ischemia reperfusion injury. Thus, we investigated the role of MBL in restenosis after eversion endarterectomy in patients with severe carotid atherosclerosis.

Methods.—In a prospective study, 123 patients who underwent carotid endarterectomy were followed-up by carotid duplex scan (CDS) sonography for 14 months. In a retrospective study, we examined 17 patients and 29 patients, respectively, who had or had not at least 50% restenosis 29 months after carotid eversion endarterectomy. MBL genotypes were analyzed by a polymerase chain reaction-based method, and MBL serum concentrations were measured.

Results.—In the prospective study in the patients homozygous for the normal MBL genotype, CDS values were significantly higher after 14 months of follow-up compared with the values measured 6 weeks after surgery ($P<0.001$). In contrast, only a slight increase was registered in patients carrying MBL variant alleles. The differences were much more pronounced in female than in male patients. Similar differences were observed when patients with high and low MBL serum concentrations were compared. In the retrospective study, a significant increase in the frequency of MBL variant genotypes was observed in patients not experiencing restenosis compared with the patients with restenosis ($P=0.007$).

Conclusions.—These results indicate that reoccurrence of stenosis after carotid endarterectomy is partially genetically determined and imply that MBL contributes significantly to the pathophysiology of this condition.

▶ The data indicate that a variant genotype compared to a normal genotype for mannose-binding lectin (MBL) may be protective with respect to development of carotid restenosis. The pathophysiologic mechanisms underlying the MBL genotype and carotid restenosis are unknown. In addition, the data make it difficult to completely separate the gender effect. Overall, there may be complicated interplay between genetic and hormonal factors in the development of carotid restenosis.

G. L. Moneta, MD

The influence of concurrent carotid endarterectomy on coronary bypass: A case-controlled study
Ricotta JJ, Wall LP, Blackstone E (State Univ of New York, Stonybrook; Cleveland Clinic Found, Ohio)
J Vasc Surg 41:397-402, 2005   11–18

Background.—Concurrent carotid endarterectomy (CEA) and coronary artery bypass grafting (CABG) are associated with an increased incidence of stroke and death compared to isolated CABG. It is unclear whether this reflects two concurrent operative procedures or the increased risk in patients with more extensive atherosclerosis.

Methods.—To address this question, a case-controlled study was performed using data from the New York State Cardiac Database from 1997 to 1998. Patients who underwent combined CEA-CABG were compared with all isolated CABG patients and a risk-matched cohort of isolated CABG patients.

Results.—The 35,539 isolated CABG patients had fewer postoperative complications than the 744 combined CEA-CABG patients, but also had a lower overall risk profile. The isolated CABG patients had a lower incidence of stroke (2% vs 5.1%), death (2% vs 4.4%), and combined stroke and death (3.7% vs 8.1%) compared with the combined group ($P < .001$). After risk-factor matching, no differences in stroke (5% vs 5.1%), death (3.9% vs 4.4%), or combined stroke and death (8.5% vs 8.1%) were observed.

Conclusions.—Although increased complications are reported after CEA-CABG, these do not differ from those of a risk-matched cohort of isolated CABG patients. Thus, the major morbidity of combined CEA-CABG is due to inherent patient risk and not the addition of CEA to CABG.

▶ It is always popular to blame the patients. I am sure that in the hands of surgeons who do a lot of combined procedures technical risks are minimized. We are, however, still waiting for the randomized trial. With the rapid emergence of carotid stents, that study will probably never happen.

G. L. Moneta, MD

Simultaneous carotid endarterectomy and coronary artery bypass surgery in Canada

Hill MD, Shrive FM, Kennedy J, et al (Univ of Calgary, Alta, Canada; Univ of Alberta, Edmonton, Canada)
Neurology 64:1435-1437, 2005   11–19

Background.—An increased risk of stroke as a complication of coronary artery bypass grafting (CABG) is associated with both previous stroke and current carotid artery stenosis. The risk of stroke with CABG overall is approximately 2%, but that risk is likely increased with the degree of carotid artery stenosis and whether 1 or both carotid arteries are involved. The risk of stroke among patients with recently symptomatic carotid artery stenosis is higher than among patients who are asymptomatic, but both groups are offered carotid endarterectomy (CEA).

A review of carotid artery surgery among Medicare patients in the United States found that of 10,561 endarterectomy procedures, 226 (2.1%) were combined CEA-CABG procedures. The crude combined stroke and death rate among this cohort was 17.7%. An expert panel examining the appropriateness of CEA concluded that CEA-CABG was an uncertain indication for CEA. This study explored the use of the combined CEA-CABG procedure in Canada, evaluated its use over time and across provinces, and also evaluated outcomes.

Methods.—The study group comprised all patients who underwent CABG at a Canadian hospital (excluding the province of Quebec) in fiscal years 1992/1993 to 2000/2001. Patients were included if a CABG code was included in any of 10 procedure fields scanned by the Canadian Classification of Procedures codes 48.11 through 48.19. In a small number of patients, the dates for both CABG and CEA were available and in 83% of these patients, the procedures occurred on the same day. Data on these admissions were reported as "combined CEA-CABG." Outcomes were in-hospital mortality and postoperative stroke.

Results.—In the 9 years of the study, 131,762 patients underwent CABG and of these patients, 669 (0.51%) underwent combined CEA-CABG. There was significant variation in use of the combined procedure by province. Use on a countrywide basis increased 2-fold in the study period.

In-hospital mortality was 4.9%, and the postoperative stroke rate was 8.5% among patients who underwent combined CEA-CABG compared with 3.3% among patients who underwent CABG alone. After adjustment, there was no statistically significant difference in the risk of death between the 2 groups, but an excess risk of stroke persisted in the combined CEA-CABG group (6.8% vs 1.8% in the CABG-only group). The adjusted combined stroke and death rate for the CABG-alone group was 4.9% compared with 13% for the combined CEA-CABG group. There was no discernible relationship between low-volume sites and increased risk.

Conclusions.—There is little evidence to support or refute the use of combined CEA-CABG to reduce the risk of stroke among patients undergoing CABG. The use of the combined procedure is increasing in Canada despite a high risk of perioperative stroke and death, but it is still 4-fold less than the 2% observed among US Medicare recipients. It is unknown what proportion of patients had symptomatic or asymptomatic carotid stenosis or how severely the arteries were stenosed.

▶ The data point out that the combination of CEA and CABG can carry a high perioperative risk of stroke and death (see Abstract 11–18). Despite this, combined CEA-CABG procedures are offered to an increasing number of Canadian CABG patients. We do not know what proportion of patients in this study had symptomatic or asymptomatic carotid stenosis or the degree of narrowing of the arteries. Clearly, there is little real evidence to support or refute the use of the combined CEA-CABG procedures.

G. L. Moneta, MD

Surgical vs medical treatment for isolated internal carotid artery elongation with coiling or kinking in symptomatic patients: A prospective randomized clinical study

Ballotta E, Thiene G, Baracchini C, et al (Univ of Padua, Padova, Italy)

J Vasc Surg 42:838-846, 2005   11–20

Background.—Whether surgically correcting symptomatic carotid elongation with coiling or kinking in the absence of an atherosclerotic lesion of the carotid bifurcation (isolated elongation) is effective in preventing stroke remains a controversial issue. The hypothesis behind this study was that surgical correction of symptomatic isolated carotid elongation with coiling or kinking could yield better results, in terms of stroke prevention and freedom from late stroke or carotid occlusion, than medical treatment.

Methods.—We conducted a prospective clinical study randomly assigning symptomatic patients with isolated carotid elongation to undergo either elective surgery or medical treatment, with surgery reserved for any new onset or worsening of symptoms. The follow-up ranged from 1 month to 10 years (median, 5.9; mean, 6.2 years) and was obtained for all patients. The study end points were perioperative (30-day) stroke and mortality, late stroke, and stroke-related death and late carotid occlusions.

Results.—Ninety-two patients were randomly assigned for surgery and 90 for medical treatment. Overall, 139 carotid surgical corrections were performed in 129 patients. All 92 patients in the surgical arm had an elective operation; 10 of these patients later developed symptoms on the opposite side (7 hemispheric and 3 retinal transient ischemic attacks) and had contralateral internal carotid artery surgery. An additional 37 patients (41.1%) randomly assigned to medical treatment crossed over to the surgical group within a mean of 16.8 months after randomization due to new hemispheric symptoms or worsening nonhemispheric complaints. There were no perioperative strokes or deaths. The incidence of late hemispheric and retinal transient ischemic attacks was significantly lower in the surgical than in the medical group, respectively, 7.6% (7 of 92) vs 21.1% (19 of 90) (*P* = .01) and

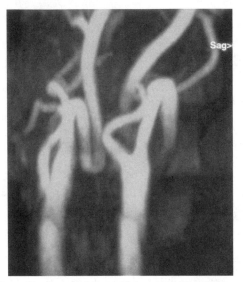

FIGURE 5A.—Angiographic picture of a left carotid elongation with kinking causing hemispheric symptoms. (Reprinted by permission of the publisher from Ballotta E, Thiene G, Baracchini C, et al: Surgical vs medical treatment for isolated internal carotid artery elongation with coiling or kinking in symptomatic patients: a prospective randomized clinical study. *J Vasc Surg* 42:838-846, 2005. Copyright 2005 by Elsevier.)

3.2% (3 of 92) vs 12.2% (11 of 90) ($P = .03$). Late strokes, 2 (2.2%) of which were fatal, occurred only in the medical group (6 of 90, 6.6%; $P = .01$). Late carotid occlusions also developed only in the medical group (5 of 90, 5.5%; $P = .02$). All surgically treated carotid elongations were analyzed histologically and 78 (56.1%) of 139 showed atypical and typical patterns of fibromuscular dysplasia.

Conclusions.—The overall results of this trial indicate that surgical correction of symptomatic isolated carotid elongations with coiling or kinking is better for stroke prevention than medical treatment (Fig 5A).

▶ Most patients with carotid coils or kinks will have other risk factors for stroke. Unless there is an associated atherosclerotic lesion or some other luminal irregularity, it is difficult to imagine how a tortuous artery could produce symptoms. However, that is why articles such as this are valuable in that they may change approaches to a particular problem, but only if others can show the same thing.

M. K. Eskandari, MD

Acute Carotid Artery Thrombosis: Description of 12 Surgically Treated Cases

Berthet J-P, Marty-Ané C-H, Picard E, et al (Arnaud de Villeneuve Hosp, Montepellier, France; Doumergue Hosp, Nimes, France)
Ann Vasc Surg 19:11-18, 2005   11–21

The morbidity and mortality of stroke secondary to acute internal carotid artery thrombosis range from 40 to 69% and from 15 to 55%, respectively, after purely medical treatment. This report describes a series of 12 patients who underwent urgent surgical treatment for primary acute carotid artery thrombosis between January 1999 and December 2002. Upon admission, all patients had severe neurologic deficits contralateral to carotid artery thrombosis. One patient experienced ongoing changes in the level of consciousness. The interval between the onset of symptoms and admission was less than 6 hr in all cases. Initial work-up in all patients included a brain computed tomographic scan with contrast injection and carotid duplex scan. The operative procedure consisted of carotid thromboendarterectomy after shunt placement with prosthetic patch closure. Intraoperative angiography was performed in all cases. Following treatment, we observed deterioration of neurologic status leading to death in one case; improvement with partial regression of initial neurologic deficit in two cases, including one patient who died from causes unrelated to carotid artery disease; and full neurologic recovery in nine cases. The delay to revascularization was longer than 6 hr in both patients who died. These data support surgical intervention for carotid artery thrombosis in selected patients without major disturbances of consciousness or hemorrhagic infarction, provided that the delay to revascularization is less than 6 hr.

▶ Re-establishment of flow to an acutely thrombosed internal carotid artery (ICA) within an average of 5 hours of symptom onset is a commendable accomplishment. If surgical revascularization can be achieved in less than 6 hours, maybe it should be considered in select cases of de novo atherosclerotic ICA occlusions?

M. K. Eskandari, MD

Carotid graft replacement: A durable option

Veldenz HC, Kinser R, Yates GN (Surgical Specialists, PSC, Elizabethtown, Ky)
J Vasc Surg 42:220-226, 2005   11–22

Background.—Carotid artery bifurcation reconstruction after endarterectomy has been refined over the years. Methods including primary closure, patch closure, and eversion endarterectomy have been proven to be durable. However, there are patients who require more complicated reconstructions in primary or recurrent disease management. Carotid replacement with a prosthetic interposition graft is potentially a durable option to reconstruct an artery that is technically unsuitable for primary or patch closure.

Methods.—The charts of all carotid endarterectomies (n = 482) performed by the authors at our institution between January 1999 and December 2003 were retrospectively reviewed. Follow-up was performed in an Intersocietal Commission for the Accreditation of Vascular Laboratories–accredited vascular laboratory. Patients were divided into two main groups: carotid replacement with 6-mm expanded polytetrafluoroethylene (ePTFE) (REP) or standard endarterectomy (CEA) with or without patch closure. The decision for REP vs CEA (as well as the type of closure) was at the discretion of the surgeon according to an assessment of the end point, the distal internal carotid artery, and the quality and length of the endarterectomy segment. Interposition grafting with a 6-mm stretch of ePTFE from the transected common carotid to the transected internal carotid artery was performed in replacement reconstruction. The external carotid was ligated. Follow-up statistical analyses were performed with the Fisher exact test and analysis of variance for nominal values and *t* tests for continuous variables. Life table analyses were performed for patency and survival.

Results.—Complete perioperative data were available for 478 of the 482 operations performed (including all REP cases) during the study. At least one duplex ultrasound scan in follow-up was documented in 84% (n = 402) of the patients. A total of 51 were in the REP group, and 427 received CEA (95.3% with patch closure). Preoperative demographics, preoperative symptoms, and degree of stenosis did not vary within the study groups. Three 30-day surgical deaths occurred. The perioperative stroke rate between groups was not statistically different (REP, 1/51 [1.9%]; CEA, 3/427 [0.70%]; P = .35). Long-term patency and stroke-free survival rates at 3 years exceeded 96% and did not vary significantly between groups. The presence of a patch in the CEA group had no influence on outcomes. Duplex follow-up scan averaged two studies for at least 14 months in each group. Significantly more REP cases were reoperative procedures.

Conclusions.—Carotid interposition reconstruction with an ePTFE graft is an acceptable alternative in cases in which the standard technique would be technically difficult or compromising to the endarterectomy closure. Carotid ePTFE interposition graft replacement seems to be safe and durable and to have no increased perioperative risk or altered intermediate-term outcomes.

▶ Carotid replacement with ePTFE and external carotid artery ligation is a safe alternative, but probably not the first choice.

M. K. Eskandari, MD

Brachiocephalic reconstruction II: Operative and endovascular management of single-vessel disease

Takach TJ, Duncan JM, Livesay JJ, et al (Texas Heart Inst, Houston)
J Vasc Surg 42:55-61, 2005   11–23

Objective.—Although the surgical management of brachiocephalic disease is well established, evolving endovascular techniques present new options for treatment. We explored the potential benefits and drawbacks of these interventions in terms of outcome.

Methods.—From 1966 to 2004, 391 consecutive patients (43.7% male; mean age, 61.9 years) with single-vessel brachiocephalic disease were treated with either operative bypass (group A; n = 229) or percutaneous transluminal angioplasty and stenting (group B; n = 162).

Results.—All patients were asymptomatic after surgery or endovascular intervention. Group A and group B had similar operative mortality (0.9% vs 0.6%) and stroke (1.3% vs 0%) rates. However, 5 years after the procedure, group A had significantly better freedom from graft or intervention failure (92.7% ± 2.1%) than did group B (83.9% ± 3.7%; P = .03, Kaplan-Meier analysis; P = .001, Cox regression analysis). At 10 years, group A had the following rates of actuarial freedom from specific events: death, 73.7% ± 4.6%; myocardial infarction, 84.2% ± 3.6%; stroke, 91.4% ± 3.4%; graft failure, 88.1% ± 3.3%; coronary revascularization, 69.8% ± 5.1%; and other vascular operation, 70.7% ± 4.6%. Endovascular intervention involved less initial cost (mean savings, $8787 per procedure), was less invasive, and did not necessitate general anesthesia. On satisfaction questionnaires, 96.5% of patients receiving an endovascular intervention and 95.1% of patients receiving operative bypass for single-vessel brachiocephalic disease subjectively rated their treatment as "good" or "very good."

Conclusions.—Operative bypass and endovascular intervention for single-vessel brachiocephalic disease are both associated with acceptably low operative morbidity and mortality. Operative bypass produces significantly better mid-term freedom from graft or intervention failure than endovascular intervention and produces excellent long-term freedom from failure. Endovascular intervention offers tangible benefits regarding cost, level of invasiveness, and subjective patient satisfaction. Undetermined are the differences between the procedures regarding long-term durability, patterns of failure, efficacy as an adjunct to coronary artery bypass grafting, need for anticoagulation, efficacy as treatment for complex (multivessel) disease, and long-term cost.

▶ Left subclavian stenosis can be associated with arm fatigue, vertebrobasilar insufficiency, or, in rare instances, coronary-subclavian steal. The authors demonstrate that both carotid-subclavian bypass and endoluminal angioplasty and stenting can alleviate these symptoms with reasonable midterm results. Alternatives include medical therapy or carotid-subclavian transposition.

M. K. Eskandari, MD

Carotid Revascularization Using Endarterectomy or Stenting Systems (CaRESS) phase I clinical trial: 1-year results

McKinlay SM, for the CaRESS Steering Committee (New England Research Insts, Inc, Watertown, Mass; et al)
J Vasc Surg 42:213-219, 2005   11–24

Objective.—Current clinical trials evaluating carotid stenting have focused on high-risk patients and may not reflect the broad population of patients with carotid stenosis who undergo treatment to prevent stroke. The Carotid Revascularization Using Endarterectomy or Stenting Systems (CaRESS) phase I study is a multicenter, prospective, nonrandomized trial designed to address the question of whether carotid stenting (CAS) with cerebral protection is comparable to carotid endarterectomy (CEA) in patients with symptomatic and asymptomatic carotid stenosis.

Methods.—Patients with symptomatic (with >50% stenosis) or asymptomatic (with >75% stenosis) carotid stenosis were entered into the study in a 2:1 ratio of carotid stent and GuardWire Plus distal protection device. This unique trial model was developed through collaboration with the International Society of Endovascular Specialists, the Food and Drug Administration, the Centers for Medicare and Medicaid Services, the National Institutes of Health, and industry representatives. The primary end points included death and stroke at 30 days and a composite 1-year end point of death, stroke, or myocardial infarction (MI) from 0 to 30 days and death or stroke from 31 days to 1 year. The secondary end points included residual stenosis, restenosis, repeat angiography, and carotid revascularization at 30 days and 1 year and quality-of-life changes at 1 year.

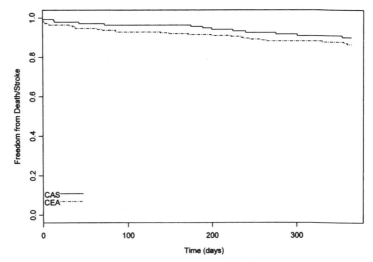

FIGURE 1.—Kaplan-Meier curves at 1 year for combined death/stroke. *CAS*, Carotid stenting; *CEA*, carotid endarterectomy. (Reprinted by permission of the publisher from McKinlay SM, for the CaRESS Steering Committee. Carotid revascularization using endarterectomy or stenting systems (CaRESS) phase I clinical trial: 1-year results. *J Vasc Surg* 42:213-219, 2005. Copyright 2005 by Elsevier.)

Results.—A total of 397 patients (254 CEA and 143 CAS) were enrolled in the study: 32% were symptomatic and 68% were asymptomatic. There were no significant differences in patient characteristics, symptoms, or surgical risk profiles between groups at baseline. Kaplan-Meier analysis revealed no significant differences in combined death/stroke rates at 30 days (3.6% CEA vs 2.1% CAS) or at 1 year (13.6% CEA vs 10.0% CAS). Similarly, there was no significant difference in the combined end point of death, stroke, or MI at 30 days (4.4% CEA vs 2.1% CAS) or at 1 year (14.3% CEA vs 10.9% CAS). There were no significant differences between CEA and CAS in the secondary end points of residual stenosis (0% CEA vs 0.9% CAS), restenosis (3.6% CEA vs 6.3% CAS), repeat angiography (2.1% CEA vs 3.6% CAS), carotid revascularization (1.0% CEA vs 1.8% CAS), or change in quality of life (−1.56 points CEA vs −4.22 points CAS).

Conclusions.—The CaRESS phase I study suggests that the 30-day and 1-year risk of death, stroke, or MI with CAS is equivalent to that with CEA in symptomatic and asymptomatic patients with carotid stenosis (Fig 1).

▶ CaRESS is a prospective nonrandomized trial comparing CEA with CAS using a distal balloon occlusion cerebral protection device. Selection into each arm was at the discretion of the physician and patient in an attempt to simulate the "real world" environment. Combined stroke/death/MI rate at 30 days after CAS for both symptomatic (32%) and asymptomatic (68%) patients is 2.1%. We, as usual, await a powered randomized trial to make definitive conclusions.

M. K. Eskandari, MD

Clinical Predictors of Transient Ischemic Attack, Stroke, or Death Within 30 Days of Carotid Angioplasty and Stenting
Kastrup A, Gröschel K, Schulz JB, et al (Univ of Tübingen, Germany; Univ of Jena, Germany)
Stroke 36:787-791, 2005   11–25

Background and Purpose.—Carotid angioplasty and stenting (CAS) is currently being assessed in the treatment of severe carotid stenosis. However, little data are available concerning patient-related factors affecting the risk of CAS. The purpose of this study was to identify potential clinical risk factors for the development of postprocedural deficits after CAS.

Methods.—The clinical characteristics of 299 patients (217 men, 82 women; mean age 69±9 years) who underwent CAS for asymptomatic (n=129, 43%) or symptomatic (n−170, 57%) stenoses and the combined 30 day complication rates (any transient ischemic attack [TIA], minor stroke, major stroke, or death) were analyzed with logistic regression analysis.

Results.—The overall 30-day TIA rate was 3.7%; the minor stroke rate was 5.3%, the major stroke rate was 0.7%, and the death rate was 0.7%. Although patients presenting with a hemispherical TIA or minor stroke had a significantly higher risk than asymptomatic patients (odds ratio [OR] 5.69;

95% confidence interval [CI], 2.03 to 19.57; $P<0.001$), the complication rates between patients presenting with a retinal TIA and asymptomatic patients was comparable (OR, 1.42; 95% CI, 0.13 to 9.09; $P=0.6$). Multivariate regression analysis revealed advanced age (OR, 1.06; 95% CI, 1 to 1.11; $P<0.05$), stroke (OR, 8; 95% CI, 2.6 to 24.4; $P<0.01$) or hemispherical TIA (OR, 4.7; 95% CI, 1.6 to 13.3) as presenting symptoms as independent clinical predictors of the combined 30-day outcome measures any TIA, stroke, or death.

Conclusions.—Aside from advanced age and symptom status, the type of presenting event predicts postprocedural complications after CAS. When evaluating the outcome of CAS and comparing this treatment modality to surgery, patients should be stratified according to their presenting event.

▶ Identification of potential risk factors for carotid artery stenting (CAS) is crucial to proper patient selection for CAS and for patient counseling. This study helps identify presenting clinical features that may be important in selecting patients for CAS. Unfortunately, angiographic features of the carotid stenoses were not reported. It is likely that a combination of angiographic and clinical features will ultimately prove most useful in the selection of patients for CAS.

G. L. Moneta, MD

Outcomes of Carotid Angioplasty and Stenting for Radiation-Associated Stenosis

Harrod-Kim P, Kadkhodayan Y, Derdeyn CP, et al (Washington Univ, St Louis)
AJNR Am J Neuroradiol 26:1781-1788, 2005   11–26

Background and Purpose.—In light of their high surgical risk, carotid angioplasty and stent placement may be preferred in patients with radiation-associated carotid stenosis. The purpose of this study was to determine the procedural complication rate, patency, and clinical outcomes after carotid angioplasty and stent placement in this small group of high-risk patients.

Methods.—Sixteen patients (mean age, 65 years; 5 women and 11 men) who received radiation therapy for head and/or neck malignancy subsequently developed carotid stenosis (mean, 84%; range, 70%-99%) in a total of 19 carotid arteries, which were treated with angioplasty and stent placement. The patients were followed for a mean time of 28 months (range, 5-78 months) with periodic Doppler studies, angiography, CT angiography, or clinically.

Results.—In the total 19 stented carotid arteries, 23 procedures were performed (22 stent placement procedures and one repeat angioplasty). The procedural stroke rate was 1/23 (4%). The procedural transient ischemic attack rate was 0/23 (0%). There was one other observed complication: a puncture site hematoma. The 30-day postprocedure complication rate was 0/23 (0%); no neurologic symptoms were reported. Fifteen of the 19 vessels (79%) developed no new stenosis throughout the follow-up period. Two of 19 (11%) vessels had repeat angioplasty and stent placement; 1/19 (5%) had

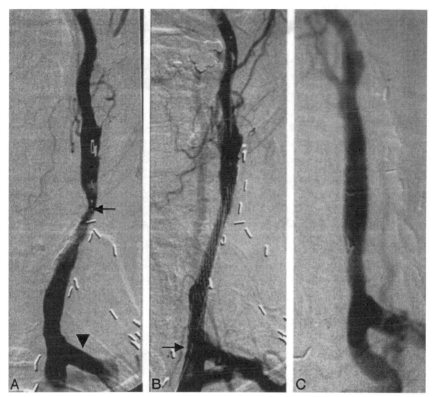

FIGURE 1.—A case of long-term stent patency in patient 4, a 68-year-old woman with thyroidectomy for carcinoma followed by postoperative radiation, bilateral radical neck dissection, and permanent tracheostomy, who experienced transient ischemic changes in the left cerebral hemisphere 21 years after radiation therapy. The patient had a history of graft placement between her left common carotid artery (CCA) and left subclavian arteries (5 years before admission) as well as a right CCA vein graft bypass (10 years before admission). A, Digital subtraction angiography (DSA) reveals a 70% stenosis (*arrow*) of the distal left CCA. Note the bypass graft (*arrowhead*) between the left CCA and left subclavian arteries. B, Successful stent placement with little residual stenosis. The proximal end of the 8 × 40 mm Wallstent (Boston Scientific, Natick, MA) extends across the origin of the left subclavian graft (*arrow*). Poststent angioplasty with an 8 × 40 mm Olbert balloon (Boston Scientific) resulted in rupture of the balloon. C, Repeat DSA 4.5 years after stent placement shows a patent carotid artery with interval auto expansion of the stent. (Courtesy of Harrod-Kim P, Kadkhodayan Y, Derdeyn CP, et al: Outcomes of carotid angioplasty and stenting for radiation-associated stenosis. *AJNR Am J Neuroradiol* 26:1781-1788, 2005. Copyright by American Society of Neuroradiology.)

a repeat angioplasty. One restented vessel has remained patent for 50 months. Another restented vessel required a third stent placement 17 months after the second. Two of 19 (11%) vessels occluded per Doppler examination 14 and 22 months postprocedure.

Conclusion.—Angioplasty and stent placement have low rates of complications and restenosis in the treatment of radiation-associated carotid occlusive disease (Fig 1).

▶ External beam radiation–induced carotid disease is typically diffuse and frequently involves the common carotid artery. Wound healing after carotid endarterectomy in an irradiated neck is always a concern. Carotid artery stenting is therefore an attractive alternative for patients with carotid radiation injury who require treatment. Early results with self-expanding bare metal stents are encouraging. Keep in mind, however, that the ability to treat a lesion does not mean the lesion needs to be treated.

M. K. Eskandari, MD

Embolic Protection Devices for Carotid Artery Stenting: Is There a Difference Between Filter and Distal Occlusive Devices?
Zahn R, for the Arbeitsgemeinschaft Leitende Kardiologische Krankenhausärzte (ALKK) (Herzzentrum, Kardiologie, Ludwigshafen, Germany; et al)
J Am Coll Cardiol 45:1769-1774, 2005   11–27

Objectives.—We sought to compare the efficacy of a filter embolic protection device (F-EPD) and a distal occlusive embolic protection device (DO-EPD) in patients undergoing carotid artery stenting (CAS).

Background.—The embolic protection device (EPD) may lower the periprocedural rate of cerebral ischemic events during CAS. However, it is unclear whether there is a difference in effectiveness between the different types of EPD.

Methods.—We analyzed data from the Carotid Artery Stent (CAS) Registry.

Results.—From July 1996 to July 2003, 1,734 patients were included in the prospective CAS Registry. Of these patients, 729 patients were treated with an EPD, 553 (75.9%) with F-EPD, and 176 (24.1%) with DO-EPD. Patients treated with DO-EPD were more likely to be treated for symptomatic stenosis (64.5% vs. 53.4%, p = 0.011). The carotid lesions in patients treated under DO-EPD seemed to be more complicated, as expressed by a higher proportion of ulcers (p = 0.035), severe calcification (p = 0.039), a longer lesion length (p = 0.025), and a higher pre-interventional grade of stenosis (p < 0.001). The median duration of the CAS intervention was 30 min in the DO-EPD group, compared with 48 min in the filter group (p < 0.001). No differences in clinical events rate between the two groups of pro-

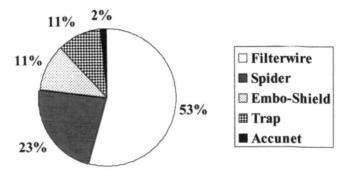

FIGURE 2.—Use of different filter devices. (Courtesy of Zahn R, for the Arbeitsgemeinschaft Leitende Kardiologische Krankenhausärzte (ALKK): Embolic protection devices for carotid artery stenting. *J Am Coll Cardiol* 45:1769-1774, 2005. Reprinted with permission from the American College of Cardiology.)

tection devices were observed. Multivariate analysis on the occurrence of the combined end point of in-hospital death or stroke found no difference between filter- and DO-EPD (4 of 176 [2.3%] for DO-EPD vs. 10 of 551 [1.8%] for F-EPD; adjusted odds ratio = 1.04, 95% confidence interval 0.24 to 4.44; p = 0.958).

Conclusions.—Filter EPD is the currently preferred method of EPD in clinical practice. Both F-EPD and DO-EPD seem to be equally effective during CAS (Fig 2).

▶ The data indicate that the filter embolic protection devices are preferred by physicians over occlusive embolic protection devices. The larger percentage of patients were treated with filter embolic protection devices in this registry. Nevertheless, both filter and occlusive embolic protection devices appear to have about the same efficacy during carotid artery stenting (CAS). What matters is keeping particulate matter out of the brain during CAS. At this point, it appears embolic protection devices can be chosen based on relative ease of use and individual operator preference.

G. L. Moneta, MD

Slow-Flow Phenomenon During Carotid Artery Intervention With Embolic Protection Devices: Predictors and Clinical Outcome

Casserly IP, Abou-Chebl A, Fathi RB, et al (Univ of Colorado, Denver; Cleveland Clinic Found, Ohio; Vancouver Gen Hosp, Canada; et al)
J Am Coll Cardiol 46:1466-1472, 2005   11–28

Objectives.—The purpose of this research was to define the predictors of the "slow-reflow" phenomenon during carotid artery intervention with filter-type embolic protection devices (EPDs) and to determine its prognostic significance.

Background.—During carotid artery intervention using filter-type EPDs, we have observed cases in which there is angiographic evidence of a significant reduction in antegrade flow in the internal carotid artery proximal to the filter device, termed "slow-flow." The predictors of this phenomenon and its prognostic significance are unknown.

Methods.—Using a single-center prospective carotid intervention registry, patients with slow-flow were compared to patients with normal flow during carotid intervention with respect to clinical, procedural, and lesion characteristics, and the 30-day incidence of death and stroke.

Results.—A total of 414 patients underwent 453 carotid artery interventions using EPDs. Slow-flow occurred in 42 patients (10.1%) undergoing 42 carotid interventions (9.3%), and most commonly occurred after post-stent balloon dilatation (71.4%). Multivariate logistic regression analysis identified the following predictors of slow-flow: recent history (<6 months) of stroke or transient ischemic attack (odds ratio [OR] 2.8, 95% confidence interval [CI] 1.4 to 5.6, p = 0.004), increased stent diameter (OR 1.4, 95% CI 1.02 to 1.94, p = 0.044), and increased patient age (OR 1.05, 95% CI 1.01

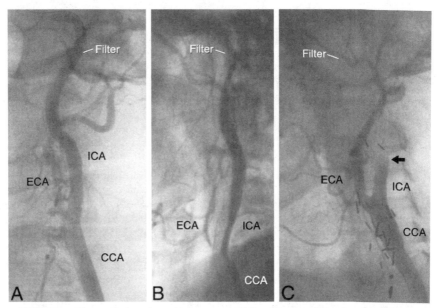

FIGURE 1.—Characteristic angiographic appearance of slow-flow (**A and B**) and no-flow (**C**) in the internal carotid artery (ICA) during carotid intervention with emboli protection devices (EPD). (**A**) Complete column of contrast in ICA with mild reduction in antegrade flow compared with the external carotid artery (ECA). (**B**) Marked reduction in antegrade flow in the ICA with incomplete filling of the lumen, but contrast does flow beyond the EPD. In **C**, there is no antegrade flow beyond the origin of the ICA (**arrow**). CCA = common carotid artery. (Courtesy of Casserly IP, Abou-Chebl A, Fathi RB, et al: Slow-flow phenomenon during carotid artery intervention with embolic protection devices. *J Am Coll Cardiol* 46:1466-1472, 2005. Reprinted with permission from the American College of Cardiology.)

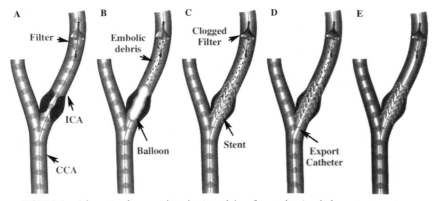

FIGURE 2.—Schematic of proposed mechanism of slow-flow and rationale for aspiration prior to retrieval of filter. (**A**) Carotid bifurcation lesion with filter placed in the distal internal carotid artery (ICA). (**B and C**) Balloon angioplasty and stenting results in distal embolization of debris from atherosclerotic plaque causing occlusion of filter pores and accumulation of debris in stagnant column of blood proximal to the filter. (**D and E**) Aspiration proximal to the filter removes the debris from the stagnant column of blood without affecting the debris causing occlusion of the filter. CCA = common carotid artery. (Courtesy of Casserly IP, Abou-Chebl A, Fathi RB, et al: Slow-flow phenomenon during carotid artery intervention with embolic protection devices. *J Am Coll Cardiol* 46:1466-1472, 2005. Reprinted with permission from the American College of Cardiology.)

to 1.09, p = 0.025). Among patients with slow-flow, the 30-day incidence of stroke or death was 9.5% compared to 2.9% in patients with normal flow (chi-square = 4.73, p = 0.03). This difference was driven by the disparity in the 30-day incidence of stroke (9.5% vs. 1.7%).

Conclusions.—Slow-flow during carotid intervention with EPDs is a frequent event that is associated with an excess risk of periprocedural stroke. The association of the phenomenon with clinically symptomatic carotid lesions and use of larger stent diameters suggests that embolization of vulnerable plaque elements may play a pathogenic role (Figs 1 and 2).

▶ It makes sense that if enough debris is trapped in a cerebral protection device that flow will be reduced through the ipsilateral internal carotid artery. However, it may be the increased debris in the protection device is also a marker of increased embolization at the time of initially crossing the lesion. The strokes therefore may be likely embolic rather than hemodynamic in origin. (See also Abstract 11–27.)

G. L. Moneta, MD

Prediction of early cerebral outcome by transcranial Doppler monitoring in carotid bifurcation angioplasty and stenting

Ackerstaff RGA, for the Antonius Carotid Endarterectomy, Angioplasty, and Stenting Study Group (St Antonius Hosp Nieuwegein, Utrecht, Netherlands; et al)
J Vasc Surg 41:618-624, 2005   11–29

Objective.—The outcomes of carotid angioplasty and stenting (CAS) are, in addition to patient baseline characteristics, highly dependent on the safety of the endovascular procedure. During the successive stages of CAS, transcranial Doppler (TCD) monitoring of the middle cerebral artery was used to assess the association of cerebral embolism and hemodynamic changes with transient (amaurosis fugax and transient ischemic attack) and persistent (minor and major stroke) cerebral deficits, and death.

Methods.—By use of a prospectively completed database of 550 patients, the association of various TCD emboli and velocity variables with periprocedural cerebral outcome ≤7 days was evaluated by univariable and multivariable logistic regression analyses in combination with receiver operating characteristic (ROC) curve analyses. The impact of basic patient characteristics, such as age, sex, preprocedural cerebral symptoms, and ipsilateral carotid endarterectomy before CAS, was also evaluated.

Results.—We observed 36 patients with amaurosis fugax (n = 6; 1.1%) or transient ischemic attack (n = 30; 5.4%), 1 patient (0.2%) with an ipsilateral retinal infarct, and 21 patients with minor (n − 15; 2.7%) or major (n = 6; 1.1%) stroke, respectively. Five patients (0.9%) died. Multiple showers of microemboli (>5) at postdilation after stent deployment (odds ratio [OR] 2.6, 95% confidence interval [CI], 1.3 to 5.1), particulate macroembolus (OR, 27.0; 95% CI, 4.5 to 157), and massive air embolism (OR, 51.4; 95%

CI, 5.4 to 492), as well as angioplasty-induced asystole and prolonged hypotension with a >70% reduction of middle cerebral artery blood flow velocities (OR, 6.4; 95% CI, 2.3 to 17.8) were independently associated with cerebral deficits. The ROC area of this model was 0.72. Of the patient characteristics, only preprocedural cerebral ischemia (OR, 5.0; 95% CI, 2.4 to 10.4) was associated with outcome. Adding this patient characteristic to the model, the area under the ROC curve increased to 0.80.

Conclusions.—In CAS, in addition to such obviously adverse events as particulate macroembolism and massive air embolism, multiple microemboli (>5 showers) at postdilation after stent deployment and angioplasty-induced asystole and hypotension with a significant reduction of middle cerebral artery blood flow velocities are associated with periprocedural cerebral deficits. In combination with the presence of preprocedural cerebral symptoms, these four TCD monitoring variables reasonably differentiate between patients with and without adverse cerebral outcome. TCD monitoring provides insight into the pathogenesis of CAS-related adverse cerebral events.

► Transcranial Doppler (TCD) is a valuable tool when attempting to judge the procedural implications of CAS. Prior reports from this group have detected more microemboli released in conjunction with the use of filter systems compared to unprotected CAS. This study extends their experience and shows that multiple microembolic showers coupled with hypotension and the presence of preprocedural neurologic symptoms predicts poorer outcomes. Perhaps flow-reversal systems of cerebral protection will be an alternative to filter systems to more effectively reduce microembolization.

M. K. Eskandari, MD

Cerebral microembolization after protected carotid artery stenting in surgical high-risk patients: Results of a 2-year prospective study
Hammer FD, Lacroix V, Duprez T, et al (Univ Hosp St Luc, Brussels, Belgium)
J Vasc Surg 42:847-853, 2005   11–30

Background.—This was a prospective single-center study to assess and analyze cerebral embolization resulting from carotid artery stenting with neuroprotective filter devices in patients considered as poor surgical candidates for surgical carotid endarterectomy.

Methods.—Fifty-three consecutive patients with an internal carotid artery stenosis were treated by placement of carotid Wallstents with two different types of temporary distal filter protection devices: the Spider filter and the FilterWire. Diffusion-weighted magnetic resonance imaging (DWI) of the brain was obtained 24 hours before the procedure and within 5 to 30 hours after the procedure to detect ischemic brain lesions resulting from the procedure. Inclusion criteria were symptomatic ($\geq$70%) or asymptomatic ($\geq$80%) stenoses in surgical high-risk patients.

Results.—Two (4%) regressive minor strokes occurred. Postprocedural DWI detected new focal ischemic lesions in 21 patients (40%). The average number of lesions was 5.9 per patient, and the mean lesion volume was 1 mL or less in 19 patients (90%). Small differences were found in the lesion distribution: homolateral anterior circulation in eight cases (15.1%), other vascular territories in seven cases (13.2%), and homolateral anterior circulation plus other vascular territories in six cases (11.3%). The microembolization risk seemed nonpredictable on the basis of clinical parameters and internal carotid artery lesion characteristics. An increased risk in the rate of ipsilateral hemispheric embolization has been observed in difficult carotid arch implantations ($P = .04$).

Conclusions.—The incidence of new focal ischemic lesions detected by DWI is higher than expected on the basis of previous reports. Embolization from the aortic arch or common carotid arteries could account for most of those events in patients considered as surgical high-risk patients. Although 90% of the events were clinically silent, this high rate of microembolization raises questions about the possible consequences on cerebral cognitive functions.

▶ DWI is a powerful tool for the detection of acute focal brain ischemia. This article demonstrated new focal ischemic lesions in 40% of patients treated with carotid artery stenting and a filter embolic protection device. The pattern of lesions was widespread: unilateral (target lesion side), contralateral, and posterior. Fortunately, the majority of lesions were clinically silent, but the long-term effects are unknown. Are we creating patients at increased risk for late multi-infarct dementia?

G. L. Moneta, MD

Leukocyte Count Predicts Microembolic Doppler Signals During Carotid Stenting: A Link Between Inflammation and Embolization
Aronow HD, Shishehbor M, Davis DA, et al (Michigan Heart PC, Ypsilanti; Cleveland Clinic Found, Ohio)
Stroke 36:1910-1914, 2005   11–31

Background and Purpose.—Protected stenting has emerged as a safe and effective alternative to endarterectomy for the treatment of carotid stenosis in patients at high operative risk. Distal microembolization occurs invariably during carotid stenting. Little is known about the relationship between systemic inflammation and embolization during carotid stenting.

Methods.—We examined 43 consecutive patients who underwent carotid stenting with simultaneous transcranial Doppler (TCD) monitoring of the ipsilateral middle cerebral artery. Embolization was quantified by measuring microembolic signals (MES) on TCD. Preprocedure leukocyte counts were related to MES.

Results.—In unadjusted analyses, preprocedure leukocyte count was positively correlated with total procedural MES ($r^2 = 0.16$; $P=0.008$). After considering age, gender, comorbidities, concomitant medical therapies, and the use of emboli prevention devices, increasing leukocyte count ($\beta = 35$ for each 1000/µL increment; $P = 0.018$) remained a significant and independent predictor of embolization (model-adjusted $r^2 = 0.365$; $P = 0.0005$).

Conclusions.—Increasing preprocedure leukocyte count independently predicted more frequent MES during carotid stenting. These data suggest that systemic inflammation may influence the degree of procedural embolization.

▶ The association of increased leukocyte count with microembolic signals during carotid stenting is interesting. However, the patients reported in this series are unlikely representative of current practice in that only 16% underwent carotid stenting with embolic protection devices. The 12% major procedural complication rate also seems high. Finally, the only marker of inflammation utilized in this retrospective study was leukocyte count. Further data using modern techniques and additional markers of inflammation are required before a link can be established between inflammation and microembolization during carotid artery stenting.

G. L. Moneta, MD

Use of Quantitative Magnetic Resonance Angiography to Stratify Stroke Risk in Symptomatic Vertebrobasilar Disease

Amin-Hanjani S, Du X, Zhao M, et al (Univ of Illinois at Chicago)
Stroke 36:1140-1145, 2005   11–32

Background and Purpose.—Symptomatic vertebrobasilar disease (VBD) carries a high risk of recurrent stroke. We sought to determine whether a management algorithm consisting of quantitative hemodynamic assessment could stratify stroke risk and guide the need for intervention.

Methods.—All patients with symptomatic VBD at our institution are evaluated by a standard protocol including quantitative magnetic resonance angiography (QMRA). Patients are stratified on the basis of the presence or absence of distal flow compromise. Those with low distal flow are offered intervention (surgical or endovascular); all patients receive standard medical therapy. We reviewed the clinical outcome of patients managed with this protocol from 1998 to 2003.

Results.—Follow-up was available for 47 of 50 patients over a mean interval of 28 months. Stroke- and combined stroke/transient ischemic attack–free survival at 2 years was calculated using the Kaplan-Meier curve. Patients with normal distal flow (n=31) had an event-free survival of 100% and 96%, respectively. Comparatively, patients with low distal flow (n=16) experienced a 71% and 53% event-free survival, demonstrating a significantly higher risk of recurrent ischemia ($P = 0.003$). Patients with low flow who subsequently underwent treatment (n=12) had an 82% event-free survival. Cox proportional hazards analysis demonstrated that flow status affected event-free survival regardless of covariates.

Conclusions.—Patients with symptomatic VBD demonstrating low distal flow on QMRA appear to have a high risk of stroke; conversely, those with normal flow seem to have a benign course and may be optimally managed with medical therapy alone.

▶ Quantitative magnetic resonance angiography (QMRA) is a slick technique. It may be able to determine the cause of symptomatic vertebrobasilar disease. Certainly, help is needed in this area. At present, anyone who says they can say with assurance which vertebral artery lesions require treatment is either naïve, lying, or both.

M. K. Eskandari, MD

NXY-059 for Acute Ischemic Stroke

Lees KR, for the Stroke–Acute Ischemic NXY Treatment (SAINT I) Trial Investigators (Gardiner Inst, Glasgow, Scotland; et al)
N Engl J Med 354:588-600, 2006   11–33

Background.—NXY-059 is a free-radical–trapping agent that is neuroprotective in animal models of stroke. We tested whether it would reduce disability in humans after acute ischemic stroke.

Methods.—We conducted a randomized, double-blind, placebo-controlled trial involving 1722 patients with acute ischemic stroke who were randomly assigned to receive a 72-hour infusion of placebo or intravenous NXY-059 within 6 hours after the onset of the stroke. The primary outcome was disability at 90 days, as measured according to scores on the modified Rankin scale for disability (range, 0 to 5, with 0 indicating no residual symptoms and 5 indicating bedbound, requiring constant care).

Results.—Among the 1699 subjects included in the efficacy analysis, NXY-059 significantly improved the overall distribution of scores on the modified Rankin scale, as compared with placebo ($P=0.038$ by the Cochran–Mantel–Haenszel test). The common odds ratio for improvement across all categories of the scale was 1.20 (95 percent confidence interval, 1.01 to 1.42). Mortality and rates of serious and nonserious adverse events were each similar in the two groups. NXY-059 did not improve neurologic functioning as measured according to the National Institutes of Health Stroke Scale (NIHSS): the difference between the two groups in the change from baseline scores was 0.1 point (95 percent confidence interval, -1.4 to 1.1; $P=0.86$). Likewise, no improvement was observed according to the Barthel index ($P=0.14$). In a post hoc analysis of patients who also received alteplase, NXY-059 was associated with a lower incidence of any hemorrhagic transformation ($P=0.001$) and symptomatic intracranial hemorrhage ($P=0.036$).

Conclusions.—The administration of NXY-059 within six hours after the onset of acute ischemic stroke significantly improved the primary outcome (reduced disability at 90 days), but it did not significantly improve other outcome measures, including neurologic functioning as measured by the NIHSS

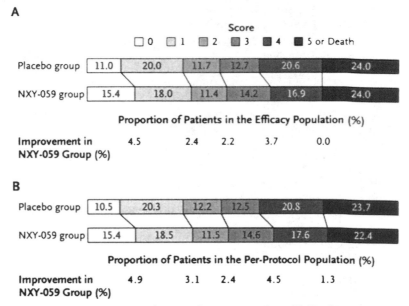

A

Score

☐ 0   ☐ 1   ☐ 2   ☐ 3   ☐ 4   ■ 5 or Death

| Placebo group | 11.0 | 20.0 | 11.7 | 12.7 | 20.6 | 24.0 |
| NXY-059 group | 15.4 | 18.0 | 11.4 | 14.2 | 16.9 | 24.0 |

Proportion of Patients in the Efficacy Population (%)

Improvement in   4.5   2.4   2.2   3.7   0.0
NXY-059 Group (%)

B

| Placebo group | 10.5 | 20.3 | 12.2 | 12.5 | 20.8 | 23.7 |
| NXY-059 group | 15.4 | 18.5 | 11.5 | 14.6 | 17.6 | 22.4 |

Proportion of Patients in the Per-Protocol Population (%)

Improvement in   4.9   3.1   2.4   4.5   1.3
NXY-059 Group (%)

FIGURE 2.—Primary outcome at 90 days, according to scores on the modified Rankin scale. P=0.038 for the comparison between patients in the two study groups included in the efficacy population (Panel A). P=0.028 for the comparison between patients in the two groups included in the per-protocol population (Panel B). Percentages are rounded to nearest decimal place. P values were calculated with the use of the Cochran–Mantel–Haenszel test. Percentages below the bars are the differences in the proportions of patients who attained a particular score or range of scores on the modified Rankin scale between the treatment group and the placebo group. (Reprinted by permission of *The New England Journal of Medicine* from Lees KR, for the Stroke–Acute Ischemic NXY Treatment (SAINT I) Trial Investigators: NXY-059 for acute ischemic stroke. *N Engl J Med* 354:588-600, 2006. Copyright 2006, Massachusetts Medical Society. All rights reserved.)

score. Additional research is needed to confirm whether NXY-059 is beneficial in ischemic stroke (Fig 2). (ClinicalTrials.gov number, NCT00119626.)

▶ This study shows a modest, but statistically significant benefit of NXY-059 for neuron-protection during ischemic stroke. With NXY-059, and using the modified Rankin scale, 4.4% more stroke patients became asymptomatic and 3.7% more patients were able to walk without help. While other parameters were not statistically significant in this study, this is the first study in humans to show a neuroprotective effect of any kind for drug therapy for ischemic stroke. Stroke is extraordinarily disabling and has huge personal and social costs. The number of patients is huge, and therefore any improvement, even if a modest percentage, is progress.

G. L. Moneta, MD

Cartoid Plaque Pathology: Thrombosis, Ulceration, and Stroke Pathogenesis
Fisher M, Paganini-Hill A, Martin A, et al (Univ of Southern California, Los Angeles; Wake Forest School of Medicine, Winston-Salem, NC; John P Roberts Research Inst, London, Ont, Canada; et al)
Stroke 36:253-257, 2005   11–34

Background and Purpose.—To determine the relationship between ulceration, thrombus, and calcification of carotid artery atherosclerotic plaques and symptoms of ipsilateral or contralateral stroke.

Methods.—We compared microscopic plaque morphology from patients with and without stroke symptoms ipsilateral or contralateral to the plaque. Plaques were characterized for ulceration, thrombus, and calcification. We analyzed plaques from 241 subjects: 170 patients enrolled in the Asymptomatic Carotid Atherosclerosis Study (ACAS) and 71 patients enrolled in the North American Symptomatic Carotid Endarterectomy Trial (NASCET); 128 subjects had no history of stroke symptoms, 80 subjects had ipsilateral symptoms, and 33 had contralateral symptoms.

Results.—Plaque ulceration was more common in plaques taken from symptomatic patients than those without symptoms (36% versus 14%; $P<0.001$); frequency of ulceration was similar for plaques associated with ipsilateral (34%) and contralateral (42%) symptoms. Thrombus was most common in plaques taken from patients with both ipsilateral symptoms and ulceration. The extent of calcification was unassociated with stroke symptoms.

Conclusions.—Carotid plaque ulceration and thrombosis are more prevalent in symptomatic patients. Ulceration is more common in symptomatic patients regardless of side of carotid symptoms, whereas thrombus is associated with ipsilateral symptoms and plaque ulceration. Preoperative identification of carotid ulceration and thrombus should lead to greater efficacy of stroke prevention by carotid endarterectomy.

▶ This is another indirect attempt trying to determine which plaques in asymptomatic patients may have a greater propensity to produce stroke. The authors' conclusions are not new, not unexpected, and add very little to what is already known or suspected. There continues to be great interest in characterizing surgically removed plaques. What is needed is a preoperative marker of plaque virulence that is sufficiently sensitive and powerful to improve the selection of asymptomatic patients with carotid stenosis for a prophylactic carotid intervention. I think we have had enough of this type of paper.

G. L. Moneta, MD

12 Vascular Trauma

Penetrating Abdominal Vena Cava Injuries
Navsaria PH, de Bruyn P, Nicol AJ (Univ of Cape Town, South Africa)
Eur J Vasc Endovasc Surg 30:499-503, 2005   12–1

Objective.—The surgical management and outcome of abdominal vena cava (AVC) injuries is presented.

Study Design, Patients, and Methods.—A retrospective record review of patients with AVC injuries treated in the Trauma Unit at Groote Schuur Hospital between January 1999 and December 2003 was undertaken. Demographic data, mechanism of injury, surgical management, associated injuries, duration of hospital stay, complications and mortality were extracted from patient records. Patients with acute peritonitis and/or shock underwent emergency laparotomy.

Results.—Forty-eight patients with AVC injuries were identified. Gunshot wounds accounted for 45 (94%) injuries. The mean weighted revised trauma score, injury severity score (ISS) and penetrating abdominal trauma index (PATI) were 6.3, 24 and 42, respectively. The AVC injury was infrarenal and suprarenal in 41 and seven patients, respectively. Thirty injuries were ligated. There were 15 deaths (31%). Significant differences between survivors and non-survivors included ISS, preoperative hypotension and blood transfusion requirements, whereas site of injury, PATI, and surgical management did not.

Conclusion.—Abdominal vena cava injuries are associated with a high mortality. Ligation of the AVC in critically ill patients is a feasible and life-saving option.

▶ The results of ligation of the inferior vena cava were surprisingly good in the short term. No fasciotomies were required, and lower-limb swelling subsided in 7 to 10 days. Inferior vena cava ligation can be considered a life-saving procedure to treat caval injury. Follow-up for late leg complications was not available in this study. No follow-up extended beyond 30 days.

G. L. Moneta, MD

The Insensate Foot Following Severe Lower Extremity Trauma: An Indication for Amputation?

Bosse MJ, for the Lower Extremity Assessment Project (*LEAP*) Study Group (Johns Hopkins Univ, Baltimore, Md)
J Bone Joint Surg Am 87-A:2601-2608, 2005   12–2

Background.—Plantar sensation is considered to be a critical factor in the evaluation of limb-threatening lower extremity trauma. The present study was designed to determine the long-term outcomes following the treatment of severe lower extremity injuries in patients who had had absent plantar sensation at the time of the initial presentation.

Methods.—We examined the outcomes for a subset of fifty-five subjects who had had an insensate extremity at the time of presentation. The patients were divided into two groups on the basis of the treatment in the hospital: an insensate amputation group (twenty-six patients) and an insensate salvage group (twenty-nine patients), the latter of which was the group of primary interest. In addition, a control group was constructed from the parent cohort so that the patients in the study groups could be compared with patients in whom plantar sensation was present and in whom the limb was reconstructed. Patient and injury characteristics as well as functional and health-related quality-of-life outcomes at twelve and twenty-four months after the injury were compared between the subjects in the insensate salvage group and those in the other two groups.

Results.—The patients in the insensate salvage group did not report or demonstrate significantly worse outcomes at twelve or twenty-four months after the injury compared with subjects in the insensate amputation or sensate control groups. Among the patients in whom the limb was salvaged (that is, those in the insensate salvage and sensate control groups), an equal proportion (approximately 55%) had normal plantar sensation at two years after the injury, regardless of whether plantar sensation had been reported to be intact at the time of admission. No significant differences were noted among the three groups with regard to the overall, physical, or psychosocial scores. At two years after the injury, only one patient in the insensate salvage group had absent plantar sensation.

Conclusions.—Outcome was not adversely affected by limb salvage, despite the presence of an insensate foot at the time of presentation. More than one-half of the patients who had presented with an insensate foot that was treated with limb reconstruction ultimately regained sensation at two years. Initial plantar sensation is not prognostic of long-term plantar sensory status or functional outcomes and should not be a component of a limb-salvage decision algorithm.

▶ The data suggest that assessment of plantar sensation after lower-extremity trauma is essentially worthless in predicting the final sensory status of the foot. These study findings do not support the widespread belief that absent initial plantar sensation in patients with a leg-threatening injury correlates with poor long-term outcome if the limb were to be salvaged. The implication from this study is that tibial nerve dysfunction at the time of presentation does not necessarily imply transsection of the tibial nerve. It is important to remember that reversible ischemic injuries to nerves and neurapraxic injuries of peripheral nerves may mimic permanent loss of peripheral nerve function.

G. L. Moneta, MD

Carotid Artery Stents for Blunt Cerebrovascular Injury: Risks Exceed Benefits
Cothren CC, Moore EE, Ray CE Jr, et al (Univ of Colorado, Denver)
Arch Surg 140:480-486, 2005   12–3

Background.—Carotid stenting has been advocated in patients with grade III blunt carotid artery injuries (hereafter referred to as "blunt CAIs") because of the persistence of the pseudoaneurysm and concern for subsequent embolization or rupture.

Hypothesis.—Carotid stenting is safe and effective for blunt CAIs.

Design.—Analysis of a prospective database of all patients with blunt CAIs.

Setting.—A state-designated, level I, urban trauma center.

Patients and Methods.—In January 1, 1996, we initiated comprehensive screening for blunt CAIs with angiography based on injury patterns. Patients without contraindications receive anticoagulation therapy immediately for documented lesions. Patients with persistent pseudoaneurysms on a second angiography at 7 to 10 days after injury are candidates for stent placement.

Results.—During the study period (January 1, 1996, to May 1, 2004), 46 patients sustained blunt carotid pseudoaneurysms; 23 (50%) underwent carotid stent placement. There were 4 complications in patients undergoing carotid stent placement: 3 strokes and 1 subclavian dissection. Follow-up angiography was performed in 38 patients (18 patients with stents who received antithrombotic agents, 20 patients who received antithrombotic agents alone); 8 patients had poststent carotid occlusion despite having received concurrent anticoagulation therapy. Carotid occlusion rates were significantly different (45% in patients with stents vs 5% in those who received antithrombotic agents alone). In the patients not undergoing stent placement, the only complication was a middle cerebral artery stroke in a patient not treated with antithrombotic therapy.

Conclusions.—Patients who have carotid stents placed for blunt carotid pseudoaneurysms have a 21% complication rate and a documented occlusion rate of 45%. In contrast, patients treated with antithrombotic agents alone had an occlusion rate of 5%; no asymptomatic patient treated with antithrombotic agents for their injury had a stroke. Antithrombotic therapy remains the recommended therapy for blunt CAIs, but the role of intraluminal stents remains to be defined.

▶ The study indicates safety and efficacy of anticoagulation therapy for patients with pseudoaneurysm after blunt carotid injury. The carotid occlusion rate in patients treated with stents was, however, alarming. The antithrombotic regimen used in the patients treated with stents was heparin. Perhaps better results may have been obtained with the use of clopidogrel or even a combination of clopidogrel and heparin. The data indicate anticoagulation alone is effective for most patients with pseudoaneurysm after CAI. If stenting must be done for pseudoaneurysm after CAI, an alternative form of periprocedure antithrombotic therapy other than heparin should be used. Clearly, the combination of heparin and stents is unacceptable.

G. L. Moneta, MD

Contemporary management of wartime vascular trauma

Fox CJ, Gillespie DL, O'Donnell SD, et al (Walter Reed Army Med Ctr, Washington, DC; Uniformed Univ of the Health Sciences, Bethesda, Md)
J Vasc Surg 41:638-644, 2005   12–4

Objective.—The treatment of wartime injuries has led to advances in the diagnosis and treatment of vascular trauma. Recent experience has stimulated a reappraisal of the management of such injuries, specifically assessing the effect of explosive devices on injury patterns and treatment strategies. The objective of this report is to provide a single-institution analysis of injury patterns and management strategies in the care of modern wartime vascular injuries.

Methods.—From December 2001 through March 2004, all wartime evacuees evaluated at a single institution were prospectively entered into a database and retrospectively reviewed. Data collected included site, type, and mechanism of vascular injury; associated trauma; type of vascular repair; initial outcome; occult injury; amputation rate; and complication. Liberal application of arteriography was used to assess these injuries. The results of that diagnostic and therapeutic approach, particularly as it related to the care of the blast-injured patient, are reviewed.

Results.—Of 3057 soldiers evacuated for medical evaluation, 1524 (50%) sustained battle injuries. Known or suspected vascular injuries occurred in 107 (7%) patients, and these patients comprised the study group. Sixty-eight (64%) patients were wounded by explosive devices, 27 (25%) were wounded by gunshots, and 12 (11%) experienced blunt traumatic injury. The majority of injuries (59/66 [88%]) occurred in the extremities. Nearly half (48/107) of the patients underwent vascular repair in a forward hospital in Iraq or Afghanistan. Twenty-eight (26%) required additional operative intervention on arrival in the United States. Vascular injuries were associated with bony fracture in 37% of soldiers. Twenty-one of the 107 had a primary amputation performed before evacuation. Amputation after vascu-

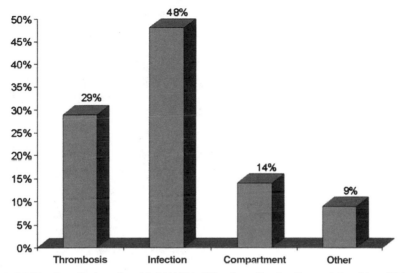

FIGURE.—Complications of repair in 21 (44%) of 48 patients. (Reprinted by permission of the publisher from Fox CJ, Gillespie DL, O'Donnell SD, et al: Contemporary management of wartime vascular trauma. *J Vasc Surg* 41:638-644, 2005. Copyright 2005 by Elsevier.)

lar repair occurred in 8 patients. Of those, 5 had mangled extremities associated with contaminated wounds and infected grafts. Sixty-seven (63%) patients underwent diagnostic angiography. The most common indication was mechanism of injury (42%), followed by abnormal examination (33%), operative planning (18%), or evaluation of a repair (7%).

Conclusions.—This interim report represents the largest analysis of US military vascular injuries in more than 30 years. Wounding patterns reflect past experience with a high percentage of extremity injuries. Management of arterial repair with autologous vein graft remains the treatment of choice. Repairs in contaminated wound beds should be avoided. An increase in injuries from improvised explosive devices in modern conflict warrants the more liberal application of contrast arteriography. Endovascular techniques have advanced the contemporary management and proved valuable in the treatment of select wartime vascular injuries (Figure).

▶ Only treated vascular injuries are reported here. In fact, only a small percentage of overall treated injuries were vascular in nature. This likely reflects use of body armor and the fatal nature of truncal vascular injuries. The main points of this article and similar articles are the same as always. Most treated vascular injuries are extremity injuries, and repair in contaminated fields should be avoided.

G. L. Moneta, MD

13 Nonatherosclerotic Conditions

The spectrum, management and clinical outcome of Ehlers-Danlos syndrome type IV: A 30-year experience
Oderich GS, Panneton JM, Bower TC, et al (Mayo Clinic, Rochester, Minn; Virginia Med School, Norfolk)
J Vasc Surg 42:98-106, 2005   13–1

Purpose.—Ehlers-Danlos syndrome type IV (EDS-IV) results from abnormal procollagen III synthesis and leads to arterial, intestinal, and uterine rupture. The purpose of this study was to review the spectrum, management, and clinical outcome of EDS-IV patients.

Methods.—We retrospectively reviewed the clinical data of 31 patients (15 male and 16 female) with a clinical diagnosis of EDS-IV treated over a 30-year period (1971 to 2001). Biochemical confirmation was obtained in 24 patients, and mutation of the *COL3A1* gene was confirmed in 11 patients. The study excluded patients with other connective tissue dysplasias.

Results.—The mean age at the time of diagnosis was 28.5 ± 11 years (range, 10 to 53 years). Twenty-four patients developed 132 vascular complications; of these, 85 were present either before or at the time of the initial evaluation, and 47 complications occurred during a median follow-up of 6.3 years (range, 0.5 to 26 years). Survival free of vascular complications was 90% at age 20 years, 39% at 40 years, and 20% at age 60 years. Fifteen patients underwent 30 operative interventions for vascular complications, including arterial reconstruction (n = 15), simple repair or ligation (n = 4), coil embolization (n = 3), splenectomy (n = 2), and abdominal decompression, nephrectomy, graft thrombectomy, vein stripping and thoracoscopy (n = 1 each). Three hospital deaths occurred from exsanguinating hemorrhage: two after operative interventions and one because of a ruptured splenic artery. Procedure-related morbidity was 46%, including a 37% incidence of postoperative bleeding and a 20% need for re-exploration. The incidence of late graft-related complications was 40% of arterial reconstructions, including 4 anastomotic aneurysms, 1 fatal anastomotic disruption, and 1 graft thrombosis. Patient survival was 68% at age 50 years and 35% at age 80 years. Of the 12 deaths during the study period, 11 were associated with vascular or graft-related complications.

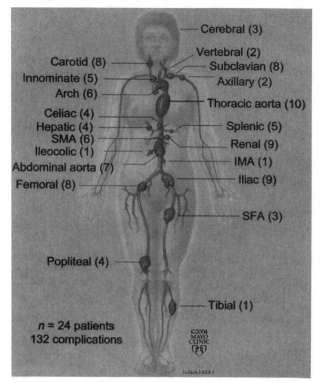

FIGURE 3.—Distribution of 132 vascular complications in 24 patients with a clinical diagnosis of Ehlers-Danlos syndrome type IV. (Reprinted by permission of the publisher from Oderich GS, Panneton JM, Bower TC, et al: The spectrum, management and clinical outcome of Ehlers-Danlos syndrome type IV: A 30-year experience. *J Vasc Surg* 42:98-106, 2005. Copyright 2005 by Elsevier.)

Conclusion.—Operative mortality in patients with vascular complications of EDS-IV was not excessively high, but the incidence of postoperative bleeding complications and late graft-related problems was significant. Despite successful repair of vascular complications, survival was shortened because of secondary vascular or graft-related complications (Fig 3).

▶ EDS-IV results from a mutation of the *COL3A1* gene that encodes for type III procollagen. Complications increase with age, with 80% of afflicted patients having a complication by the age of 40 years. Vascular procedures are unpredictable in these patients, with some doing well and others doing poorly. However, even if the patient gets through a vascular reconstruction, many (40%) will have a late graft-related complication. Late deaths are overwhelmingly caused by vascular or graft complications. Proceed when necessary, but proceed with caution, and be prepared to see the patient again!

G. L. Moneta, MD

Influence of Traditional Risk Factors of Atherosclerosis in the Development of Severe Ischemic Complications in Giant Cell Arteritis

Gonzalez-Gay MA, Piñeiro A, Gomez-Gigirey A, et al (Hosp Xeral-Calde, Lugo, Spain; Univ of Cantabria, Santander, Spain)
Medicine 83:342-347, 2004   13–2

Because the prognosis of giant cell arteritis (GCA) is related to the development of ischemic complications, we sought to assess the possible influence of traditional risk factors of atherosclerosis in the development of severe ischemic complications of GCA. We conducted a retrospective study of patients with biopsy-proven GCA diagnosed from 1981 to 2001 at the single hospital for a well-defined population of almost 250,000 people. Patients were considered to have severe ischemic manifestations if they suffered visual manifestations, cerebrovascular accidents, jaw claudication, or signs of occlusive changes in large arteries of the extremities. Patients were assessed for the presence of hypercholesterolemia, hypertension, diabetes mellitus, and heavy smoking at the time of GCA diagnosis. The presence of traditional risk factors of atherosclerosis at the time of GCA diagnosis in this series of 210 patients increased significantly the risk of developing at least 1 of the severe ischemic complications (odds ratio [OR], 1.79; 95% confidence intervals [CI], 1.03-3.11; p − 0.04). Patients with traditional atherosclerosis risk factors had fever less commonly than the rest of GCA patients (5.2% vs. 16.0%; p = 0.01). GCA patients with hypertension exhibited a significantly increased risk of developing severe ischemic complications (OR, 1.80; 95% CI, 1.00-3.25; p = 0.05). The current study suggests that the presence of atherosclerosis risk factors at the time of diagnosis of GCA may influence the development of severe ischemic manifestations of the disease.

▶ There has long been a suggestion that atherosclerosis and GCA may share a common pathway.[1] If the authors' findings are correct, patients with GCA should be assessed for atherosclerotic risk factors, and those risk factors should be vigorously treated along with the usual treatment for GCA.

G. L. Moneta, MD

Reference

1. Machado EBV, Gabriel SE, Beard CM, et al: A population-based case-control study of temporal arteritis: Evidence for an association between temporal arteritis and degenerative vascular disease? *Int J Epidemiol* 18:836-841, 1989.

Surgical treatment of atypical aortic coarctation complicating Takayasu's arteritis—experience with 33 cases over 44 years

Taketani T, Miyata T, Morota T, et al (Univ of Tokyo)
J Vasc Surg 41:597-601, 2005

13–3

Purpose.—This study was conducted to evaluate the long-term outcomes of surgical treatment for atypical aortic coarctation due to Takayasu's arteritis and to elucidate the factors that affected outcome.

Methods.—The outcomes of surgical treatment for atypical aortic coarctation complicating Takayasu's arteritis in 33 consecutive patients over the previous 44 years at our institution were reviewed retrospectively. Preoperatively, 29 patients had coarctation proximal to the renal arteries and hypertension in the upper half of the body. Four hospital deaths occurred, and the remaining 29 patients were followed from 0.5 to 42.0 years (median, 17.9 years). The impacts of several risk factors on survival as well as cardiac and vascular events were analyzed.

Results.—Among 27 initial survivors who had hypertension preoperatively, 15 did not show normalization of blood pressure. The overall cumulative survival and event-free survival rate at 20 years were 62.3% and 58.4%, respectively. Serious long-term complications were anastomotic aneurysms, congestive heart failure, cerebrovascular accident, graft deterioration, abdominal aortic aneurysms, and renal failure. Among several risk factors analyzed, only the presence of postoperative hypertension had an effect on event-free survival.

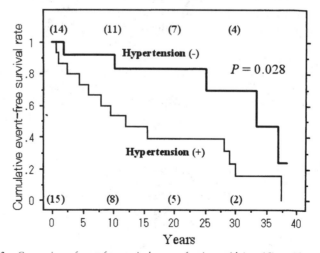

FIGURE 3.—Comparison of event-free survival curves of patients with (n = 15) or without (n = 14) postoperative hypertension. A log-rank test showed a significant difference between the two groups. The number of patients alive at the beginning of each follow-up period is given in parentheses. (Reprinted by permission of the publisher from Taketani T, Miyata T, Morota T, et al: Surgical treatment of atypical aortic coarctation complicating Takayasu's arteritis—experience with 33 cases over 44 years. *J Vasc Surg* 41:597-601, 2005. Copyright 2005 by Elsevier.)

Conclusions.—The long-term survival after surgery for atypical aortic co-arctation was satisfactory. However, our study showed that complications associated with cardiovascular system or the operation could occur at any time after surgery; thus, life-long follow-up is mandatory. Further, the absence of normalization of blood pressure after surgery was a poor prognostic factor. Our results demonstrate the need for an intimate preoperative evaluation of renal and carotid artery lesions, which often coexist and may also cause secondary hypertension, to fully manage hypertension by surgery (Fig 3).

▶ The message is to look beyond the aortic coarctation in patients with Takayasu's arteritis and aortic coarctation with secondary hypertension. Some of the patients with aortic coarctation will also have renal artery lesions that lead to postoperative continued hypertension. Deal with the renal artery lesions to avoid the severe adverse affects of continued hypertension in these patients.

G. L. Moneta, MD

Takayasu's arteritis: Operative results and influence of disease activity
Fields CE, Bower TC, Cooper LT, et al (Mayo Clinic, Rochester, Minn; Univ of Virginia, Charlottesville)
J Vasc Surg 43:64-71, 2006   13–4

Objectives.—To determine the short- and long-term outcomes of patients treated operatively for Takayasu's arteritis and the effect of disease activity on results.

Methods.—Forty-two (17%) of the 251 patients enrolled in our Takayasu's arteritis registry between 1975 and 2002 required operation for symptomatic disease. Data were obtained from the registry, patient records, phone correspondence, and written surveys.

Results.—There were 38 females and 4 males with a median age of 29 years (range, 12 to 56 years), and 32 (76%) were white. Sixty operations were performed for symptomatic disease. The mean duration of symptoms before operation was 5.6 months (range, 0 to 25 months). Thirteen (31%) patients had active disease and underwent operation for acute presentation or failure of medical management. Thirty-nine patients (93%) had operation for occlusive disease. Twenty-two (52%) patients had involvement of both the great and abdominal aortic branch vessels; 10 (24%) had great vessel disease alone; 9 (21%) had involvement of abdominal arteries; and 1 (2%) had coronary artery disease. There was no operative death, myocardial infarction, major stroke, or renal failure. Three patients had early graft thrombosis, two had a minor stroke, and two developed hyperperfusion syndrome. The median follow-up was 6.7 years (range, 1 month to 19.3 years). Eleven (26%) patients required 15 graft revisions; five of the patients had active disease at the time of initial operation. All early revisions (<1 year) were in patients with active disease. By Kaplan-Meier analysis, freedom from revision at 5 and 10 years was 100% in patients with quiescent disease

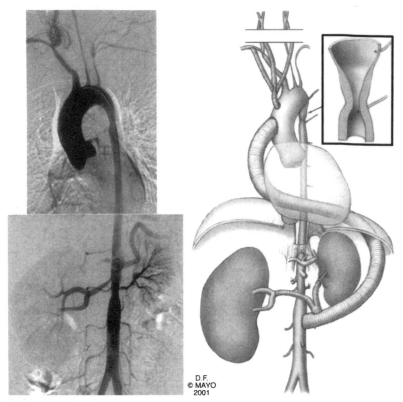

FIGURE 1.—Complex reconstruction performed in a patient with combined great vessel, thoracic aorta, and renal occlusive disease. *Arrows* at areas of revascularization. (Reprinted by permission of Mayo Foundation for Medical Education and Research. All rights reserved.) (Courtesy of Fields CE, Bower TC, Cooper LT, et al: Takayasu's arteritis: Operative results and influence of disease activity. *J Vasc Surg* 43:64-71, 2006.)

not requiring steroids (group I, n = 5, 12%), 95% and 81% in patients whose disease was quiescent on steroids (group II, n = 24, 57%), 57% in patients with active disease on steroids (group III, n = 7, 17%), and 33% in patients with active disease and no long-term steroids (group IV, n = 6, 14%) ($P < .006$). The rate of revision or progression of disease at another site in 5 years was 0% in group 1, 10% in group 2, 57% in group 3, and 67% in group 4 ($P < .001$) The differences were even more pronounced when an analysis was done on the basis of disease activity alone, irrespective of steroid use. During the follow-up period, 3 of 39 great vessel, 2 of 18 mesenteric/renal, and 1 of 9 aortofemoropopliteal reconstructions occluded. The predicted mortality for patients was 4% at both 5 and 10 years (95% CI) respectively (confidence interval [CI], 0% to 11%) and 10 (CI, 0% to 14%) years, respectively.

Conclusions.—The minority of patients with Takayasu's arteritis require operation. In our predominantly white female patient population, occlusive symptoms were the most common indication for operation. Operation for these selected patients was safe, with no operative mortality, myocardial infarction, major stroke, or renal failure. Patients with active disease requiring operation are more likely to require revision or develop progressive symptomatic disease at another site. Long-term survival is excellent, regardless of disease activity at the time of operation (Fig 1).

▶ The computers at Mayo are always humming, generating reasonably large series of patients with rare disorders seen over many years (see Abstract 13–1). Some of the authors of this study were likely still in diapers when the first patients were treated. Nevertheless, this approach of records-based research has some validity when dealing with rare disorders. There are no surprises horc; patients operated on with active disease did not do as well as those operated on with quiescent disease. Survival is, however, quite high at 10 years. That is a nice bit of information to communicate to any patient with Takayasu's arteritis. Always remember to treat the hypertension (see Abstract 13–3).

G. L. Moneta, MD

Oral bacteria in the occluded arteries of patients with Buerger disease
Iwai T, Inoue Y, Umeda M, et al (Tokyo Med and Dental Univ)
J Vasc Surg 42:107-115, 2005   13–5

Objective.—Recent studies have suggested that infectious organisms play a role in vascular diseases. In this study, to explore a possible link between oral infection and Buerger disease, we investigated whether oral (periodontal) bacteria were present in occluded arteries removed from patients with characteristic Buerger disease.

Methods.—Fourteen male patients with a smoking history who had developed characteristics of Buerger disease before the age of 50 years were included in this study. Occluded arteries, including superficial femoral (n = 4), popliteal (n = 2), anterior tibial (n = 4), and posterior tibial (n = 4) arteries, were removed and studied. A periodontist performed a periodontal examination on each patient and collected dental plaque and saliva samples from them at the same time. The polymerase chain reaction method was applied to detect whether seven species of periodontal bacteria—*Porphyromonas gingivalis, Tannerella forsythensis, Treponema denticola, Campylobacter rectus, Actinobacillus actinomycetemcomitans, Prevotella intermedia,* and *Prevotella nigrescens*—were present in the occluded arteries and oral samples. In addition, arterial specimens from seven control patients were examined by polymerase chain reaction analysis.

Results.—DNA of oral bacteria was detected in 13 of 14 arterial samples and all oral samples of patients with Buerger disease. *Treponema denticola* was found in 12 arterial and all oral samples. *Campylobacter rectus, Porphyromonas gingivalis, Prevotella intermedia, Tannerella forsythensis,* and *Prevotella nigrescens* were found in 14% to 43% of the arterial samples and 71% to 100% of the oral samples. A pathologic examination revealed that arterial specimens showed the characteristics of an intermediate-chronic-stage or chronic-stage lesion of Buerger disease. All 14 patients with Buerger disease had moderate to severe periodontitis. None of the control arterial samples was positive for periodontal bacteria.

Conclusions.—This is the first study to identify oral microorganisms in the lesions of Buerger disease. Our findings suggest a possible etiologic link between Buerger disease and chronic infections such as oral bacterial infections.

▶ People keep trying to implicate oral bacteria as important in development of arterial disease. This article, like those before it, suffers from the "chicken and egg" problem; that is, are the bacteria in the blood vessels a cause of the blood vessel disease or are the bacteria there because of the blood vessel disease? In either case, it will not hurt to get your patients with Buerger's disease to brush their teeth.

G. L. Moneta, MD

Successful Treatment of Buerger's Disease with Intramedullary K-wire: The Results of the First 11 Extremities
Inan M, Alat I, Kutlu R, et al (Inönü Univ, Malatya, Turkey)
Eur J Vasc Endovasc Surg 29:277-280, 2005   13–6

Objective.—This study describes a new technique for treatment of Buerger's disease, developed to stimulate angiogenesis, using a Kirschner wire placed in the medullary canal of the tibia. The aim of the study was to evaluate clinical and radiological effects of this technique in patients where medical and surgical therapy had failed.

Material and Methods.—Eleven extremities (six patients) with Buerger's disease were treated with the intramedullary Kirschner wire technique. Inclusion criteria were chronic critical ischemia, Rutherford Grade II or III, with major arterial occlusion shown by Doppler examination and angiography; failure to respond to non-surgical and surgical treatment; and the need for strong analgesics.

Results.—The mean follow-up time was 19 months (range, 13-25 months). Satisfactory remission in each patient was obtained within 6 weeks of intervention. A significant improvement in clinical manifestations including reduced rest pain and increased claudication distance was observed. Foot ulcers completely healed after Kirschner wire intervention.

Conclusion.—Despite short-term follow-up and small patient series, the intramedullary Kirschner wire technique can be expected to achieve relief of pain and a decrease in major amputations in patients with Buerger's disease in whom medical and surgical therapy had failed. However, comparative studies with longer follow-up should be done to confirm the benefits of this new treatment.

▶ It is hard to know why placement of a wire in the tibia should stimulate angiogenesis. The patients appeared to improve, but they also all stopped smoking. Patients with Buerger's disease will virtually never lose their limbs if they stop smoking. The patients belong in a stop-smoking program. I doubt the orthopedic clinic is where they should be.

G. L. Moneta, MD

The role of epidural spinal cord stimulation in the treatment of Buerger's disease
Donas KP, Schulte S, Ktenidis K, et al (Univ of Cologne, Germany)
J Vasc Surg 41:830-836, 2005   13–7

Purpose.—This clinical, retrospective study evaluated the effect of epidural spinal cord stimulation (SCS) in the treatment of Buerger's disease.

Methods.—The clinical criteria of Shionoya were used to diagnose 29 patients (22 men, 7 women; mean age 33.7 years) with Buerger's disease. The patients underwent SCS. Complete physical examination and vascular laboratory data were available and recorded for all patients. Questions regarding the improvement of symptoms, in lifestyle, and in physical activities were asked direct interview or by telephone during mean follow-up of 4 years.

Results.—The regional perfusion index (RPI), the ratio between the foot and chest transcutaneous oxygen pressure at baseline (before SCS treatment) was 0.27 ± 0.25. Three months after SCS implantation the RPI increased to 0.41 ± 0.22. During the follow-up period, a sustained improvement in microcirculation was recorded: the RPI at 1-year follow-up was 0.49 ± 0.34 and at 3-year follow-up was 0.52 ± 0.21. The most pronounced improvement in the RPI values was found in the subgroup of 13 patients with trophic lesions. In this group, the RPI increased significantly from 0.17 ± 0.21 to 0.4 ± 0.18 ($P < .023$) after a mean follow-up of 5.7 years. Two pa-

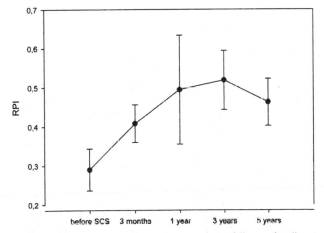

FIGURE 1.—Course of the regional perfusion index (*RPI*) during follow-up for all patients with Buerger's disease treated with spinal cord stimulation (*SCS*). Graphed values are presented as the mean ± SE. (Reprinted by permission of the publisher from Donas KP, Schulte S, Ktenidis K, et al: The role of epidural spinal cord stimulation in the treatment of Buerger's disease. *J Vasc Surg* 41:830-836, 2005. Copyright 2005 by Elsevier.)

tients underwent major amputation of the lower target limb. The limb survival rate was 93.1%. During the follow-up period of 4 years, 21 of the 29 patients continued to smoke, and only five patients stopped nicotine exposure.

Conclusions.—We recorded a significant benefit in the microcirculation, a good limb survival rate, and the absence of new trophic lesions. During the follow-up period, no severe complications related to the implanted devices occurred. Because of the diffuse, distal, segmental nature of the disease, SCS should be considered as an alternative treatment modality in patients with Buerger's disease (Fig 1).

▶ SCS has for years been advocated by selected centers as treatment for unreconstructable arterial disease. The articles are generally favorable but always uncontrolled and, essentially, anecdotal. However, complications are minimal, and no one suggests it makes things worse. The principle drawback is expense. It all depends on where one wishes to spend money. One can buy a lot of SCSs for the price of 1 tank.

G. L. Moneta, MD

The surgical treatment of arterial aneurysms in Behçet disease: A report of 16 patients

Kalko Y, Basaran M, Aydin U, et al (Vakif Gureba Hosp, Istanbul, Turkey)
J Vasc Surg 42:673-677, 2005   13–8

Objective.—The aim of this article is to report our experience in the surgical treatment of arterial aneurysms in patients with Behçet disease.

Methods.—From October 2001 through May 2004, 18 arterial aneurysms were diagnosed in 16 Behçet patients. All patients were male. The patients ranged in age from 24 to 52 years (mean, 37.4 ± 5.2 years). There were six abdominal aortic, three common femoral, two iliac, two popliteal, two superficial femoral, and two anterior tibial aneurysms and one subclavian artery aneurysm. All patients but four were in remission at the time of diagnosis. Those 4 patients received immunosuppressive therapy before the surgical intervention to induce remission. After hospital discharge, all patients were followed up regularly at 3-month intervals. The mean duration of follow-up was 17 ± 4.2 months (range, 6-24 months).

Results.—All patients underwent a successful surgical intervention. During the study period, we performed five aortic tube graft interpositions, two aortofemoral bypasses, one aortobifemoral bypass, three common femoral artery graft interpositions, and two femoropopliteal bypasses. The popliteal artery (n = 2), anterior tibial artery (n = 2), and subclavian artery (n = 1) aneurysms were repaired primarily. There was no in-hospital mortality. One patient with an abdominal aortic aneurysm had to undergo reoperation because of postoperative bleeding. The postoperative hospital stay was 8.5 ± 4.3 days. Two patients were lost to follow-up. During the follow-up period, two false aneurysms of the common femoral artery were repaired with a graft interposition procedure. Another patient who had undergone an aortic tube graft interposition was readmitted 9 months later with an external iliac artery aneurysm. The external iliac artery was ligated through a retroperitoneal approach, and femorofemoral bypass was performed. In addition, one femoropopliteal interposition graft was occluded, without disabling ischemia.

Conclusions.—Although aneurysmal disease is rare in Behçet disease, it can complicate the clinical picture and cause life-threatening complications. We believe that the establishment of remission before the surgical intervention decreases the incidence of postoperative complications. Because recur-

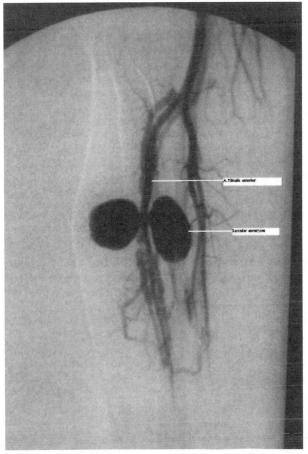

FIGURE 3.—Digital subtraction angiography image of a tibialis anterior artery aneurysm. (Reprinted by permission of the publisher from Kalko Y, Basaran M, Aydin U, et al: The surgical treatment of arterial aneurysms in Behçet disease: A report of 16 patients. *J Vasc Surg* 42:673-677, 2005. Copyright 2005 by Elsevier.)

rence at the site of anastomosis is possible, prolonged monitoring is required (Fig 3).

▶ Behçet disease is a vasculitis characterized by genital ulcers, oral aphthous ulcers, and ocular lesions. It is strongly associated with HLA-B51. Most patients with Behçet disease do not have large artery problems. Such problems are, however, the main cause of death in patients with Behçet disease. It therefore makes sense, when feasible, to repair such lesions. The authors' suggestion to induce remission before arterial repair seems logical, but there is, of course, no convincing data one way or the other.

G. L. Moneta, MD

Long-term outcome after surgical treatment of arterial lesions in Behçet disease

Hosaka A, Miyata T, Shigematsu H, et al (Univ of Tokyo)
J Vasc Surg 42:116-121, 2005
13–9

Objective.—Surgical treatment of arterial lesions associated with Behçet disease (BD) is often complicated by graft occlusion and recurrence of aneurysms. The purpose of this study was to clarify the long-term outcome of surgical intervention for arterial involvement in BD.

Methods.—Ten patients with BD (9 men, 1 woman) who underwent surgical treatment for arterial aneurysms between 1980 and 2004 were included in the study. The age of patients at the first operation ranged from 36 to 69 years (mean, 50.4 ± 9.0 years). The mean period between the onset of BD and that of arterial manifestations was 8.0 ± 5.0 years. We retrospectively reviewed their postoperative courses, including survival, graft occlusion, formation of anastomotic false aneurysms, and the development of aneurysms at different sites. The Kaplan-Meier method was used to calculate the chronologic incidence of complications after surgery.

Results.—The mean follow-up period was 133 ± 92 months, ranging from 5 to 285 months. One patient died of rupture of a dissecting aortic aneurysm after undergoing several surgical interventions for multiple aneurysms. There were five graft occlusions among 21 grafts. The cumulative primary graft patency rate in the infrainguinal region was 83.9% at 3 years. Five anastomotic false aneurysms formed among 49 anastomoses between grafts and host arteries. The overall cumulative incidence of formation of anastomotic pseudoaneurysm was 12.9% at 5 and 10 years. All of them formed within 18 months after surgery. Development of new aneurysms in different arteries was observed in two patients.

Conclusions.—Early occurrence of anastomotic false aneurysm is characteristic of BD. Further investigation is necessary to establish effective postoperative treatment.

▶ This and the previous abstract (Abstract 13–8) highlight the problems of anastomotic false aneurysms after aneurysm repair in patients with BD. While the rate of false aneurysm formation is greater than that after repair for atherosclerotic aneurysm, it is not so high as to preclude indicated repairs. In follow-up, the patients need to be monitored for development of new aneurysms in addition to false aneurysms. Why the occasional patient with BD is an "aneurysm former" is unknown.

G. L. Moneta, MD

Endovascular treatment for superior vena cava obstruction in Behçet disease
Castelli P, Caronno R, Piffaretti G, et al (Univ of Insubria, Varese, Italy)
J Vasc Surg 41:548-551, 2005   13–10

Background.—Vascular involvement in patients with Behçet disease has been thought to result from systemic vasculitis, which most frequently affects veins and occurs in 5% to 10% of these patients. However, involvement of the superior vena cava (SVC) is rare, accounting for only 6% of these cases. Presented was a case of SVC recanalization through the use of fibrinolysis and self-expanding stents as treatment of life-threatening SVC syndrome in a young patient with Behçet disease.

Case Report.—Man, 25, from North Africa with Behçet disease was seen with a history of persistent dyspnea and chest pain. Physical examination showed acneiform nodules and swelling of his arms and

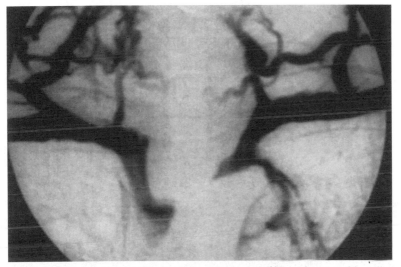

FIGURE 2.—Digital venography of the upper extremities confirmed bilateral patency of the axillary and subclavian veins, with thrombosis of the superior vena cava and innominate veins. (Reprinted by permission of the publisher from Castelli P, Caronno R, Piffaretti G, et al: Endovascular treatment for superior vena cava obstruction in Behçet disease. *J Vasc Surg* 41:548-551, 2005. Copyright 2005 by Elsevier.)

neck. Medical treatment had consisted of 6 months of immunosuppressive and steroid therapy.

Venous collateral structures were detected in his neck and anterior thoracic wall. An ophthalmologic examination confirmed the presence of uveitis. CT angiography (CTA) excluded the presence of a mediastinal mass and showed obstruction of the SVC, which was confirmed by bilateral upper arm digital venography. The venography also showed patency of the axillary and subclavian veins and obstruction of the innominate veins (Fig 2). US examination did not show any other localization of vein thrombosis.

An endovascular recanalization procedure of the SVC was scheduled. Postoperative digital venography showed bilateral recanalization of the innominate veins with persistent obstruction of the SVC;

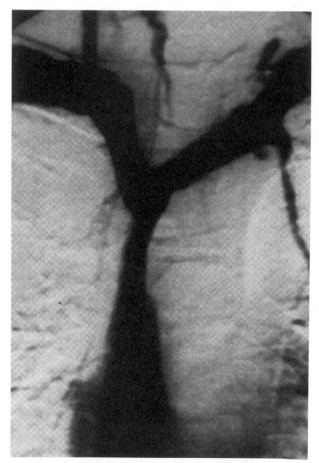

FIGURE 3.—Final digital venography control after fibrinolysis and stenting of the superior vena cava. (Reprinted by permission of the publisher from Castelli P, Caronno R, Piffaretti G, et al: Endovascular treatment for superior vena cava obstruction in Behçet disease. *J Vasc Surg* 41:548-551, 2005. Copyright 2005 by Elsevier.)

thereafter the SVC was stented with an 18-mm balloon-expandable stent. The final digital venography control confirmed the complete recanalization of the SVC (Fig 3). The patient was discharged with warfarin, imunosuppressive drugs, and steroids. CTA control examinations were scheduled at 1, 3, and 6 months after the procedure and then yearly. The final CTA control at 36 months confirmed the patency of both the stent and the SVC, and the patient had no symptoms of venous disease.

Conclusions.—The use of stents as a first choice for patients with nonmalignant SVCs is still debatable because of the need for repeated interventions. However, in this case, the clinical outcome was satisfactory. The placement of stents in patients with nonmalignant SVC obstruction could be an effective and viable procedure when performed by an experienced surgeon.

▶ Veins are more commonly involved than arteries in Behçet disease. I wonder if endolumenal techniques as applied to the SVC in this case might help eliminate the false aneurysms associated with arterial aneurysm repair in Behçet disease. (See also Abstracts 13–8 and 13–9.)

G. L. Moneta, MD

Role of computed tomographic angiography in the detection and comprehensive evaluation of persistent sciatic artery

Jung AY, Lee W, Chung JW, et al (Seoul Natl Univ College of Medicine, Republic of Korea; Hanyan Univ Hosp, Seoul, Republic of Korea)
J Vasc Surg 42:678-683, 2005   13–11

Purpose.—To define the role of computed tomographic (CT) angiography in the evaluation of persistent sciatic artery and to identify its potential advantages as a diagnostic modality.

Methods.—Between July 2002 and August 2004, 307 consecutive patients underwent CT angiography for suspected lower-extremity arterial insufficiency. All CT angiograms were retrospectively reviewed to determine the presence and laterality of persistent sciatic artery and its associated vascular abnormalities, such as aneurysm, thrombus, distal thromboembolism, and atherosclerotic change. The relationship of persistent sciatic artery with adjacent structures, such as sciatic nerve, muscle, accompanying vein, and femoral artery, as well as the presence of other anomalies, was analyzed. Clinical data regarding the presenting symptoms and hospital course were obtained from patient charts.

Results.—Six persistent sciatic arteries, with or without occlusion, were identified in five female patients (age range, 54 to 80 years). CT angiography revealed unilateral persistent sciatic artery in four patients (left, 3; right, 1) and bilateral persistent sciatic artery in one patient. Aneurysm was present in two (mean size, 26 mm × 20 mm), thrombosis in three, and distal thromboembolism in all six persistent sciatic arteries. All persistent sciatic arteries

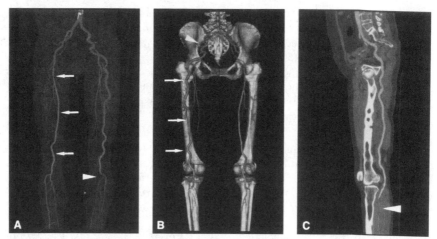

FIGURE 1.—Computed tomographic angiography of a left persistent sciatic artery (PSA) in a 66-year-old woman with left leg claudication and pain. **A,** Maximum intensity projection image after bone segmentation shows the typical appearance of a left PSA as an abnormal tortuous extension of the left internal iliac artery that continues as the popliteal artery. The left superficial femoral artery is hypoplastic, and distal thromboembolism is present in the tibioperoneal trunk and anterior tibial artery (*arrowhead*). The contralateral side shows the normal anatomy of lower-extremity arteries (*arrows*). **B,** Posterior view of volume rendering image shows the left PSA (*arrows*) passing through the sciatic notch (*arrowhead*) and running posteriorly to ischial bone. **C,** Curved multiplanar image shows the cross section of the entire lumen of the PSA and the presence of thromboembolism at the tibioperoneal trunk (*arrowhead*). (Reprinted by permission of the publisher from Jung AY, Lee W, Chung JW, et al: Role of computed tomographic angiography in the detection and comprehensive evaluation of persistent sciatic artery. *J Vasc Surg* 42:678-683, 2005. Copyright 2005 by Elsevier.)

coursed along the sciatic nerve and continued as popliteal artery. Characteristically, in all these instances, the superficial femoral arteries were hypoplastic and tapered smoothly. Anomalous popliteal venous drainage was noted in all ipsilateral limbs with persistent sciatic artery and even in contralateral limbs with normal superficial femoral artery in all but one.

Conclusion.—CT angiography enables the detection of persistent sciatic artery even in the presence of complete occlusion and is useful in the comprehensive evaluation of various complications and associated venous anomalies. It can potentially be used as the sole imaging modality for persistent sciatic artery (Fig 1).

▶ There are no new insights into the arterial side of persistent sciatic artery presented in this article. However, I was not aware of associated venous abnormalities. The imaging presented here is impressive and was obtained with only 4- and 8-detector row scanners. A potential advantage of CT scanning over catheter-based angiography in the evaluation of sciatic artery is the ability to identify with a single procedure venous abnormalities associated with the persistent sciatic artery.

G. L. Moneta, MD

Accelerated atherosclerosis in patients with Wegener's granulomatosis

de Leeuw K, Sanders J-S, Stegeman C, et al (Univ Hosp, Groningen, Netherlands)

Ann Rheum Dis 64:753-759, 2005   13–12

Background.—Several autoimmune disorders are complicated by excess cardiovascular disease. In addition to traditional risk factors, non-traditional risk factors such as endothelial activation and excessive vascular remodelling might be determinants of the progression of atherosclerosis in patients with an autoimmune disease.

Objective. –To evaluate whether patients with Wegener's granulomatosis (WG) have an increased prevalence of atherosclerosis and to determine predisposing factors.

Methods.—29 WG patients (19 men; mean (SD) age, 53 (14) years) with inactive disease and 26 controls (16 men; age 53 (15) years) were studied. Common carotid intima-media thickness (IMT) was measured by ultrasound. In all individuals traditional risk factors for cardiovascular disease were determined. High sensitivity C reactive protein (hsCRP) was measured. Endothelial activation was assessed by measuring thrombomodulin, vascular cell adhesion molecule-1, and von Willebrand factor. As a marker of vascular remodelling matrix metalloproteinases (MMP-3 and MMP-9) and TIMP-1 were measured.

Results.—IMT was increased in WG patients compared with controls ($p<0.05$). No differences in traditional risk factors and endothelial activation markers between patients and controls were found. Levels of hsCRP, MMPs, and TIMP-1 were increased in WG patients ($p<0.05$).

Conclusions.—Increased IMT found in WG patients cannot be explained by an increased prevalence of traditional risk factors. Although endothelial activation markers in WG patients with inactive disease were not increased, the raised levels of hsCRP, MMPs, and TIMP-1 suggest that enhanced inflammation and excessive vascular remodelling are contributing factors in the development of accelerated atherosclerosis in WG.

▶ Inflammation is a strong component of autoimmune disorders. Atherosclerosis, clearly, also has some component of inflammation. The inflammatory markers measured in the patients with WG were only weakly correlated with IMT levels, but the patients were relatively young. Given more time, increase in IMT in the patients with WG may have been more profound. At present, I doubt the atherogenic tendency ascribed to the associated inflammation of WG is likely to have clinical significance. It serves more as another bit of evidence supporting the role of inflammation in atherosclerosis.

G. L. Moneta, MD

Brief Communication: High Incidence of Venous Thrombotic Events among Patients with Wegener Granulomatosis: The Wegener's Clinical Occurrence of Thrombosis (WeCLOT) Study

Merkel PA, for the Wegener's Granulomatosis Etanercept Trial Research Group (Boston Univ; et al)
Ann Intern Med 142:620-626, 2005   13–13

Background.—Venous thrombotic events (VTEs) have been observed in Wegener granulomatosis, but the incidence rate is not known.

Objective.—To measure the incidence of VTEs in patients with Wegener granulomatosis.

Design.—Prospective, observational cohort study.

Setting.—A multicenter, randomized, double-blind, placebo-controlled treatment trial for Wegener granulomatosis.

Patients.—180 patients with Wegener granulomatosis enrolled during periods of active disease.

Measurements.—Venous thrombotic events (deep venous thromboses or pulmonary emboli) were documented and confirmed prospectively. Incidence rates were calculated on the basis of time to first VTE.

Results.—Thirteen patients had VTEs before enrollment. During 228 person-years of prospective follow-up, 16 VTEs occurred in 167 patients

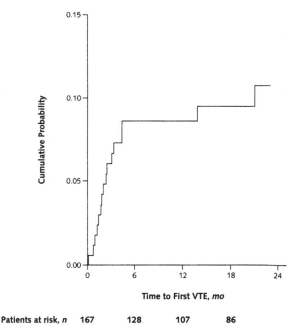

FIGURE.—Time to first venous thrombotic event (VTE) among patients with Wegener granulomatosis. All patients had active disease at time 0. (Courtesy of Merkel PA, for the Wegener's Granulomatosis Etanercept Trial Research Group: Brief communication: High incidence of venous thrombotic events among patients with Wegener granulomatosis: The Wegener's Clinical Occurrence of Thrombosis (WeCLOT) Study. *Ann Intern Med* 142:620-626, 2005.)

with no history of VTE. Median time from enrollment to VTE for patients with an event was 2.1 months. The incidence of VTE among patients with Wegener granulomatosis was 7.0 per 100 person-years (95% CI, 4.0 to 11.4).

Limitations.—Although prospectively recorded, screening for VTEs did not occur.

Conclusions.—The incidence rate of VTEs in Wegener granulomatosis is high when compared with available rates in the general population, patients with lupus, and patients with rheumatoid arthritis. These results have important implications for clinical care of patients with Wegener granulomatosis (Figure).

▶ It is unclear why there is increased incidence of VTE in patients with Wegener granulomatosis (WG). Whether the inflammation associated with WG can damage venous endothelium or patients with WG have an as-yet undefined hypercoagulable state is anyone's guess. I suspect a procoagulant state in patients with WG. Other autoimmune disorders associated with inflammation do not produce the incidence of VTE documented by this report in patients with WG.

G. L. Moneta, MD

Results of limb-sparing surgery with vascular replacement for soft tissue sarcoma in the lower extremity

Schwarzbach MHM, Hormann Y, Hinz U, et al (Inst of Pathology, Heidelberg, Germany; Univ of Heidelberg, Germany)
J Vasc Surg 42:88-97, 2005   13–14

Objective.—To evaluate limb-salvage surgery with vascular resection for lower extremity soft tissue sarcomas (STS) in adult patients and to classify blood vessel involvement.

Methods.—Subjects were consecutive patients (median age, 56 years) who underwent vascular replacement during surgery of STS in the lower limb between January 1988 and December 2003. Blood vessel involvement by STS was classified as follows: type I, artery and vein; type II, artery only; type III, vein only; and type IV, neither artery nor vein (excluded from the analysis). Patient data were prospectively gathered in a computerized database.

Results.—Twenty-one (9.9%) of 213 patients underwent vascular resections for lower limb STS. Besides 17 type I tumors (81.0%), 3 (14.3%) type II and 1 (4.7%) type III STS were diagnosed. Arterial reconstruction was performed for all type I and II tumors. Venous replacement in type I and III tumors was performed in 66.7% of patients. Autologous vein (n = 8) and synthetic (Dacron and expanded polytetrafluoroethylene; n = 12) bypasses were used with comparable frequency for arterial repair, whereas expanded polytetrafluoroethylene prostheses were implanted in veins. Morbidity was 57.2% (hematoma, thrombosis, and infection), and mortality was 5% (em-

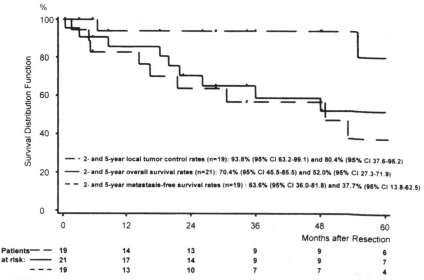

FIGURE 5.—Local tumor control, survival, and metastasis-free survival after complete resection with vascular reconstructions in 19 patients for lower-limb extremity soft tissue sarcoma. The median follow-up was 34 months (interquartile range, 20-62 months). Censored patients are marked (as a vertical line); patients at risk and the 95% confidence interval are shown. (Reprinted by permission of the publisher from Schwarzbach MHM, Hormann Y, Hinz U, et al: Results of limb-sparing surgery with vascular replacement for soft tissue sarcoma in the lower extremity. *J Vasc Surg* 42:88-97, 2005. Copyright 2005 by Elsevier.)

bolism). At a median follow-up of 34 months, the primary and secondary patency rates of arterial (venous) reconstructions were 58.3% (54.9%) and 78.3% (54.9%). Limb salvage was achieved in 94.1% of all cases. The 5-year local control rate and survival rate were 80.4% and 52%, respectively. We observed a 5-year metastasis-free survival rate of 37.7% and found vessel infiltration and higher tumor grade (low-grade vs intermediate grade and high grade tumors) to be negative prognostic factors at univariate and multivariate analysis.

Conclusions.—Long-term bypass patency rates, the high percentage of limb salvage, and the oncologic outcome underline the efficacy of en bloc resection of STS involving major vessels in the lower limb. Disease-specific morbidity must be anticipated. The classification of vascular involvement (type I to IV) is useful for surgical management (Fig 5).

▶ The authors used prosthetic grafts frequently for above-knee arterial and venous reconstructions but bypass infections developed in 19% of patients after hospital discharge (including 1 venous bypass). This infection rate is unacceptably high and may relate to the long procedures and presumed associated wound complications. I think that the rationale of using prosthetic to "shorten an otherwise long operation" is a bit bogus. Harvesting saphenous vein does not take much time, and prosthetic graft infections cause much trouble. I would recommend autogenous reconstruction, even if it takes a bit longer.

G. L. Moneta, MD

Renal artery stenosis and aneurysms associated with neurofibromatosis
Han M, Criado E (State Univ of New York at Stony Brook)
J Vasc Surg 41:539-543, 2005   13–15

Renal artery lesions associated with neurofibromatosis may involve stenosis and aneurysm formation at all levels of the renal artery to the intraparenchymal branches, and usually are associated with hypertension. A 13-year-old boy with type I neurofibromatosis and severe hypertension presented with multiple aneurysms and multiple stenotic lesions in the renal artery and segmental arteries. The patient underwent ex-vivo renal artery repair with autologous hypogastric artery and autotransplantation to the iliac fossa and was clinically improved. The characteristic histologic findings are presented. A review of the recent literature comparing different treatment modalities for renovascular hypertension in children with neurofibromatosis suggests that surgery remains the best treatment alternative.

► This article was included in the YEAR BOOK to remind everyone that neurofibromatosis can be associated with proliferative lesions of the arterial wall in both large and small arteries. The histogenesis of such lesions is unknown.

G. L. Moneta, MD

Palmar hyperhidrosis—which is the best level of denervation using video-assisted thoracoscopic sympathectomy: T2 or T3 ganglion?
Yazbek G, Wolosker N, Milanez de Dampos JR, et al (Univ of São Paulo, Brazil)
J Vasc Surg 42:281-285, 2005   13–16

Purpose.—This study compares early results of video-assisted thoracoscopic sympathectomy (VTS) at the thoracic T2 versus T3 ganglion denervation levels for the treatment of palmar hyperhidrosis (PH).

Methods.—Sixty patients with PH were prospectively randomized for VTS at the thoracic T2 or T3 ganglion denervation levels. The patients underwent postoperative evaluation on three occasions: before surgery, and 1 and 6 months after the operation. Endpoints included the absence of PH, the presence, location, and severity of compensatory hyperhidrosis (CH), and a quality-of-life assessment.

Results.—Fifty-nine of 60 patients reported complete resolution of PH after surgery. One failure occurred in the T3 group. CH was observed in 26 patients (86.66%) in the T2 group and in 27 patients (90%) in the T3 group at 1 month. At 6 months, 30 of 30 patients in the T2 group and 29 of 30 in the T3 group experienced CH, although in the T3 group, CH was less severe at both 1 and 6 months ($P < .05$). Quality of life was very poor in both groups before surgery. One month after operation, quality of life was improved similarly in both groups. This improvement was maintained at 6 months in both groups.

Conclusion.—PH is well treated by VTS at either the T2 or T3 levels. Denervation at the T3 level appears associated with less severe CH in the early postoperative period. Quality of life improved significantly in both groups.

▶ Compensatory hyperhydrosis (CH) is common after VTS. CH is defined as the postoperative appearance of perspiration in body areas not previously affected by sweating, usually the abdomen and back. The definition of severe CH is a bit vague in this study; that is, new sweating necessitating "more than one change of clothes during the day." It seems the denervations at either the T2 or T3 level were both effective in alleviating symptoms of PH. CH may be a bit less severe with the denervation at T3. I am not sure how these results would translate elsewhere. It is hot in Brazil, and deciding what is normal versus what is excessive sweating may be difficult to discern.

G. L. Moneta, MD

Sildenafil in the Treatment of Raynaud's Phenomenon Resistant to Vasodilatory Therapy

Fries R, Shariat K, von Wilmowsky H, et al (Universitätsklinikum des Saarlandes, Homburg/Saar, Germany; Knappschaftskrankenhaus, Püttlingen, Germany)

Circulation 112:2980-2985, 2005   13–17

Background.—Vasodilatory therapy of Raynaud's phenomenon represents a difficult clinical problem because treatment often remains inefficient and may be not tolerated because of side effects.

Method and Results.—To investigate the effects of sildenafil on symptoms and capillary perfusion in patients with Raynaud's phenomenon, we performed a double-blinded, placebo-controlled, fixed-dose, crossover study in 16 patients with symptomatic secondary Raynaud's phenomenon resistant to vasodilatory therapy. Patients were treated with 50 mg sildenafil or placebo twice daily for 4 weeks. Symptoms were assessed by diary cards including a 10-point Raynaud's Condition Score. Capillary flow velocity was measured in digital nailfold capillaries by means of a laser Doppler anemometer. While taking sildenafil, the mean frequency of Raynaud attacks was significantly lower (35 ± 14 versus 52 ± 18, $P=0.0064$), the cumulative attack duration was significantly shorter (581 ± 133 versus 1046 ± 245 minutes, $P=0.0038$), and the mean Raynaud's Condition Score was significantly lower (2.2 ± 0.4 versus 3.0 ± 0.5, $P=0.0386$). Capillary blood flow velocity increased in each individual patient, and the mean capillary flow velocity of all patients more than quadrupled after treatment with sildenafil (0.53 ± 0.09 versus 0.13 ± 0.02 mm/s, $P=0.0004$). Two patients reported side effects leading to discontinuation of the study drug.

Conclusions.—Sildenafil is an effective and well-tolerated treatment in patients with Raynaud's phenomenon.

▶ Sildenafil has a half life of about 4 hours. Clearly, functional effects exceeded the half-life in this study population. Although sildenafil has an established effect on erectile dysfunction, it also has been used successfully in the treatment of pulmonary hypertension and now may represent the first reasonably effective therapy for secondary Raynaud's syndrome.

G. L. Moneta, MD

Thoracic outlet syndrome: Pattern of clinical success after operative decompression
Altobelli GG, Kudo T, Haas BT, et al (Univ of California at Los Angeles)
J Vasc Surg 42:122-128, 2005   13–18

Objective.—To evaluate the pattern of clinical results in patients with neurogenic thoracic outlet syndrome (N-TOS) after operative decompression and longitudinal follow-up.

Methods.—From May 1994 to December 2002, 254 operative sides in 185 patients with N-TOS were treated by the same operative protocol: (1) transaxillary first rib resection and the lower part of scalenectomy for the primary procedure with or without (2) the subsequent upper part of scalenectomy with supraclavicular approach for patients with persistent or recurrent symptoms. This retrospective cohort study included 38 men and 147 women with an age range of 19 to 80 years (mean, 40 years). Evaluated were primary success, defined as uninterrupted success with no procedure performed, and secondary success, defined as success maintained by the secondary operation after the primary failure. Success was defined as ≥50% symptomatic improvement judged by the patient using a 10-point scale, returning to preoperational work status, or both.

Results.—Follow-up was 2 to 76 months (mean, 25 months). Eighty sides underwent a secondary operation for the primary clinical failure. No technical failures and no deaths occurred ≤30 days after the operations. The complication rate was 4% (13/334) and consisted of 7 pneumothoraxes, 3 subclavian vein injuries, 1 nerve injury, 1 internal mammary artery injury, and 1 suture granuloma. Of 254 operative sides, the primary and secondary success was 46% (118/254) and 64% (163/254). Most the primary failures (90%, 122/136) and the secondary failures (66%, 23/35) occurred <18 months after the respective operation.

Conclusions.—The long-term results of operations for TOS in this study were much worse than those initially achieved, and most of the primary and secondary failures occurred <12 months of the respective operations. A minimum of 18-month follow-up on patients and standardized definition of

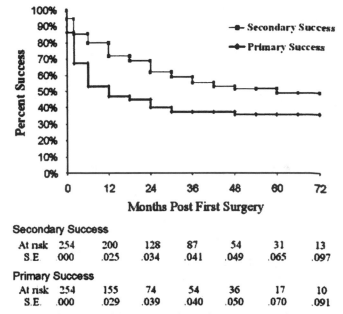

Secondary Success						
At risk 254	200	128	87	54	31	13
S.E 000	.025	.034	.041	.049	.065	.097

Primary Success						
At risk 254	155	74	54	36	17	10
S.E. .000	.029	.039	.040	.050	.070	.091

FIGURE 4.—Life-table analysis of the primary and secondary success rates after operative decompression for neurogenic thoracic outlet syndrome. (Reprinted by permission of the publisher from Altobelli GG, Kudo T, Haas BT, et al: Thoracic outlet syndrome: Pattern of clinical success after operative decompression. *J Vasc Surg* 42:122-128, 2005. Copyright 2005 by Elsevier.)

the outcomes are necessary to determine the true effectiveness and outcome of operative treatment of N-TOS (Fig 4).

▶ The results reported here for treatment of N-TOS are considerably worse than what we have come to expect from first-rib enthusiasts. I doubt this reflects poor surgical technique; complications were minimal in this study. Those of us who doubt the efficacy of first-rib resection for N-TOS are not surprised by these results. The first-rib enthusiasts will point out that more than 50% of patients were patients with worker's compensation, patients with pain for an average of 3 years before surgery, and one third had previous neck, shoulder, wrist, or elbow operations. All of these are factors that are associated with worse outcomes of N-TOS surgery. The effectiveness of first-rib resection for N-TOS remains controversial. It is hard to know who will do well; it is clear many do not do well.

G. L. Moneta, MD

Ethanol Embolization of Arteriovenous Malformations: Interim Results

Do YS, Yakes WF, Shin SW, et al (Sungkyunkwan Univ, Seoul, Korea; Vascular Malformation Ctr, Englewood, Colo)
Radiology 235:674-682, 2005   13–19

Purpose.—To assess retrospectively the interim results and the complications of ethanol embolization treatment of arteriovenous malformations (AVMs).

Materials and Methods.—Institutional review board approval was obtained for a retrospective review of patient medical and imaging records. Informed consent was not required by the institutional review board. Written

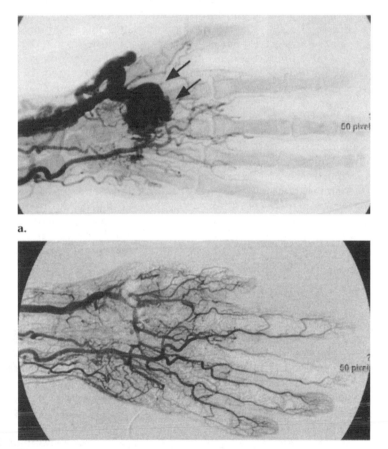

a.

b.

FIGURE 2.—Patient 8. A 33-year-old- woman with painful pulsating mass in left hand. (a) Pretreatment posteroanterior angiogram shows AVM (arrows) with dilated outflow vein in palm of left hand. (b) Posteroanterior arteriogram shows that AVM was obliterated completely after two sessions of embolization with 20mL and 3.5 mL of ethanol by using direct puncture of the dilated outflow vein. (Courtesy of Do YS, Yakes WF, Shin SW, et al: Ethanol embolization of arteriovenous malformations: Interim results. *Radiology* 235:674-682, 2005. Reprinted by permission, Radiological Society of North America.)

consent for the procedure was obtained from all patients after a discussion about the advantages and risks of the procedure. After a general anesthetic was administered, 40 patients (16 male, 24 female; age range, 9-53 years) with inoperable AVMs in the body and extremities underwent staged ethanol embolizations (range, 1-24; median, 3). Pulmonary artery pressure and arterial blood pressure were monitored as ethanol was injected. Ethanol embolizations (50%-100% ethanol mixed with nonionic contrast material) were performed by using transcatheter and/or direct puncture techniques. Ten patients underwent additional coil deployment during ethanol embolization. Clinical follow-up (range, 2-48 months; mean, 14.6 months; median, 12 months) was performed in all patients, and results from imaging follow-up (range, 0-48 months; mean, 8.4 months; median, 6 months) were available from the last treatment session in 28 patients. Therapeutic outcomes were established by evaluating the clinical outcome of symptoms and signs, as well as the degree of devascularization at follow-up angiography.

Results.—One hundred seventy-five ethanol embolizations were performed in 40 patients. Sixteen (40%) of 40 patients were cured, 11 (28%) had partial remission, seven (18%) had no remission, and one (2%) experienced aggravation. Treatment failed in five patients (12%). Ethanol embolization was considered effective (cure, 16 patients; partial remission, 11 patients) in 27 patients (68%). Eleven patients will need further treatment sessions for residual AVMs. Twenty-one patients (52%) experienced complications. Twenty-seven minor complications (skin and transient peripheral nerve injuries) (27 [15%] of 175 procedures) occurred in 18 (45%) of 40 patients. All minor complications were healed with wound dressing and observation. Five major complications (five [3%] of 175 procedures) occurred in five (12%) of 40 patients, and four patients recovered completely.

Conclusion.—Ethanol embolization has the potential for cure in the management of AVMs of the body and extremities but with acceptable risk of minor and major complications (Fig 2).

▶ This article indicates ethanol embolization of AVMs has a reasonable chance of helping selected patients with difficult AVMs. Complications occur and can be severe. Therefore, the presence of an AVM is not an indication for embolization. It would have been interesting to know how many patients were considered for embolization but were unsuitable for the procedure because of inappropriate anatomy or risk of complication. It is often just as important to understand when not to treat as when to treat. The article therefore does not adequately define the role of ethanol embolization in the overall management of patients with AVMs. All it tells us is that it can be done, and the outcomes can be good in selected cases.

G. L. Moneta, MD

An injectable tissue-engineered embolus prevents luminal recanalization after vascular sclerotherapy
Smithers CJ, Vogel AM, Kozakewich HPW, et al (Harvard Med School, Boston)
J Pediatr Surg 40:920-925, 2005   13–20

Background/Purpose.—Sclerotherapy for vascular malformations is often limited by luminal recanalization. This study examined whether an injectable tissue-engineered construct could prevent this complication in a rabbit model of venous sclerotherapy.

Methods.—Ethanol sclerotherapy of a temporarily occluded jugular vein segment was performed in 46 rabbits, which were then divided into 3 groups. Group I (n = 16) had no further manipulations. In groups II (n = 15) and III (n = 15), 0.5 mL collagen hydrogel was injected intraluminally, respectively, devoid of and seeded with autologous fibroblasts. At 1, 4, and 20 to 24 weeks postoperatively, vein segments were examined for patency and resected for histological evaluation. Statistical analysis was by Fisher's Exact test.

Results.—All vein segments were occluded at 1 and 4 weeks in all groups, despite histological evidence of progressive endothelial ingrowth. However, at 20 to 24 weeks, angiography demonstrated restoration of vessel patency in groups I (3/6) and II (3/5), but not in group III (0/6; *P* = .043), in which histology confirmed an obliterated lumen for all vessels.

Conclusion.—An injectable, fibroblast-based, engineered construct prevents midterm to long-term recanalization in a leporine model of vascular sclerotherapy. This novel therapeutic approach may prevent recurrence of vascular malformations after sclerotherapy, thus reducing the need for repeated procedures and morbid operative resections.

▶ Rabbit jugular veins are a long way from human vascular malformations. But, there are no animal models of vascular malformations. Despite reasonable short-term efficacy of sclerotherapy for vascular malformations (see Abstract 13–19), eventual recurrence remains a problem. The approach outlined here focuses on recurrences secondary to recanalization of treated areas. Opening of new, previously present, but minimally perfused portions of arteriovenous malformations may also be a mechanism of "recurrence."

G. L. Moneta, MD

14 Venous Thrombosis and Pulmonary Embolization

Malignancies, Prothrombotic Mutations, and the Risk of Venous Thrombosis

Blom JW, Doggen CJM, Osanto S, et al (Leiden Univ, The Netherlands)

JAMA 293:715-722, 2005   14–1

Context.—Venous thrombosis is a common complication in patients with cancer, leading to additional morbidity and compromising quality of life.

Objective.—To identify individuals with cancer with an increased thrombotic risk, evaluating different tumor sites, the presence of distant metastases, and carrier status of prothrombotic mutations.

Design, Setting, and Patients.—A large population-based, case-control (Multiple Environmental and Genetic Assessment [MEGA] of risk factors for venous thrombosis) study of 3220 consecutive patients aged 18 to 70 years, with a first deep venous thrombosis of the leg or pulmonary embolism, between March 1, 1999, and May 31, 2002, at 6 anticoagulation clinics in the Netherlands, and separate 2131 control participants (partners of the patients) reported via a questionnaire on acquired risk factors for venous thrombosis. Three months after discontinuation of the anticoagulant therapy, all patients and controls were interviewed, a blood sample was taken, and DNA was isolated to ascertain the factor V Leiden and prothrombin 20210A mutations.

Main Outcome Measure.—Risk of venous thrombosis.

Results.—The overall risk of venous thrombosis was increased 7-fold in patients with a malignancy (odds ratio [OR], 6.7; 95% confidence interval [CI], 5.2-8.6) vs persons without malignancy. Patients with hematological malignancies had the highest risk of venous thrombosis, adjusted for age and sex (adjusted OR, 28.0; 95% CI, 4.0-199.7), followed by lung cancer and gastrointestinal cancer. The risk of venous thrombosis was highest in the first few months after the diagnosis of malignancy (adjusted OR, 53.5; 95% CI, 8.6-334.3). Patients with cancer with distant metastases had a higher risk vs patients without distant metastases (adjusted OR, 19.8; 95% CI, 2.6-

149.1). Carriers of the factor V Leiden mutation who also had cancer had a 12-fold increased risk vs individuals without cancer and factor V Leiden (adjusted OR, 12.1; 95% CI, 1.6-88.1). Similar results were indirectly calculated for the prothrombin 20210A mutation in patients with cancer.

Conclusions.—Patients with cancer have a highly increased risk of venous thrombosis especially in the first few months after diagnosis and in the presence of distant metastases. Carriers of the factor V Leiden and prothrombin 20210A mutations appear to have an even higher risk.

▶ The data raise questions as to whether patients with cancer should be screened for factor V Leiden and prothrombin 20210A mutation and treated with prophylactic anticoagulation therapy if a mutation is present. The cost effectiveness of such strategies and the ultimate ability of such strategies to prolong life or improve quality of life is clear in patients with cancer who are undergoing surgery or active chemotherapy.[1]

There are currently no data to suggest that routine prophylaxis for venous thromboembolism in all cancer patients would be effective. However, the results of the current study suggest that certain subgroups of patients with cancer should be studied more closely for possible routine venous thromboembolism prophylaxis.

G. L. Moneta, MD

Reference

1. Thodiyil PA, Walsh DC, Kakkar AK: Thromboprophylaxis in the cancer patient. *Acta Haematol* 106:73-80, 2001.

Risk factors for venous thrombosis in Swedish children and adolescents
Rask O, Berntorp E, Ljung R (Univ Hosp, Malmö, Sweden)
Acta Paediatr 94:717-722, 2005   14–2

Aim.—To identify prothrombotic risk profiles in children and adolescents referred to a regional coagulation centre in southern Sweden for a first thrombotic event.

Methods.—One hundred and twenty-eight consecutive children and adolescents (newborn to 20 y) referred for evaluations of a first episode of venous thrombosis were investigated. Clinical data were collected retrospectively, and the following variables were investigated: protein C, protein S, antithrombin; resistance to activated protein C; the genotypes FV-G1691A, F II-G20210A, MTHFR-C677T, MTHFR-A1298C; coagulation factors VIII and XI.

Results.—104/128 subjects (81%) had identifiable acquired risk factors, most often indwelling catheters and hormone therapy. Predisposing genetic factors related to thromboembolic events were revealed in 53/83 (64%) of subjects who agreed to follow-up blood sampling, and 17/83 (20%) had two or more inherited risk factors. Combinations of genetic and acquired risk factors were identified in 45/83 (54%) of the subjects, and 77/83 (93%) had

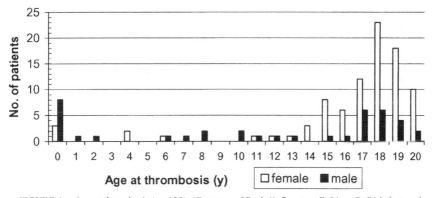

FIGURE 1.—Age at thrombosis (*n*=128). (Courtesy of Rask O, Berntorp E, Ljung R: Risk factors for venous thrombosis in Swedish children and adolescents. *Acta Paediatr* 94:717-722, 2005. Published by Taylor & Francis, Ltd. at http://www.tandf.cc.uk/journals/jsp.htm.)

at least one such risk factor. Both sexes had one peak in frequency at less than 1 y of age and then an increase during adolescence, more in females than in males. Plasma values for coagulation factors VIII and XI were age appropriate and showed a normal Gaussian distribution.

Conclusion.—This study identified prothrombotic risk profiles in almost all children and adolescents with venous thrombosis, which underlines the importance of careful evaluation of genetic and acquired risk factors (Fig 1).

▶ While venous thromboembolism (VTE) is unusual in children and adolescents, the data here suggest that a VTE event in a child should be investigated with a detailed hypercoagulable panel. The yield is high enough to make this routine in children with VTE.

G. L. Moneta, MD

Thrombophilic abnormalities and recurrence of venous thromboembolism in patients treated with standardized anticoagulant treatment

Santamaria MG, Agnelli G, Taliani MR, et al (Università di Perugia, Italy; Università di Padova, Italy; IRCCS Ospedale Maggiore, Milan, Italy; et al)
Thromb Res 116:301-306, 2005   14–3

Introduction.—Whether patients with hereditary or acquired thrombophilia have an increased risk for recurrence of venous thromboembolism (deep vein thrombosis and/or pulmonary embolism) is still controversial. The aim of this study was to evaluate the incidence of recurrence of venous thromboembolism in patients with and without thrombophilic abnormalities treated with standardized anticoagulant treatment.

Material and Methods.—Database was from a prospective multicenter randomized study aimed at evaluating the long-term clinical benefit of extending to 1 year the 3-month oral anticoagulant treatment after a first episode of idiopathic proximal deep vein thrombosis. The screening for throm-

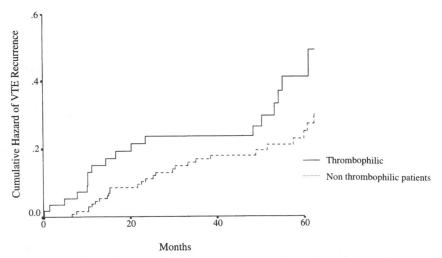

Months

FIGURE 1.—Cumulative hazard of VTE recurrence in thrombophilic and non-thrombophilic patients. (Reprinted from Santamaria MG, Agnelli G, Taliani MR, et al: Thrombophilic abnormalities and recurrence of venous thromboembolism in patients treated with standardized anticoagulant treatment. *Thromb Res* 116:301-306, 2005. Copyright 2005, with kind permission from Elsevier Science Ltd, The Boulevard, Langford Lane, Kidlington OX5 1GB, UK.)

bophilia included antithrombin, protein C, protein S deficiencies, resistance to activated protein C and/or factor V R506Q mutation, the mutation 20210GA of the prothrombin gene, hyperhomocysteinemia and antiphospholipid antibodies. The diagnosis of venous thromboembolism recurrence was done by objective tests and adjudicated by a panel unaware of the results of the thrombophilia screening.

Results.—A screening for thrombophilic abnormalities was performed in 195 patients. Twenty of 57 (35.1%) thrombophilic patients experienced a recurrence of venous thromboembolism as compared with 29 of 138 (21.0%) patients without thrombophilia (HR=1.78, 95% CI 1.002-3.140, p=0.046). The difference in VTE recurrence between patients with and without thrombophilia was accounted for by those who received 3 months of oral anticoagulation (HR=3.21, 95% CI 1.349-7.616, p=0.008). No difference between thrombophilic and non-thrombophilic patients was observed in the time interval from the index episode to recurrent venous thromboembolism (29.1±23.9 and 30.6±19.8 months, respectively).

Conclusions.—Thrombophilic abnormalities are associated with an increased risk of venous thromboembolism recurrence. The role of thrombophilia in the long-term management of venous thromboembolism should be addressed in prospective management studies (Fig 1).

▶ This study, like others before it, suggests longer durations of treatment for patients with idiopathic venous thromboembolism (VTE). There are too few patients in this study to allow precise recommendations for duration of therapy based on the thrombophilic abnormality identified. Nevertheless, it is now quite clear that not all VTE is the same. Patients with thrombophilia should be considered at higher risk of recurrence and probably treated for at least 1 year with warfarin after their initial VTE event.

G. L. Moneta, MD

Thrombophilia, Clinical Factors, and Recurrent Venous Thrombotic Events
Christiansen SC, Cannegieter SC, Koster T, et al (Leiden Univ, The Netherlands)
JAMA 293:2352-2361, 2005   14–4

Context.—Data on the recurrence rate of venous thrombotic events and the effect of several risk factors, including thrombophilia, remain controversial. The potential benefit of screening for thrombophilia with respect to prophylactic strategies and duration of anticoagulant treatment is not yet known.

Objectives.—To estimate the recurrence rate of thrombotic events in patients after a first thrombotic event and its determinants, including thrombophilic abnormalities.

Design, Setting, and Patients.—Prospective follow-up study of 474 consecutive patients aged 18 to 70 years without a known malignancy treated for a first objectively confirmed thrombotic event at anticoagulation clinics in the Netherlands. The Leiden Thrombophilia Study (LETS) was conducted from 1988 through 1992 and patients were followed up through 2000.

Main Outcome Measures.—Recurrent thrombotic event based on thrombophilic risk factors, sex, type of initial thrombotic event (idiopathic or provoked), oral contraceptive use, elevated levels of factors VIII, IX, XI, fibrinogen, homocysteine, and anticoagulant deficiencies.

Results.—A total of 474 patients were followed up for mean (SD) of 7.3 (2.7) years and complete follow-up was achieved in 447 (94%). Recurrence of thrombotic events occurred in 90 patients during a total of 3477 patient-years. The rate of thrombotic event recurrence was 25.9 per 1000 patient-years (95% confidence interval [CI], 20.8-31.8 per 1000 patient-years). The incidence rate of recurrence was highest during the first 2 years (31.9 per 1000 patient-years; 95% CI, 20.3-43.5 per 1000 patient-years). The risk of thrombotic event recurrence was 2.7 times (95% CI, 1.8-4.2 times) higher in men than in women. Patients whose initial thrombotic event was idiopathic had a higher risk of a thrombotic event recurrence than patients whose initial event was provoked (hazard ratio [HR], 1.9; 95% CI, 1.2-2.9). Women who used oral contraceptives during follow-up had a higher thrombotic event recurrence rate (28.0 per 1000 patient-years; 95% CI, 15.9-49.4 per 1000 patient-years) than those who did not (12.9 per 1000 patient-years; 95% CI, 7.9-21.2 per 1000 patient-years). Recurrence risks of a thrombotic event by laboratory abnormality ranged from an HR of 0.6 (95% CI, 0.3-1.1) in patients with elevated levels of factor XI to an HR of 1.8 (95% CI, 0.9-3.7) for patients with anticoagulant deficiencies.

Conclusions.—Prothrombotic abnormalities do not appear to play an important role in the risk of a recurrent thrombotic event. Testing for prothrombotic defects has little consequence with respect to prophylactic strategies. Clinical factors are probably more important than laboratory abnormalities in determining the duration of anticoagulation therapy.

▶ This article has the potential to significantly influence practice. The authors found that a thrombophilic defect discovered after an initial venous thromboembolic event does not influence recurrence of venous thromboembolism to any significant extent. The obvious implication is that after a first-time venous thromboembolic event (even if the event appeared unprovoked), workup for a thrombophilic defect is unlikely to convey any benefit to the patient. This is a bit of a paradigm shift for me. I think I will need additional data to change this aspect of my practice.

G. L. Moneta, MD

Randomized clinical trial of postoperative fondaparinux *versus* perioperative dalteparin for prevention of venous thromboembolism in high-risk abdominal surgery

Agnelli G, for the PEGASUS investigators (Univ of Perugia, Italy; et al)
Br J Surg 92:1212-1220, 2005   14–5

Background.—The aim of this study was to assess whether the synthetic factor Xa inhibitor fondaparinux reduced the risk of venous thromboembolism more efficiently than the low molecular weight heparin dalteparin in patients undergoing major abdominal surgery.

Methods.—In a double-blind double-dummy randomized study, patients scheduled for major abdominal surgery under general anaesthesia received once-daily subcutaneous injections of fondaparinux 2.5 mg or dalteparin 5000 units for 5-9 days. Fondaparinux was started 6 h after surgery. The first two doses of dalteparin, 2500 units each, were given 2 h before surgery and 12 h after the preoperative administration. The primary outcome measure was a composite of deep vein thrombosis detected by bilateral venography and symptomatic, confirmed deep vein thrombosis or pulmonary embolism up until day 10. The main safety outcome measure was major bleeding during treatment.

Results.—Among 2048 patients evaluable for efficacy, the rate of venous thromboembolism was 4.6 per cent (47 of 1027) with fondaparinux compared with 6.1 per cent (62 of 1021) with dalteparin, a relative risk reduction of 24.6 (95 per cent confidence interval -9.0 to 47.9) per cent ($P = 0.144$), which met the predetermined criterion for non-inferiority of fondaparinux. Major bleeding was observed in 49 (3.4 per cent) of 1433 patients given fondaparinux and 34 (2.4 per cent) of 1425 given dalteparin ($P = 0.122$).

Conclusion.—Postoperative fondaparinux was at least as effective as perioperative dalteparin in patients undergoing high-risk abdominal surgery.

▶ Fondaparinux has been found to be at least as good as low molecular weight heparin in preventing deep venous thrombosis in virtually every study in which it has been tested. The fact that it can be started postoperatively should make it attractive for use following urgent or emergent procedures or those procedures where an epidural is desirable.

G. L. Moneta, MD

Cost-effectiveness of prophylactic low molecular weight heparin in pregnant women with a prior history of venous thromboembolism

Johnston JA, Brill-Edwards P, Ginsberg JS, et al (Veterans Affairs Med Ctr, Cincinnati, Ohio; Univ of Cincinnati, Ohio; McMaster Univ, Hamilton, Ont, Canada; et al)

Am J Med 118:503-514, 2005   14–6

Purpose.—Women with a history of prior venous thromboembolism have an increased risk for recurrence during pregnancy. Although thromboprophylaxis reduces this risk, recent evidence suggests that, in many cases, prophylaxis can be safely withheld because the estimated recurrence risk is very low. The balance of risks and benefits in women with different recurrence risks has not been examined.

Methods.—We developed a Markov state transition decision analytic model to compare prophylactic low molecular weight heparin to expectant management for pregnant women with a single prior venous thromboembo-

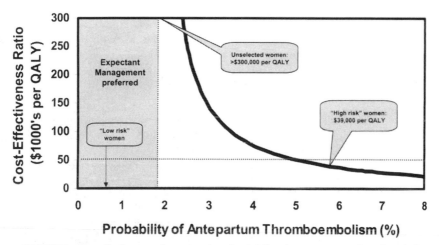

FIGURE 3.—Cost-effectiveness ratio as a function of probability of recurrent venous thromboembolism. This figure shows the cost-effectiveness ratio on the *y* axis as a function of the probability of recurrent venous thromboembolism during pregnancy on the *x*-axis. As depicted by the *gray area to the left of the dotted vertical line*, expectant management is preferred when the probability of recurrent venous thromboembolism is less than 1.8%. Prophylaxis has a cost-effectiveness ratio of less than $50 000 per QALY at a probability of recurrent venous thromboembolism greater than 5.0%. The 3 base case scenarios are represented by the 3 dialogue bubbles. (Reprinted from Johnston JA, Brill-Edwards P, Ginsberg JS, et al. Cost effectiveness of prophylactic low molecular weight heparin in pregnant women with a prior history of venous thromboembolism. *Am J Med* 118:503-514, 2005. Copyright 2005, with permission from Excerpta Medica Inc.)

lism. A lifetime time horizon and societal perspective were assumed. Input data were obtained by literature review. Outcomes were expressed as U.S. dollars per quality-adjusted life-year (QALY).

Results.—For "low-risk" women with a prior venous thromboembolism associated with a transient risk factor and no known thrombophilic condition (recurrence risk 0.5%), expectant management was both more effective and less costly than prophylaxis. For "high-risk" women with prior idiopathic venous thromboembolism or known thrombophilic condition (recurrence risk 5.9%), prophylaxis was associated with a reasonable cost-effectiveness ratio (USD 38,700 per QALY) given a risk of bleeding complications <1.0% (base case 0.5%).

Conclusion.—For low-risk women with prior venous thromboembolism, expectant management during pregnancy leads to better outcomes than administration of prophylactic low molecular weight heparin. For high-risk women, antepartum thromboprophylaxis is a cost-effective use of resources (Fig 3).

▶ There is no randomized clinical trial specifically examining the role of venous prophylaxis in pregnant women with prior episodes of venous thromboembolism (VTE). Articles such as this, therefore, are the best that are available for guiding therapy in pregnant women with previous VTE. The article suggests that significant risk stratification can guide management and improve patient outcome and is consistent with the current trend of individualization of management of VTE.

G. L. Moneta, MD

Continuous passive motion in the prevention of deep-vein thrombosis: a randomised comparison in trauma patients
Fuchs S, Heyse T, Rudofsky G, et al (Univ of Münster, Germany)
J Bone Joint Surg Br 87-B:1117-1122, 2005   14–7

There is a high risk of venous thromboembolism when patients are immobilised following trauma. The combination of low-molecular-weight heparin (LMWH) with graduated compression stockings is frequently used in orthopaedic surgery to try and prevent this, but a relatively high incidence of thromboembolic events remains. Mechanical devices which perform continuous passive motion imitate contractions and increase the volume and velocity of venous flow.

In this study 227 trauma patients were randomised to receive either treatment with the Arthroflow device and LMWH or only with the latter. The Arthroflow device passively extends and plantarflexes the feet. Patients were assessed initially by venous-occlusion plethysmography, compression ultrasonography and continuous wave Doppler, which were repeated weekly without knowledge of the category of randomisation. Those who showed evidence of deep-vein thrombosis underwent venography for confirmation. The incidence of deep-vein thrombosis was 25% in the LMWH group com-

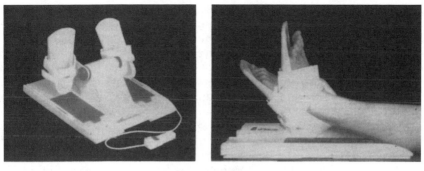

Fig. 1a   Fig. 1b

FIGURE 1.—a, Photograph of the Arthroflow device, a means of mechanical thromboprophylaxis. b, Photograph showing the Arthroflow device in action. (Courtesy of Fuchs S, Heyse T, Rudofsky G, et al: Continuous passive motion in the prevention of deep-vein thrombosis: A randomized comparison in trauma patients. *J Bone Joint Surg Br* 87-B:1117-1122, 2005.)

pared with 3.6% in those who had additional treatment with the Arthroflow device (p < 0.001). There were no substantial complications or problems of non-compliance with the Arthroflow device. Logistic regression analysis of the risk factors of deep-vein thrombosis showed high odds ratios for operation (4.1), immobilisation (4.3), older than 40 years of age (2.8) and obesity (2.2) (Fig 1).

▶ It makes sense that the combination of mechanical and chemical prophylaxis will be more effective than that of chemical prophylaxis alone. The additional effectiveness of the device studied in this article in combination with LMWH is quite impressive. However, I really can't see anything special about this particular device. It obviously should be tested against other methods of mechanical prophylaxis. As with any form of mechanical prophylaxis, the primary issue is likely to be getting patients and nurses to be compliant with use of the device.

G. L. Moneta, MD

Deep Venous Thrombosis: Withholding Anticoagulation Therapy after Negative Complete Lower Limb US Findings

Subramaniam RM, Heath R, Chou I, et al (Waikato Hosp, Hamilton, New Zealand; Univ of Auckland, Hamilton, New Zealand)
Radiology 237:348-352, 2005   14–8

Purpose.—To establish the safety of withholding anticoagulation therapy after negative findings at a complete lower limb ultrasonographic (US) examination of the symptomatic leg for suspected deep venous thrombosis (DVT).

Materials and Methods.—Regional ethics committee approval and patient consent were obtained. A total of 542 consecutive ambulatory patients presented to the emergency department and were prospectively recruited from April 2001 to May 2003. Of these patients, 16 were excluded, and radiology residents and sonographers performed a complete lower limb US examination by means of compression and Doppler US in 526 patients. Patients with negative US findings received no anticoagulation therapy, and they were observed for occurrence of any thromboembolic event for 3 months. Patients with progressive or new symptoms that were indicative of thromboembolism within the follow-up period underwent objective testing with US, computed tomographic (CT) pulmonary angiography, or both.

Results.—There were 413 patients (78.5%) with US findings that were negative for DVT and 113 patients (21.5%) with findings that were positive. There were 64 patients (56.6%) with DVT isolated to the calf and 49 (43.4%) with proximal DVT. Of the 413 patients with negative initial US findings, 16 (3.9%) underwent a second US examination for new or progressive symptoms of DVT, one patient (0.25%) underwent CT pulmonary angiography for suspected pulmonary embolism, and one patient (0.25%) underwent both US and CT pulmonary angiography during the 3-month follow-up period. One of these patients (0.24%; 95% confidence interval: 0.01%, 1.3%) developed pulmonary embolism, which was diagnosed with CT pulmonary angiography. DVT was not diagnosed in any patient, and no patient died during follow-up. The negative predictive value of a complete single lower limb US examination to exclude clinically important DVT is 99.6% (95% confidence interval: 98.4%, 99.9%).

Conclusion.—A single negative complete lower limb US examination is sufficient to exclude clinically important DVT, and it is safe to withhold anticoagulation therapy after negative complete lower limb US findings were obtained in patients suspected of having symptomatic lower limb DVT. New or progressive symptoms require further objective imaging.

▶ This is clearly what people do in the "real" world. If a US exam that includes the calf veins is negative, there is no need to treat.

There are some important details: (1) the examination must visualize the veins well for the entire length of the extremity; (2) new symptoms require repeat study; and (3) if the initial examination does not exclude calf vein thrombosis, a repeat examination in 5 to 7 days in indicated. Those reporting venous US studies must clearly indicate to the referring physician the technical adequacy of the examination and whether the examination has excluded calf vein thrombosis.

G. L. Moneta, MD

A Randomized Trial of Diagnostic Strategies after Normal Proximal Vein Ultrasonography for Suspected Deep Venous Thrombosis: D-Dimer Testing Compared with Repeated Ultrasonography

Kearon C, Ginsberg JS, Douketis J, et al (McMaster Univ, Hamilton, Ont, Canada; Henderson Research Centre, Hamilton, Ont, Canada)

Ann Intern Med 142:490-496, 2005   14–9

Background.—With suspected deep venous thrombosis and normal results on proximal vein ultrasonography, a negative D-dimer result may exclude thrombosis and a positive D-dimer result may be an indication for venography.

Objective.—To evaluate and compare the safety of 2 diagnostic strategies for deep venous thrombosis.

Design.—Randomized, multicenter trial.

Setting.—Four university hospitals.

Patients.—810 outpatients with suspected deep venous thrombosis and negative results on proximal vein ultrasonography.

Interventions.—Erythrocyte agglutination D-dimer testing followed by no further testing if the result was negative and venography if the result was positive (experimental) or ultrasonography repeated after 1 week in all patients (control).

Measurements.—Symptomatic deep venous thrombosis diagnosed initially and symptomatic venous thromboembolism during 6 months of follow-up.

Results.—Nineteen of 408 patients (4.7%) in the D-dimer group and 3 of 402 patients (0.7%) in the repeated ultrasonography group initially received a diagnosis of deep venous thrombosis ($P < 0.001$). During follow-up of patients without a diagnosis of deep venous thrombosis on initial testing, 8 patients (2.1% [95% CI, 0.9% to 4.0%]) in the D-dimer group and 5 patients (1.3% [CI, 0.4% to 2.9%]) in the repeated ultrasonography group developed symptomatic venous thromboembolism (difference, 0.8 percentage point [CI, −1.1 to 2.9 percentage points]; $P < 0.2$). Venous thromboembolism occurred in 1.0% (CI, 0.2% to 2.8%) of those with a negative D-dimer result.

Limitations.—Seventy patients (8.6%) deviated from the diagnostic protocols, and 9 patients (1.1%) had inadequate follow-up.

Conclusion.—In outpatients with suspected deep venous thrombosis who initially had normal results on ultrasonography of the proximal veins, a strategy based on D-dimer testing followed by no further testing if the result was negative and venography if the result was positive had acceptable safety and did not differ from the safety of a strategy based on withholding anticoagulant therapy and routinely repeating ultrasonography after 1 week.

▶ This study is good news for those who wish to avoid examination of the calf veins with venous US. The authors' strategy essentially uses D-dimer testing as a substitute for calf vein imaging. One can consider utilizing this strategy in patients in whom examination of the calf veins with US is technically difficult.

In patients in whom an adequate calf vein US examination can be obtained, it really doesn't make much sense to stop with the proximal examination only.

Overall, based on this study, it would appear to be safe to use proximal venous US in combination with D-dimer testing for patients whose calf veins cannot be well examined with US. If the proximal US is negative and the D-dimer test is negative, no additional follow-up studies appear to be required.

G. L. Moneta, MD

Exclusion of venous thromboembolism: evaluation of D-Dimer PLUS for the quantitative determination of D-dimer

Vermeer HJ, Ypma P, van Strijen MJL, et al (Leyenburg Hosp, The Hague, The Netherlands)

Thromb Res 115:381-386, 2005   14–10

The objective of this study was to evaluate if D-Dimer PLUS (Dade Behring, USA), a rapid fully automated assay, could be used as an initial screening test in the diagnosis of venous thromboembolism (VTE). Samples from 274 consecutive symptomatic patients with suspected pulmonary embolism ($n=229$; 79% outpatients, 21% inpatients), deep venous thrombosis ($n=37$; 84% outpatients, 16% inpatients) or suspected for both complications ($n=8$) were tested with this D-dimer assay with a Sysmex CA-1500 Coagulation Analyzer. Clinical probability for pulmonary embolism (PE) or deep venous thrombosis (DVT) was staged according to a pretest risk score proposed by Wells. Final diagnosis of PE and/or DVT was established by spiral-computed tomography of the pulmonary arteries or compression ul-

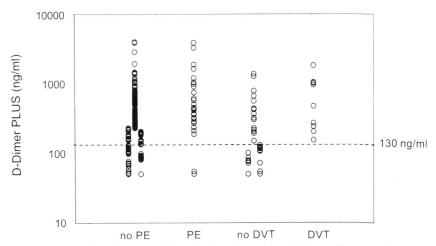

FIGURE 1.—Individual D-Dimer PLUS results for patients with and without pulmonary embolism (*PE*) or deep venous thrombosis (*DVT*). The *broken line* represents the decision threshold (=cut-off value). (Reprinted from Vermeer HJ, Ypma P, van Strijen MJL, et al: Exclusion of venous thromboembolism evaluation of D-dimer PLUS for the quantitative determination of D-dimer. *Thromb Res* 115:381-386, 2005. Copyright 2005, with kind permission from Elsevier Science Ltd, The Boulevard, Langford Lane, Kidlington OX5 1GB, UK.)

trasonography, respectively. PE was diagnosed in 13.5% of the patients, whereas DVT was confirmed in 17.7% of the patients. The optimal cut-off value for exclusion of venous thromboembolism was 130 µg/l, and sensitivity, specificity and negative predictive value (NPV) were 95.0% (95% CI: 92.4-97.6), 30.4% (95% CI: 25.0-35.8) and 97.2% (95% CI: 95.2-99.2), respectively. In fact, two patient with PE were missed using D-Dimer PLUS; both cases were outpatients. In conclusion, this assay appears to be safe when implemented in an algorithm based on clinical assessment, D-dimer concentration, and radiological diagnostic techniques to stratify the risk for PE or DVT. However, higher sensitivities and negative predictive values were claimed in the scarce published reports for the D-Dimer PLUS assay than found in this study. (Fig 1).

▶ The point is that D-dimer is a good test but may not be good enough as a stand-alone test to exclude DVT. The NPV is not perfect and D-dimer testing probably should be used in conjunction with clinical risk assessment. When D-dimer and clinical risk are discordant, an imaging study is required.

That study should be a US if DVT is suspected and a CT scan if PE is suspected. Also, the different D-dimer assays have different cutoffs to suggest VTE. The whole thing is a bit complicated and probably explains why so many outpatient venous ultrasounds are still being performed.

G. L. Moneta, MD

Oral anticoagulation strategies after a first idiopathic venous thromboembolic event

Aujesky D, Smith KJ, Roberts MS (Univ of Pittsburgh, Pa; VA Pittsburgh Healthcare System, Pa)
Am J Med 118:625-635, 2005   14–11

Purpose.—The optimal duration and intensity of warfarin therapy after a first idiopathic venous thromboembolic event are uncertain. We used decision analysis to evaluate clinical and economic outcomes of different anticoagulation strategies with warfarin.

Methods.—We built a Markov model to assess 6 strategies to treat 40- to 80-year-old men and women after their first idiopathic venous thromboembolic event: 3-month, 6-month, 12-month, 24-month, and unlimited-duration conventional-intensity anticoagulation (International Normalized Ratio, 2-3) and unlimited-duration low-intensity anticoagulation (International Normalized Ratio, 1.5-2). The model incorporated age- and sex-specific clinical parameters, utilities, and costs. Using a societal perspective, we compared strategies based on quality-adjusted life-years (QALYs), lifetime costs, and incremental cost-effectiveness ratios.

Results.—In our baseline analysis, incremental cost-effectiveness ratios were lower in younger patients and in men, reflecting the higher bleeding risk at older ages, and the lower risk of recurrence among women. Based on a willingness-to-pay of <$50 000/QALY, the 24-month strategy was most cost-effective in 40-year-old men ($48 805/QALY), while the 6-month strategy was preferred in 40-year-old women ($35 977/QALY) and 60-year-old men ($29 878/QALY). In patients aged ≥80 years, 3-month anticoagulation was less costly and more effective than other strategies. Cost-effectiveness results were influenced by the risks associated with recurrent venous thromboembolism, the major bleeding risk of conventional-intensity anticoagulation and the disutility of taking warfarin.

Conclusion.—Longer initial conventional-intensity anticoagulation is cost-effective in younger patients while 3 months of anticoagulation is preferred in elderly patients. Patient age, sex, clinical factors, and patient preferences should be incorporated into medical decision making when selecting an appropriate anticoagulation strategy.

▶ Treatment of venous thromboembolism (VTE) is becoming more individualized. The strategies outlined in the article make sense in that they incorporate recent findings concerning the natural history and treatment of idiopathic VTE. By taking into account sex, age, risk of bleeding, and the cost and difficulties of warfarin therapy, the authors have proposed a reasonable outline for treatment of idiopathic VTE in both men and women.

G. L. Moneta, MD

Effect of Physical Activity after Recent Deep Venous Thrombosis: A Cohort Study

Shrier I, Kahn SR (Lady Davis Inst for Med Research; SMBD-Jewish Gen Hosp, Montréal)
Med Sci Sports Exerc 37:630-634, 2005   14–12

Purpose.—To determine whether increased physical activity 1 month after deep vein thrombosis (DVT) led to worsening of venous symptoms and signs within the subsequent 3 months.

Methods.—By a multicenter prospective cohort study of patients with acute DVT, we used validated questionnaires at baseline, 1 month, and 4 months post-DVT for each exposure, using the Godin Questionnaire to measure physical activity, the VEINES-QOL to measure disease severity, and the postthrombotic syndrome (PTS) scale to measure symptoms and signs usually attributed to sequelae of DVT.

Results.—Of 301 patients followed for 4 months, 25% were inactive and 25% were only mildly active before their DVT. In univariate analysis, physical activity at 1 month was not associated with a change in PTS score between 1 month and 4 months ($P = 0.42$). After adjusting for the potential confounders of age, sex, pre-DVT physical activity, and disease severity at 1 month, the results suggested that higher physical activity levels at 1 month may be protective against worsening of the PTS score over the subsequent 3 months. Compared with those who were inactive at 1 month, the adjusted OR was 0.93 (95%CI: 0.47, 1.87) for mildly to moderately active persons, and 0.52 (95%CI: 0.24, 1.15) for highly active persons. Among patients who were active pre-DVT (N = 220), 55.5% had returned to their previous levels of physical activity or greater within 4 months.

Conclusions.—For most persons, exercise at 1 month post-DVT does not appear to worsen venous symptoms and signs over the subsequent 3 months, and more than 50% resume their usual level of activity within 4 months.

▶ This study suggests that restriction of physical activity 1 month following DVT is unnecessary. Other studies have suggested that physical activity immediately following DVT does not increase the risk of pulmonary embolism. The overall message is that there does not appear to be any reason to limit patients' physical activity after an episode of DVT. There may, in fact, be a benefit to increased physical activity following DVT.

G. L. Moneta, MD

Catheter Directed Thrombolysis for Treatment of Ilio-femoral Deep Venous Thrombosis is Durable, Preserves Venous Valve Function and May Prevent Chronic Venous Insufficiency
Sillesen H, Just S, Jørgensen M, et al (Gentofte Univ, Hellerup, Denmark)
Eur J Vasc Endovasc Surg 30:556-562, 2005   14–13

Objectives.—To investigate the results of catheter directed thrombolysis offered to patients with acute femoro-iliac deep venous thrombosis (DVT).

Design.—Retrospective analysis of all patients treated with this modality at Gentofte Hospital until December 2003.

Material.—Forty-five consecutive patients treated between June 1999 and December 2003 with a median age of 31 years. All patients had femoro-iliac DVT with an average anamnesis of 6 days.

Methods.—All patients were treated by catheter directed infusion of alteplase into the popliteal vein. After thrombolysis residual venous stenoses were treated by percutaneous balloon angioplasty (PTA) and stenting. Patients were followed with color-duplex scanning for assessment of venous patency and reflux.

Results.—Forty-two of 45 (93%) of cases were treated successfully with reopening of the thrombosed vein segments. In 30 of 45 cases a residual stenosis was treated by PTA and stenting. Only one serious complication was observed: Compartment syndrome of the forearm where arterial punctures had been taken. After an average of 24 months follow-up were no cases of re thrombosis among the 42 patients discharged with open veins. Only two of 41 with presumed normal venous valve function prior to DVT developed reflux during follow-up.

Conclusion.—In this selected patient group, catheter directed thrombolysis seems effective in treating acute DVT, it appears durable and preserves venous valve function in the majority. The method needs to be tested in a randomised controlled trial.

▶ Little single-center series keep cropping up here and there, suggesting benefit for catheter-directed lytic therapy of iliofemoral DVT. Patients in such series are always highly selected and this makes it difficult to evaluate long-term results. Certainly, patients with successful lytic therapy can have a more rapid resolution of acute symptoms.

However, given the highly selective nature of the patients, perhaps many patients would do well long term without lytic therapy. A randomized trial is surely needed. I hope someone at the NIH is thinking about this.

G. L. Moneta, MD

Fatal pulmonary embolism in hospitalised patients: a necropsy review
Alikhan R, Peters F, Wilmoft R, et al (Royal United Hosp, Bath, England; Guy's, King's, and St Thomas's School of Medicine, London)
J Clin Pathol 57:1254-1257, 2004   14–14

Aims.—To carry out a retrospective review of all postmortem reports during the period 1991 to 2000 at King's College Hospital, London, as an extension of a previous analysis performed for the period 1965 to 1990.

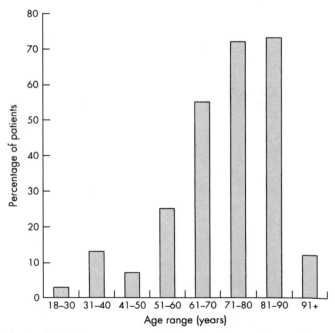

FIGURE 1.—Age distribution of necropsy-confirmed fatal pulmonary embolism. (Courtesy of Alikhan R, Peters F, Wilmoft R, et al: Fatal pulmonary embolism in hospitalised patients: A necropsy review. *J Clin Pathol* 57:1254-1257, 2004, with permission from the BMJ Publishing Group.)

Methods.—The number of deaths resulting from necropsy confirmed fatal pulmonary embolism in hospitalised patients was determined, and a limited analysis of the clinical characteristics of those patients who died was performed.

Results.—During the 10 year period, 16 104 deaths occurred and 6833 (42.4%) necropsies were performed. The outcome measure, fatal pulmonary embolism, was recorded as cause of death in 265 cases (3.9% of all necropsies; 5.2% of adult cases). No deaths from pulmonary embolism occurred in patients under 18 years of age; 80.0% occurred in patients older than 60 years. Of the fatal emboli, 214 of 265 (80.8%) occurred in patients who had not undergone recent surgery. Of these patients, 110 (51.4%) had suffered an acute medical illness in the six weeks before death, most often an acute infectious episode (26 cases).

Conclusions.—Thromboembolic events remain a relatively common cause of death in hospitalised patients and appear to occur more frequently in non-surgical than in surgical patients (Fig 1).

▶ This is a follow-up of a previous study from King's College that examined the period from 1965 to 1990. At that time, the investigators had determined that deaths from pulmonary embolism in surgical patients appeared to be decreasing. The current report validates the previous report and documents a continuing decrease in the proportion of overall pulmonary embolism deaths in patients who have had surgical procedures.

Advances in surgical care and thromboprophylaxis appear to have had some effect. There is a need for greater emphasis on thromboprophylaxis in patients hospitalized for medical conditions.

G. L. Moneta, MD

Multidetector-Row Computed Tomography in Suspected Pulmonary Embolism
Perrier A, Roy P-M, Sanchez O, et al (Geneva Univ; Angers Univ, France; Hôpital Européen Georges-Pompidou, Paris)
N Engl J Med 352:1760-1768, 2005   14–15

Background.—Single-detector-row computed tomography (CT) has a low sensitivity for pulmonary embolism and must be combined with venous-compression ultrasonography of the lower limbs. We evaluated whether the use of D dimer measurement and multidetector-row CT, without lower-limb ultrasonography, might safely rule out pulmonary embolism.

Methods.—We included 756 consecutive patients with clinically suspected pulmonary embolism from the emergency departments of three teaching hospitals and managed their cases according to a standardized sequential diagnostic strategy. All patients were followed for three months.

Results.—Pulmonary embolism was detected in 194 of the 756 patients (26 percent). Among the 82 patients with a high clinical probability of pulmonary embolism, multidetector-row CT showed pulmonary embolism in

78, and 1 patient had proximal deep venous thrombosis and a CT scan that was negative for pulmonary embolism. Of the 674 patients without a high probability of pulmonary embolism, 232 (34 percent) had a negative D-dimer assay and an uneventful follow-up; CT showed pulmonary embolism in 109 patients. CT and ultrasonography were negative in 318 patients, of whom 3 had a definite thromboembolic event and 2 died of possible pulmonary embolism during follow-up (three-month risk of thromboembolism, 1.7 percent; 95 percent confidence interval, 0.7 to 3.9). Two patients had proximal deep venous thrombosis and a negative CT scan (risk, 0.6 percent; 95 percent confidence interval, 0.2 to 2.2). The overall three-month risk of thromboembolism in patients without pulmonary embolism would have been 1.5 percent (95 percent confidence interval, 0.8 to 3.0) if the D-dimer assay and multidetector-row CT had been the only tests used to rule out pulmonary embolism and ultrasonography had not been performed.

Conclusions.—Our data indicate the potential clinical use of a diagnostic strategy for ruling out pulmonary embolism on the basis of D-dimer testing and multidetector-row CT without lower-limb ultrasonography. A larger outcome study is needed before this approach can be adopted.

▶ This study is an important addition to previous studies demonstrating a low yield for finding deep venous thrombosis with venous US in patients in whom pulmonary symptoms prompted the venous US examination. The message here is that if you suspect pulmonary embolism, get a CT and if it is negative adding a US study will detect a deep venous thrombosis less than 2% of the time.

The algorithm, unfortunately, is a bit complex and begins with clinical assessment for venous thromboembolism (see also Abstracts 14–9 and 14–10). This article should not be interpreted as indicating everyone with pulmonary symptoms needs a CT scan. Clinical assessment in determining the possibility of venous thromboembolism is making a comeback but only as part of an algorithm employing selective use of imaging studies.

G. L. Moneta, MD

The Effect of Screening for Deep Vein Thrombosis on the Prevalence of Pulmonary Embolism in Patients With Fractures of the Pelvis or Acetabulum: A Review of 973 Patients

Borer DS, Starr AJ, Reinert CM, et al (Univ of Texas, Dallas)
J Orthop Trauma 19:92-95, 2005   14–16

Objectives.—In patients with pelvic or acetabular fractures, to compare the prevalence of pulmonary embolism in a time period without screening for deep vein thrombosis to that seen when a screening protocol was in place.

Design.—Retrospective.

Setting.—County hospital.

Patients.—All patients with closed fractures of the pelvis or acetabulum treated during the study periods.

Intervention.—Prophylaxis for deep vein thrombosis was the same for both groups. From November 1, 1997 though November 31, 1999, a screening protocol for deep vein thrombosis was employed using ultrasound and magnetic resonance venography. From January 1, 2000 through December 1, 2001, no screening was used.

Main Outcome Measurement.—Pulmonary emboli were recorded.

Results.—The 1997 to 1999 time period included 486 patients with fractures of the pelvis or acetabulum; the 2000 to 2001 time period included 487. In the period when a screening protocol was in place, 10 patients (2%) were diagnosed with pulmonary embolism by pulmonary arteriogram, autopsy, or ventilation perfusion scan. All but 2 who were diagnosed with pulmonary embolism had undergone screening for deep vein thrombosis, and none of the screening tests were positive. In the 2000 to 2001 time period, when no screening for deep vein thrombosis was done, 7 patients (1.4%) were diagnosed with pulmonary embolism, by pulmonary arteriogram, autopsy, spiral computed tomography scan, or high clinical suspicion. There was no significant difference between the prevalence of pulmonary embolism seen in 1997 to 1999 and that seen in 2000 to 2001 ($P = 0.48$).

Conclusion.—Discontinuation of screening for the diagnosis of deep vein thrombosis did not change the rate of pulmonary embolism.

▶ The authors' technique for assessing calf vein thrombosis is inadequate in that calf veins are not directly imaged. This study indicates that a poorly designed protocol doesn't work. A protocol that used direct imaging of the calf veins may have been more effective. Fortunately, this study can only conclude that the protocol utilized was ineffective. It does not exclude possible effectiveness of different screening protocols in the patients at high risk for deep venous thrombobis.

G. L. Moneta, MD

Management of pulmonary embolism in the home
Ong BS, Karr MA, Chan DKY, et al (Bankstown-Lidcombe Hosp, Bankstown, Australia)
Med J Aust 183:239-242, 2005   14–17

Aim.—To describe the characteristics, outcomes and treatment complications of patients with pulmonary embolism (PE) who were treated at home and as outpatients in an ambulatory care program.

Methods.—Retrospective descriptive study of patients with PE who were treated in the ambulatory care unit during 2003. Ambulatory care unit data and medical record information were reviewed. Data collected included demographic and clinical data, standard clinical indicators of unplanned admission during treatment program, incidence of major bleeding, recurrent venous thromboembolism (VTE), and death within 3 months of admission into the ambulatory care program.

Results.—130 patients with PE were treated: 46% were treated totally as outpatients and 54% as early discharge patients. Mean age was 66.4 years; 61% were women. The program was successfully completed for 89% of patients; one patient was lost to follow-up. There were three episodes of major bleeding (2%; 95% CI, 0.5%-7%), all in patients aged > 70 years. Four patients died (3%; 95% CI, 0.8%-8%) within 3 months of admission into the program, but none in the first week, no death being directly attributable to PE. There were seven episodes of recurrent VTE (5%; 95% CI, 2%-11%).

Conclusion.—Appropriately selected patients with sub-massive PE can be treated as outpatients and in the home. Although the outcome is good in most patients, a significant proportion will require admission, emphasising the need for a well defined protocol and close medical supervision. Further study will more closely define at-risk patients and refine the care pathways.

▶ Submassive PE can be treated as an outpatient when the patient can adhere to the protocol. Older patients may have more difficulty, as suggested by the fact that 13% could not complete the protocol in this study. However, older patients often don't do as well no matter what treatment is utilized. Age itself should not exclude outpatient treatment of submassive PE.

G. L. Moneta, MD

Bed Rest or Ambulation in the Initial Treatment of Patients With Acute Deep Vein Thrombosis or Pulmonary Embolism: Findings From the RIETE Registry

Monreal M, for the RIETE Investigators (Hosp Universitari Germans Trias i Pujol, Badalona, Spain; et al)
Chest 127:1631-1636, 2005   14–18

Background.—Traditionally, many patients with acute deep vein thrombosis (DVT) are treated not only by anticoagulation therapy but additionally by strict bed rest, which is aimed at reducing the risk of pulmonary embolism (PE) events. However, this risk has not been subjected to empirical verification.

Patients and Methods.—The Registro Informatizado de la Enfermedad TromboEmbolica is a Spanish registry of consecutively enrolled patients with objectively confirmed, symptomatic acute DVT or PE. In this analysis, the clinical characteristics, details of anticoagulant therapy, and clinical outcomes of enrolled patients with and without strict bed rest prescribed during the first 15 days were compared. Patients in whom ambulation was not possible were not included in this analysis.

Results.—A total of 2,650 patients entered the study (DVT, 2,038 patients; PE, 612 patients). Of these patients, 1,050 DVT patients (52%) and 385 PE patients (63%) were prescribed strict bed rest. New events of symptomatic, objectively confirmed PE developed during the 15-day study period in 11 patients with DVT (0.5%) and 4 patients with PE (0.7%). Five of these 15 patients (33%) died as a result of their PE. Age < 65 years (odds ratio

[OR], 3.1; 95% confidence interval [CI], 0.98 to 11) and cancer (OR, 3.0; 95% CI, 0.98 to 9.1) were associated with an increased rate of new PEs. There were not significant differences between bedridden and ambulant patients in terms of new PE events, fatal PE, or bleeding complications.

Conclusions.—Our findings confirm those from previous reports suggesting that bed rest has no influence on the risk of developing PE among patients with acute DVT of the lower limbs. In addition, our findings show for the first time the lack of influence of bed rest even in patients presenting with acute submassive PE.

▶ Patients with venous thromboembolism do not need to be put to bed and, in fact, bed rest may be harmful. On the other hand, some patients are too uncomfortable to ambulate much initially. Encourage the venous thromboembolism patient to ambulate with a compression device, but don't demand so much ambulation as to put the patient in agony.

G. L. Moneta, MD

Risk factors for mortality in patients with upper extremity and internal jugular deep venous thrombosis
Hingorani A, Ascher E, Markevich N, et al (Maimonides Med Ctr, Brooklyn, NY)
J Vasc Surg 41:476-478, 2005   14–19

Objective.—To elucidate the natural history of upper extremity deep venous thrombosis (UEDVT), we examined factors that may contribute to the high mortality associated with UEDVT.

Methods.—Five hundred forty-six patients were diagnosed with acute internal jugular/subclavian/axillary deep venous thrombosis from January 1992 to June 2003 by duplex scanning at our institution. There were 329 women (60%). The mean age ± SD was 68 ± 17 years (range, 1-101 years). Risk factors for UEDVT were the presence of a central venous catheter or pacemaker in 327 patients (60%) and a history of malignancy in 119 patients (22%). Risk factors for mortality within 2 months of the diagnosis of UEDVT that were analyzed included age, sex, presence of a central venous catheter or pacemaker, history of malignancy, location of UEDVT, concomitant lower extremity deep venous thrombosis, systemic anticoagulation, placement of a superior vena caval filter, and pulmonary embolism.

Results.—The overall mortality rate at 2 months was 29.6%. The number of patients diagnosed with pulmonary embolism by positive ventilation/perfusion scan or computed tomographic scan was 26 (5%). The presence of a central venous catheter or pacemaker ($P < .001$), concomitant lower extremity deep venous thrombosis ($P = .04$), not undergoing systemic anticoagulation ($P = .002$), and the placement of a superior vena caval filter ($P = .02$) were associated with mortality within 2 months of the diagnosis of UEDVT by univariate analysis. Pulmonary embolism ($P = .42$), sex ($P = .65$), and a history of malignancy ($P = .96$) were not.

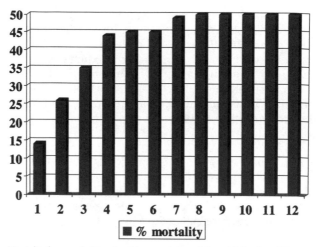

FIGURE.—Mortality by month. (Reprinted by permission of the publisher from Hingorani A, Ascher E, Markevich N, et al: Risk factors for mortality in patients with upper extremity and internal jugular deep venous thrombosis. *J Vasc Surg* 41:479-478, 2005. Copyright 2005 by Elsevier.)

Conclusions.—These data suggest that the high associated mortality of UEDVT may be due to the underlying characteristics of the patients' disease process and may not be a direct consequence of the UEDVT itself(Figure).

▶ Dr Ascher's group has finally figured it out. UEDVT is annoying but death from UEDVT basically only happens in patients with extremely severe cardio-pulmonary compromise. Upper extremity venous thrombi are just not big enough to kill people. Do not put vena cava filters in patients for the mere presence of a UEDVT. Strongly evaluate the risk/benefit ratio of any treatment for a patient with UEDVT.

G. L. Moneta, MD

15 Chronic Venous and Lymphatic Disease

Randomized clinical trial of routine preoperative duplex imaging before varicose vein surgery
Blomgren L, Johansson G, Bergqvist D (Capio St Göran's Hosp, Stockholm; Univ Hosp, Uppsala, Sweden)
Br J Surg 92:688-691, 2005   15–1

Background.—Duplex imaging is used increasingly for preoperative evaluation of varicose veins, but its value in terms of the long-term results of surgery is not clear.

Methods.—Patients with primary varicose veins were randomized to operation with or without preoperative duplex imaging Reoperation rates, clinical and duplex findings were compared at 2 months and 2 years after surgery.

Results.—Two hundred and ninety-three patients (343 legs) had varicose vein surgery after duplex imaging (group 1; 166 legs) or no imaging (group 2; 177 legs). In 44 legs (26.5 per cent), duplex examination suggested a different surgical procedure than had been considered on clinical grounds; the procedure was changed accordingly for 29 legs. At 2 months, incompetence was detected at the saphenofemoral or saphenopopliteal junction (or both) in 14 legs (8.8 per cent) in group 1 and in 44 legs (26.5 per cent) in group 2 ($P < 0.001$). At 2 years, two legs (1.4 per cent) had undergone or were awaiting reoperation in group 1, and 14 legs (9.5 per cent) in group 2 ($P = 0.002$). In the remainder, major incompetence was found in 19 legs (15.0 per cent) in group 1 and in 53 (41.1 per cent) in group 2 ($P < 0.001$).

Conclusion.—Routine preoperative duplex examination led to an improvement in results 2 years after surgery for patients with primary varicose veins.

▶ New technologies are frequently introduced into everyday surgical practice. This if often done without adequate scientific basis. Duplex scanning has rapidly become near standard of care in the preoperative evaluation of varicose vein patients. However, prior to this study, its effect on the long-term outcome of varicose vein surgery was unknown. Hopefully, as suggested by this study, routine preoperative duplex evaluation of patients undergoing varicose vein surgery will lower the high recurrence rates of varicosities after varicose vein surgery.

G. L. Moneta, MD

Randomized clinical trial comparing surgery with conservative treatment for uncomplicated varicose veins
Michaels JA, Brazier JE, Campbell WB, et al (Univ of Sheffield, England; Exeter Hosp, England)
Br J Surg 93:175-181, 2006

15–2

Background.—Surgical treatment of medically uncomplicated varicose veins is common, but its clinical effectiveness remains uncertain.

Methods.—A randomized clinical trial was carried out at two large acute National Health Service hospitals in different parts of the UK (Sheffield and Exeter). Some 246 patients were recruited from 536 consecutive referrals to vascular outpatient clinics with uncomplicated varicose veins suitable for surgical treatment. Conservative management, consisting of lifestyle advice, was compared with surgical treatment (flush ligation of sites of reflux, stripping of the long saphenous vein and multiple phlebectomies, as appropriate). Changes in health status were measured using the Short Form (SF) 6D and EuroQol (EQ) 5D, quality of life instruments based on SF-36 and EuroQol, complications of treatment, symptomatic measures, anatomical extent of varicose veins and patient satisfaction.

Results.—In the first 2 years after treatment there was a significant quality of life benefit for surgery of 0.083 (95 per cent confidence interval (c.i.) 0.005 to 0.16) quality-adjusted life years (QALYs) based on the SF-6D score and 0.13 (95 per cent c.i. 0.016 to 0.25) based on the EQ-5D score. Significant benefits were also seen in symptomatic and anatomical measures.

Conclusion.—Surgical treatment provides symptomatic relief and significant improvements in quality of life in patients referred to secondary care with uncomplicated varicose veins.

▶ This is an important study evaluating surgery versus medical care in patients with uncomplicated varicose veins. Three points are emphasized. (1) Reported symptom relief was greater at 1 year in the surgical group than in the conservative group. (2) Seventy percent of patients undergoing surgery had no further varicose veins at 1 year. In the conservative group, there was no change. (3) More than half of the patients in the conservative group requested surgery within 3 years. There was improved quality of life in the surgical group and higher functional and social scores assessed by SF-36 at 1 and 2 years. Such studies are also required in comparing endovenous ablation with surgery and whether stab phlebectomy should be staged or concomitant.

J. D. Raffetto, MD, MS

Randomized clinical trial comparing multiple stab incision phlebectomy and transilluminated powered phlebectomy for varicose veins

Chetter IC, Mylankal KJ, Hughes H, et al (Hull Royal Infirmary, England; Univ of Adelaide, South Australia)
Br J Surg 93:169-174, 2006   15–3

Background.—The aim was to compare early postoperative subjective outcome measures in a randomized trial of multiple stab incision phlebectomy (MSIP) and transilluminated powered phlebectomy (TIPP) for the treatment of varicose veins.

Methods.—Patients having surgery for varicose veins were randomized to receive either MSIP or TIPP for local avulsion of varicose veins. Operating time, number of incisions and postoperative outcome were analysed in both groups. Quality of life (QoL) was analysed before and 1 and 6 weeks after surgery using domain-specific (Burford pain scale), disease-specific (Aberdeen Varicose Vein Questionnaire) and generic (Short Form 36 and EuroQol 5D) instruments.

Results.—Sixty-six patients consented to participate in the trial but four withdrew before surgery, so 33 patients underwent MSIP and 29 patients had TIPP. All patients had symptomatic or complicated varicose veins. There was no significant difference between groups in the total duration of surgery or the time taken for the avulsions. The number of incisions was significantly lower with TIPP. However, skin bruising at 1 and 6 weeks, and Burford pain score at 6 weeks were significantly higher in the TIPP group ($P < 0.01$ for bruising and $P = 0.019$ for pain). TIPP also had a greater adverse impact on generic QoL, resulting in a more prolonged recovery.

Conclusion.—TIPP had the advantage of fewer surgical incisions, but was associated with more extensive bruising, prolonged pain and reduced early postoperative QoL.

▶ In this randomized trial of TIPP versus standard MSIP for varicose vein treatment, the only advantage of TIPP was a decreased number of incisions. Surprisingly, there was no difference in operative time. If rapid patient recovery is the issue, it appears standard MSIP provides a better outcome. If the patient is interested in fewer incisions for cosmetic concerns, TIPP will provide this but at the expense of a more prolonged recovery.

G. L Moneta, MD

Can phlebectomy be deferred in the treatment of varicose veins?

Monahan DL (Vein Surgery & Treatment Ctr of Northern California, Roseville)
J Vasc Surg 42:1145-1149, 2005   15–4

Objective.—This study was designed to observe the clinical sequelae of varicose veins after great saphenous vein (GSV) ablation and to assess possible predictability of spontaneous varicose vein regression.

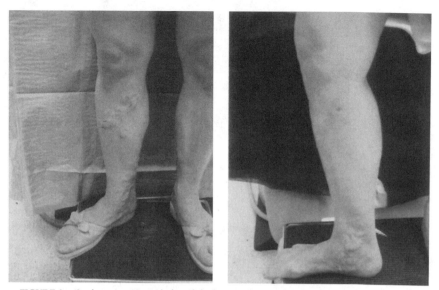

FIGURE 3.—Study patient No 16 before (*left photo*) and 6 months after (*right photo*) radiofrequency ablation, without any additional interventions for treatment of the visible varicose veins. Note the resolution of veins in the anterior and medial upper calf. (Reprinted by permission of the publisher from Monahan DL: Can phlebectomy be deferred in the treatment of varicose veins? *J Vasc Surg* 42:1145-1149, 2005. Copyright 2005 by Elsevier.)

Methods.—Patients with symptomatic varicose veins secondary to GSV insufficiency treated with radiofrequency ablation (RFA) were enrolled in the study. Up to five of the largest varicose veins in each limb were mapped, sized, and documented before RFA. No varicose vein was treated either at the time of RFA or within 6 months postoperatively. Varicose vein status was recorded at follow-up visits.

Results.—Fifty-four limbs in 45 patients were included. A total of 222 varicose veins were documented before RFA (4.1 ± 1.1 varicose veins per limb) with an average size of 11.4 ± 3.7 mm. During the follow-up period, complete resolution of visible varicose veins was seen in 13% of limbs after RFA alone, and 63 (28.4%) varicose veins spontaneously resolved. A further 88.7% (141/159) of varicose veins decreased in size an average of 34.6% (4.3 ± 3.4 mm). Preoperatively, 19.4% of varicose veins were above the knee and 75.7% were below the knee. Complete varicose vein resolution was 41.9% (18/43) above the knee and 25.6% (43/168) below the knee. For the above-knee varicose veins, 88.4% (38/43) were located medially, and all the resolved ones (47.4%, 18/38) were medial varicose veins. Resolution rates of the 168 below-knee varicose veins were 30.6% (33/108) of medial, 23.1% (6/26) of anterior, 20.0% (3/15) of lateral, and 5.3% (1/19) of posterior.

Conclusions.—Great saphenous vein ablation resulted in subsequent resolution or regression of many lower-limb visible varicose veins. With further study, the predictability of varicose vein regression may perhaps be increased, which can then direct the treatment strategy to further leverage the advantages of minimally invasive endovenous procedures (Fig 3).

▶ The regression of varicosities after GSV ablation is interesting and potentially important in development of treatment strategies for varicose veins. The study suffers from potential observer bias, as I assume data were collected and analyzed only by Dr Monahan. Nevertheless, give Dr Monahan some serious credit. Here is a guy working alone in a small California town who keeps close track of his patients and publishes his results. Good for him.

G. L. Moneta, MD

A prospective study of the fate of venous leg perforators after varicose vein surgery
van Rij AM, Hill G, Gray C, et al (Univ of Otago, Dunedin, New Zealand)
J Vasc Surg 42:1156-1162, 2005   15–5

Objective.—To describe the fate of perforator veins after surgical treatment of varicose veins and factors that influence this.

Methods.—This prospective study of 104 patients assessed perforator veins by using duplex ultrasound scanning in 145 limbs before superficial vein surgery for varicose veins. Veins were marked preoperatively with ultrasound guidance and ligated with an open procedure; those missed were later treated with sclerotherapy. Duplex ultrasound scans and air plethysmography were used to confirm surgical success within 1 month and to monitor recurrence at 6 months, 1 year, and 3 years.

Results.—A total of 850 incompetent perforators were treated, but 5.7% were missed and required further ablation. After 3 years, 75.8% of the limbs had developed further incompetent perforators for a total of 380 incompetent perforators. The number of ultrasound-detectable competent perforators had also increased from 356 to 1047 in that time. The incompetent perforators arose by (1) new vessel formation at the site of previous ligation in 152 (40.4%), (2) changes in pre-existing perforator vessels at other sites in 225 (59.2%), and (3) vessels missed at treatment (<1%). The diameter of the neovascular channels (3.0 ± 1.0 mm) was greater than the other incompetent perforators (2.7 ± 1.0 mm; $P < .001$). The anatomic distribution of the neovascular recurrences was also different, with 63% found in the paratibial region. The number of new incompetent perforators in a limb was associated with the clinical and physiologic severity of venous disease before surgery, but not to body mass index, gender, or age ($P < .01$).

Conclusion.—This study shows that incompetent perforator recurrence after surgery is far more common than previously recognized and is primarily due to either neovascularization of previously ligated perforators or the development of incompetence in newly detected perforators in association with persistent venous disease rather than due to poor surgery.

▶ A very elegant study following the evolution of perforators in patients undergoing saphenofemoral ligation, great saphenous vein stripping, and perforator ligation surgery. Important is how perforators "reform": (1) new (neovascular) perforators at ligated site (40.4%), (2) change in a preexisting perforator from competent to incompetent (59.2%), and (3) missed perforator (<1%). Worsening venous reflux severity (venous filling index >2 mL/s) was associated with development of recurrent incompetent perforators. These recurrent neovascular channels were larger in diameter, with the majority located in the paratibial region. In addition, during a 3-year follow-up, there were also many new competent perforators identified.

J. D. Raffetto, MD, MS

Changes in superficial and perforating vein reflux after varicose vein surgery
Blomgren L, Johansson G, Dahlberg-Åkerman A, et al (Capio St Göran's Hosp, Stockholm; Univ Hosp, Uppsala, Sweden)
J Vasc Surg 42:315-320, 2005   15–6

Objectives.—This prospective duplex study was conducted to study the effect of current surgical treatment for primary varicose veins on the development of venous insufficiency ≤2 years after varicose vein surgery.

Methods.—The patients were part of a randomized controlled study where surgery for primary varicose veins was planned from a clinical examination alone or with the addition of preoperative duplex scanning. Postoperative duplex scanning was done at 2 months and 2 years.

Results.—Operations were done on 293 patients (343 legs), 74% of whom were women. The mean age was 47 years. In 126 legs, duplex scanning was done preoperatively, at 2 months and 2 years, and at 2 months and 2 years in 251 legs. Preoperative perforating vein incompetence (PVI) was present in 64 of 126 legs. Perforator ligation was not done on 42 of these; at 2 months, 23 of these legs (55%) had no PVI, and at 2 years, 25 legs (60%) had no PVI. Sixty-one legs had no PVI preoperatively, 5 (8%) had PVI at 2 months, and 11 (18%) had PVI at 2 years In the group of 251 legs, reversal of PVI between 2 months and 2 years was found in 28 (41%) of 68 and was more common than new PVI, which occurred in 41 (22%) of 183 ($P = .003$). After 2 years, the number of legs without venous incompetence in which perforator surgery was not performed was 11 (26%) of 42 legs with preoperative PVI and 18 (30%) of 61 legs without preoperative PVI, ($P = .713$). After 2 years, new vessel formation was more common in the surgically obliterated saphenopopliteal junction (SPJ), 4 (40%) of 10, than in the saphenofemoral junction (SFJ), 17 (11%) of 151 ($P = .027$), and new incompetence in a previously normal junction was more common in the SFJ, 11 (18%) of 63, than in the SPJ, 3 (1%) of 226 ($P < .001$). Reflux in the great saphenous vein (GSV) below the knee was abolished after stripping above the knee in 17 (34%) of 50 legs at 2 months and in 22 legs (44%) after 2 years.

Conclusions.—Varicose vein surgery induces changes in the remaining venous segments of the legs that continue for several months. In most patients, perforators and the GSV below the knee can be ignored at the primary surgery. A substantial number of recurrences in the SFJ and SPJ are unavoidable with present surgical knowledge because they stem from new vessel formation and progression of disease.

▶ Perforator contribution to the overall clinical severity of chronic venous insufficiency is debated. This study suggests PVI is not important. In limbs in which PVI was not treated, PVI was abolished in 60% 2 years after saphenous ligation and stripping. New PVI was seen in only 18% of limbs. Treated limbs also appeared to undergo dynamic changes with respect to the incompetent perforator location and character. Neovascular formation (11%) and new reflux (18%) at a previously normal SFJ can be expected after GSV ligation and stripping. Understanding what factors cause these processes will be essential in our understanding of the development of venous insufficiency.

J. D. Raffetto, MD, MS

Patient characteristics and physician-determined variables affecting saphenofemoral reflux recurrence after ligation and stripping of the great saphenous vein
Fischer R, Chandler JG, Stenger D, et al (Ctr for Vascular Diseases, St Gallen, Switzerland; Univ of Colorado, Denver; Phlebologische Gemeinschaftspraxis, Saarlouis, Germany; et al)
J Vasc Surg 43:81-87, 2006   15–7

Objective.—To identify patient and physician-controlled treatment variables that might predict the persistence or redevelopment of saphenofemoral junction (SFJ) reflux.

Methods.—Thirteen European centers, with substantial lower extremity venous disease practices, examined their experience with SFJ ligation and GSV stripping for primary varicose veins in patients followed for ≥2 years, entering their data into a protocol-driven matrix that stipulated duplex Doppler imaging as an essential component of follow-up examinations and required a complete review of all peri-operative examinations, as well as all operative procedure and anesthesia notes. Matrix entries were centrally audited for consistency and credibility, and queried for correction or clarification before being accepted into the study database. Presence or absence of Doppler-detectable SFJ reflux was the dependent variable and principal outcome measure.

Results.—Among 1,638 limbs, 315 (19.2%) had SFJ reflux. After adjustment for follow-up length and inputting for missing values, multivariable analysis identified seven significant predictors. Ultrasonic groin mapping (odds ratio [OR], 0.28; 95% confidence interval [CI], 0.20 to 0.40) and <3-

cm groin incisions at or immediately below the groin crease (OR, 0.50; 95% CI, 0.32 to 0.78) were both uniquely associated with diminished probability of follow-up SFJ reflux. Prior parity (OR, 2.69; 95% CI, 1.45 to 4.97), body mass index >29 kg/m² (OR, 1.65; 95% CI, 1.12 to 2.43), <3-cm suprainguinal incisions (OR, 3.71; 95% CI, 1.70 to 5.88), stripping to the ankle (OR, 2.43; 95% CI, 1.71 to 3.46), and interim pregnancy during follow-up (OR, 4.74; 95% CI, 2.47 to 9.12), were each independent predictors of a greater probability of having SFJ reflux.

Conclusions.—The findings suggest that ultrasound groin mapping, reticence for short suprainguinal or longer groin incisions and extended stripping, and counseling women about the effect of future pregnancy are prudent clinical choices, especially for obese or previously parous patients.

▶ This study's contribution is in determining factors that contribute to recurrent reflux at the SFJ after ligation and stripping of the great saphenous vein. We need to know if recurrent reflux at the SFJ has any implications on global venous physiology and quality of life, and if modifying the risk factors (eg, obesity) associated with recurrent SFJ reflux leads to reversibility. Interestingly, interim pregnancy was an independent predictor of recurrence, indicating the importance of hormone homeostasis in the pathophysiology of venous insufficiency.

J. D. Raffetto, MD, MS

Four-Year Follow-up on Endovascular Radiofrequency Obliteration of Great Saphenous Reflux

Merchant RF, Pichot O, Myers KA (Reno Vein Clinic, Nev; CHU de Grenoble, France; Monash Med Centre, Melbourne)
Dermatol Surg 31:129-134, 2005   15–8

Background.—Endovascular radiofrequency obliteration has been used since 1998 as an alternative to conventional vein stripping surgery for elimination of saphenous vein insufficiency.

Objective.—To demonstrate the long-term efficacy of this treatment modality.

Methods.—Data were prospectively collected in a multicenter ongoing registry. Only great saphenous vein above-knee treatments were included in this study. Eight hundred ninety patients (1,078 limbs) were treated prior to November 2003 at 32 centers. Clinical and duplex ultrasound follow-up was performed at 1 week, 6 months, and 1, 2, 3, and 4 years.

Results.—Among 1,078 limbs treated, 858 were available for follow-up within 1 week, 446 at 6 months, 384 at 1 year, 210 at 2 years, 114 at 3 years, and 98 at 4 years. The vein occlusion rates were 91.0%, 88.8%, 86.2%, 84.2%, and 88.8%, respectively; the reflux-free rates were 91.0%, 89.3%, 86.2%, 86.0%, and 85.7%, respectively; and the varicose vein recurrence rates were 7.2%, 13.5%, 17.1%, 14.0%, and 21.4%, respectively, at each follow-up time point at 6 months, and 1, 2, 3, and 4 years. Patient symptom improvement persisted over 4 years.

Conclusions.—Endovascular temperature-controlled radiofrequency obliteration of saphenous vein reflux exhibits an enduring treatment efficacy clinically, anatomically, and hemodynamically up to 4 years following treatment.

▶ A long-term follow-up study for venous ablation is important to evaluate technical success and quality of life. It is also important to understand if various factors are contributing to clinically relevant recanalization. Unfortunately, the conclusions of this study are premature. Out of 1078 limbs treated, only 384 (35.6%) were evaluated at 1 year and only 98 (9%) at 4 years. Of interest is the 21.4% varicose vein recurrence rate in the 98 limbs at 4 years. Long-term, randomized, multicenter trials evaluating ligation and stripping versus endovenous ablation are required before equivalency or superiority can be determined for these treatment modalities.

J. D. Raffetto, MD, MS

Double-Blind Prospective Comparative Trial between Foamed and Liquid Polidocanol and Sodium Tetradecyl Sulfate in the Treatment of Varicose and Telangiectatic Leg Veins

Rao J, Wildemore JK, Goldman MP (Dermatology/Cosmetic Laser Associates of La Jolla, Inc, Calif; Thomas Jefferson Univ, Philadelphia)
Dermatol Surg 31:631-635, 2005   15-9

Background.—Twenty subjects were treated with either polidocanol (POL) or sodium tetradecyl sulfate (STS) to compare the efficacy and adverse sequelae of each agent.

Objective.—To determine the safety and efficacy of two widely used sclerosing agents.

Methods.—After the exclusion of saphenofemoral junction incompetency, each subject's leg veins were categorized by size (< 1, 1–3, and 3–6 mm in diameter). Each leg was then randomized to be treated with 0.5%, 1%, or 1% foam of POL or 0.25%, 0.5%, or 0.5% foam of STS according to vein size. An independent panel of four physicians, blinded to treatment, performed randomized photographic evaluations obtained pretreatment and 12 weeks post-treatment. Subject satisfaction index and overall clinical improvement assessment were also obtained.

Results.—An average 83% improvement was noted for all vein sizes in all subjects with both POL and STS after a single treatment. Subjects were satisfied with treatment, regardless of the sclerosing agent used or the vein size treated. There was no statistically significant difference in adverse effects between each group.

Conclusion.—Both POL and STS are safe and effective sclerosing agents in the treatment of varicose and telangiectatic leg veins. Both are very tolerable and demonstrate similar post-treatment sequelae.

▶ This is a well-designed, albeit small, study comparing 2 types of detergent-based sclerosing agents. The clinical results were assessed blindly by 4 different evaluators. Both sclerosing agents were well tolerated and effective for telangiectatic vessels less than 1 mm and varicose veins less than 6 mm in diameter. There were few side effects and high patient satisfaction.

J. D. Raffetto, MD, MS

Hemochromatosis C282Y gene mutation increases the risk of venous leg ulceration

Zamboni P, Tognazzo S, Izzo M, et al (Univ of Ferrara, Italy)
J Vasc Surg 42:309-314, 2005

15–10

Objective.—Chronic venous disease (CVD) is the most common vascular disorder, progressing in approximately 10% of cases toward chronic venous leg ulceration, whereas the hemochromatosis gene (HFE) C282Y mutation is the most common recognized genetic defect in iron metabolism. Because CVD leads to local iron overload in the affected legs, we investigated whether two common HFE mutations could increase the risk of chronic venous leg ulceration.

Methods.—This was a case-control study at the Vascular Diseases Center, University of Ferrara, Italy. From a cohort of 980 consecutive patients affected by severe CVD (CEAP clinical classes C4 to C6) we selected 238 cases with the exclusion of any other comorbidity factor potentially involved in wound etiology (group A). They were subdivided into group B, including 137 patients with ulcer (classes C5 and C6: 98 primary and 39 postthrombotic cases), and group C, including 101 cases with no skin lesions (class C4). They were completely matched for sex, age, and geographic origin with 280 healthy controls (group D). A total of 518 subjects were polymerase chain reaction genotyped for HFE mutations (C282Y and H63D). We assessed the risk of ulceration by comparing the prevalence of ulcer in homogenous cases with and without the HFE variants. Other main outcome measures were the sensitivity, specificity, and predictive values of the genetic test in CVD cases.

Results.—C282Y mutation significantly increases the risk of ulcer in primary CVD by almost seven times (odds ratio, 6.69; 95% confidence interval, 1.45-30.8; $P = .01$). Application of the HFE test in primary CVD demonstrated increased specificity and positive predictive values (98% and 86%, respectively), with negligible sensitivity and negative predictive values.

Conclusions.—The overlap of primary CVD and the C282Y mutation consistently increases the risk of developing venous leg ulceration. These data, which have been confirmed in other clinical settings, suggest new strategies for preventing and treating primary CVD.

Clinical Relevance.—The number of patients affected by primary CVD is so great that the vast majority of ulcers are also related to this common problem. On the other hand, there is not a reliable way for identifying in advance, from the broad base of primary CVD patients (20–40% of the general population), the high risk minority (10% of primary CVD cases) who will develop a venous ulcer. In such cases, a simple C282Y blood genetic test demonstrated an elevated specificity in predicting ulcer development (98%, CI 95%, 92.8–99.7). The genetic test could be applied starting from the C2 class, varicose veins, the most common situation observed in clinical practice. In perspective, the presence of the C282Y mutation would strengthen the indications and priorities for surgical correction of superficial venous insufficiency.

▶ This study suggests an association between gene mutation (C2829) and susceptibility to a venous ulcer, especially in patients with primary venous insufficiency. Further studies are needed to determine if early intervention to correct venous reflux in patients with the C282Y gene mutation reduces the risk of ulcer development.

J. D. Raffetto, MD, MS

Effectiveness of an extracellular matrix graft (OASIS Wound Matrix) in the treatment of chronic leg ulcers: A randomized clinical trial
Mostow EN, for the OASIS Venus Ulcer Study Group (Northeastern Ohio Univ, Akron; et al)
J Vasc Surg 41:837-843, 2005   15–11

Background.—Venous leg ulcers are a major cause of morbidity, economic loss, and decreased quality of life in affected patients. Recently, biomaterials derived from natural tissue sources have been used to stimulate wound closure. One such biomaterial obtained from porcine small-intestine submucosa (SIS) has shown promise as an effective treatment to manage full-thickness wounds. Our objective was to compare the effectiveness of SIS wound matrix with compression vs compression alone in healing chronic leg ulcers within 12 weeks.

Methods.—This was a prospective, randomized, controlled multicenter trial Patients were 120 patients with at least 1 chronic leg ulcer. Patients were randomly assigned to receive either weekly topical treatment of SIS plus compression therapy (n = 62) or compression therapy alone (n = 58). Ulcer size was determined at enrollment and weekly throughout the treatment. Healing was assessed weekly for up to 12 weeks. Recurrence after 6 months was recorded. The primary outcome measure was the proportion of ulcers healed in each group at 12 weeks.

Results.—After 12 weeks of treatment, 55% of the wounds in the SIS group were healed, as compared with 34% in the standard-care group ($P = .0196$) (Fig 2). None of the healed patients treated with SIS wound matrix and seen for the 6-month follow-up experienced ulcer recurrence.

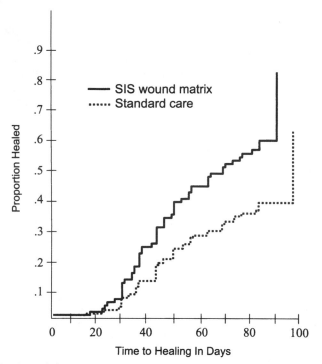

FIGURE 2.—Survival plot analysis for the small intestine submucosa (*SIS*) wound matrix group and the standard-care group. Success was defined as 100% healing. Patients treated with SIS wound matrix were more likely to heal by 12 weeks than those in the standard-care group (*P* = .0226). (Reprinted by permission of the publisher from Mostow EN, for the OASIS Venus Ulcer Study Group: Effectiveness of an extracellular matrix graft (OASIS Wound Matrix) in the treatment of chronic leg ulcers: A randomized clinical trial. *J Vasc Surg* 41:837-843, 2005. Copyright 2005 by Elsevier.)

Conclusions.—The SIS wound matrix, as an adjunct therapy, significantly improves healing of chronic leg ulcers over compression therapy alone.

▶ In this multicenter randomized study of venous ulcer wound care, the authors demonstrated improved effectiveness of complete healing with SIS as an adjuvant to compression therapy. The implication is that a biologic wound matrix improves ulcer healing.

J. D. Raffetto, MD, MS

Efficacy of the treatment with prostaglandin E-1 in venous ulcers of the lower limbs
Milio G, Miná C, Cospite V, et al (Univ of Palermo, Italy)
J Vasc Surg 42:304-308, 2005   15–12

Background.—Venous ulcers represent an important medical problem because of their high prevalence and consequent sanitary costs. In this study, we evaluated the effect of prostaglandin E-1 (PGE-1), a drug that improves district ischemia, on the healing of venous ulcers.

Methods.—We performed a randomized, placebo-controlled, single blind study in which 87 patients who had venous leg ulcers homogeneous for dimensions and characteristics were treated for 20 days with an infusion of prostaglandin E-1 or placebo, in association with topical therapy. The dimension and the number of the ulcers were determined at the beginning of the treatment and then every 20 days up to 4 months, or until total recovery. The main outcome of the study was the recovery percentage of the ulcers at the end of the 120-day period of observation and the referred healing time. The reduction in the extension of ulcers from the baseline measurement to the last observation was also evaluated.

Results.—The baseline characteristics of the treatment and control groups were similar. The reduction in the size of the ulcers was faster in the patients treated with PGE-1. In this group, 100% of the ulcers healed ≤ 100 days, whereas in the placebo group, only 84.2% did so by the end of the 120-day observation period ($P < .05$). The estimated healing times of 25%, 50%, and 75% of the patients treated with PGE-1 were 23, 49, and 72 days, respectively, compared with 52, 80, and 108 for the patients in the placebo group. Only one serious event occurred in the treated group.

Conclusions.—This study demonstrates the effectiveness of PGE-1 in reducing the healing time of venous ulcers, suggesting that venous ulcers should also be considered ischemic.

▶ Another randomized placebo-controlled trial of adjuvant treatment for venous ulcers. The effectiveness of PGE-1 is clearly documented, but the authors raise the interesting point that ischemia may have an important role in venous ulcer pathophysiology. This is based primarily on known actions of PGE-1. This interesting hypothesis deserves further evaluation.

J. D. Raffetto, MD, MS

Randomized clinical trial of compression plus surgery *versus* compression alone in chronic venous ulceration (ESCHAR study) – haemodynamic and anatomical changes
Gohel MS, Barwell JR, Earnshaw JJ, et al (Cheltenham Gen Hosp, England; Gloucestershire Royal Hosp, Gloucester, England; Southmead Hosp, Bristol, England)
Br J Surg 92:291-297, 2005   15–13

Background.—The aim of this study was to evaluate the anatomical and haemodynamic effects of superficial venous surgery and compression on legs with chronic venous ulceration.

Methods.—Legs with open or recently healed ulceration and saphenous reflux were treated with multilayer compression bandaging or superficial venous surgery plus compression as part of a clinical trial. Venous duplex imaging was performed before treatment and at 1 year. Legs were stratified before surgery as having no deep reflux, segmental deep reflux or total deep reflux. Venous refill times (VRTs) were calculated before treatment and at 1 year using photoplethysmography, with and without a narrow below-knee cuff inflated to 80 mmHg.

Results.—Of 214 legs investigated, 112 were treated with compression and 102 with compression plus surgery. Saphenous surgery abolished deep reflux in ten of 22 legs with segmental deep reflux and three of 17 with total deep reflux. Overall median (range) VRT increased from 10 (3–48) to 15 (4–48) s 1 year after surgery (*P* < 0.001). Preoperative change in VRT on application of a below-knee tourniquet correlated with actual change in VRT following surgery.

Conclusion.—Superficial venous surgery resulted in a significant haemodynamic benefit for legs with venous ulceration despite co-existent deep reflux; residual saphenous reflux was common.

▶ This study emphasizes that the venous system can undergo dynamic changes with respect to sites of reflux. Correcting superficial reflux often corrects deep segmental reflux, especially that isolated to the common femoral vein. Importantly, hemodynamic improvement measured by venous refill times was only achieved in patients undergoing surgical correction of superficial reflux. This was irrespective of the pattern of venous reflux. Close follow-up is required to determine if improved VRT translates into increased healing rates and less recurrences of venous ulcers.

J. D. Raffetto, MD, MS

Efficacy of topical pale sulfonated shale oil in the treatment of venous leg ulcers: A randomized, controlled, multicenter study
Beckert S, Warnecke J, Zelenkova H, et al (Univ Hosp, Tübingen and Hamburg, Germany; DOST Svinik; Slovakia; Univ Hosp, Düsseldorf, Germany)
J Vasc Surg 43:94-100, 2006   15–14

Background.—Venous leg ulcers are a growing socioeconomic burden. Pale sulfonated shale oils (PSSO) are used for therapy of inflammatory skin diseases and have been shown to enhance wound healing in vitro and in vivo. The aim of this study was to investigate whether PSSO is capable of enhancing venous ulcer healing beyond compression therapy alone.

Methods.—One hundred nineteen patients were enrolled in this randomized, multicenter, observer-blind study. In the treatment group, PSSO 10% was applied daily for 20 weeks, and the control group received the vehicle only. Wounds were covered by a nonadherent gauze dressing, and compression therapy with short-stretch elastic bandages was performed in an outpatient setting. The primary study end point was defined as cumulative reduction in wound area; the secondary study end point was treatment success as assessed by both physicians and patients. Additionally, adverse events, including changes with respect to physical examination and vital signs, were documented.

Results.—At the end of the study period, ulcer size was significantly more reduced in the PSSO group compared with the vehicle group (15 ± 15.9 to 6.2 ± 12.9 cm² vs 11.4 ± 14.5 to 10.8 ± 15.7 cm²; $P = .0005$). The cumulative relative reduction in ulcer area was significantly higher in the PSSO group (-4391 ± 4748.7 vs $-231.9 \pm 6283.6\%$ × days; $P < .0001$). Relative reduction in wound area was significantly greater in the PSSO group as early as 6 weeks after the beginning of treatment (-47.4 ± 28.4 vs $-23.8 \pm 42.2\%$; $P < .001$). PSSO was judged successful both by physicians and patients. There were no significant differences in adverse events (PSSO, 9 [12.2%]; vehicle, 7 [11.1%]. Similarly, tolerability of PSSO was equal to the tolerability of the vehicle.

Conclusion.—Pale sulfonated shale oils were capable of favoring venous ulcer healing in addition to compression therapy. PSSO should be considered for future wound care protocols for treatment of venous leg ulcers.

▶ Despite the ever-increasing multibillion-dollar wound care industry, well-designed randomized clinical trials evaluating the effectiveness of venous ulcer wound care are rare. I applaud Beckert et al for a much-needed contribution in venous ulcer wound care. Although there was no difference in the number of healed ulcers with PSSO versus vehicle, unless randomized studies are performed we will continue to base much of our wound care on personal observations instead of sound clinical evidence.

J. D. Raffetto, MD, MS

Mid-term results of endovascular treatment for symptomatic chronic nonmalignant iliocaval venous occlusive disease
Hartung O, Otero A, Boufi M, et al (Centre Hospitalier Universitaire Nord, Marseille, France)
J Vasc Surg 42:1138-1144, 2005   15–15

Background.—The goal of this article is to present clinical and patency results of endovascular treatment of nonmalignant, iliocaval venous obstructive disease and to discuss the evolution of technical details.

Methods.—From November 1995 to June 2004, 44 patients (female-male ratio, 3.9:1; left-right lower limb ratio, 8.6:1; median age, 42 years; range, 21-80 years) had treatment for chronic disabling obstructive venous insufficiency with iliocaval stenosis or occlusion. The clinical class of CEAP was 2 in 11 limbs, 3 in 31, 4 in 4, 5 in 1, and 6 in 1; etiology was primary in 32 patients, secondary in 10, and congenital in 2. Anatomic involvement included superficial veins in 16 patients and perforator veins in 11. Obstruction was associated with superficial reflux in 4 patients, deep reflux in 13, and both in 13. Ten patients had occlusion. All procedures were performed in the operating room with perioperative angiography and angioplasty with or without self-expanding stent implantation (Fig 1). Venous clinical severity and disability scores were obtained before and after treatment. Patency and restenosis were evaluated by duplex Doppler ultrasonography.

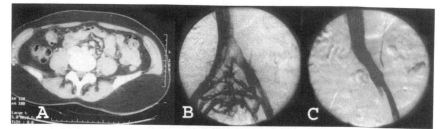

FIGURE 1.—Perioperative angiography in a patient with pelvic congestion syndrome caused by May-Thurner syndrome. A, Computed tomographic scan showing left common iliac vein stenosis. B, Angiography: tight stenosis of the left common iliac vein with large transversal collateral pathways. C, After angioplasty and stenting, the collateral pathways are no longer opacified. (Reprinted by permission of the publisher from Hartung O, Otero A, Boufi M, et al: Mid-term results of endovascular treatment for symptomatic chronic nonmalignant iliocaval venous occlusive disease. *J Vasc Surg* 41:285-290, 2005. Copyright 2005 by Elsevier.)

Results.—No perioperative death or pulmonary embolism occurred. The technical success rate was 95.5% (two recanalization failures), and two (4.5%) perioperative stent migrations occurred. One early thrombosis (2.4%) was treated by thrombectomy and creation of an arteriovenous fistula. One late death and one thrombosis occurred. Restenoses were found in five patients and were all treated successfully (four needed iterative stenting). Median follow-up was 27 months (range, 2-103 months). Median venous clinical severity score improved from 8.5 to 2, and median venous disability score improved from 2 to 0. Cumulative primary, assisted primary, and secondary patency rates of the venous segments at 36 months were 73%, 88%, and 90%, respectively, in intention to treat. The survival rate was 100% at 12 months and 97.3% at 60 months.

Conclusions.—Endovascular treatment of benign iliocaval occlusive disease is a safe and efficient minimally invasive technique with good mid-term patency rates. Moreover, it improves cases with obstruction only, as well as cases with associated reflux and obstruction. Primary stenting should always be performed by using self-expanding stents deployed under general anesthesia to avoid lumbar pain. In case of failure, the endovascular procedure does not preclude further surgical reconstruction.

▶ This study reaffirms the importance of proper preoperative imaging and planning in patients with symptomatic iliocaval venous occlusive disease. Obstructions in the venous system can be effectively treated with excellent 36-month results. Adequate follow-up is mandatory to treat restenosis (13% of patients). The article emphasizes the importance of using large (16 mm), long (60 mm), and self-expanding stents that cross into the inferior vena cava. There was dramatic improvement in the venous clinical severity score and venous disability score after treatment.

J. D. Raffetto, MD, MS

Subclavian vein obstruction without thrombosis

Sanders RJ, Hammond SL (Univ of Colorado, Denver; Uniformed Services Univ of the Health Sciences, Denver)
J Vasc Surg 41:285-290, 2005   15–16

Background.—Unilateral arm swelling caused by subclavian vein obstruction without thrombosis is an uncommon form of venous thoracic outlet syndrome (TOS). In 87 patients with venous TOS, only 21 patients had no thrombosis. We describe the diagnosis and treatment of these patients.

Material and Methods.—Twenty-one patients with arm swelling, cyanosis, and venograms demonstrating partial subclavian vein obstruction were treated with transaxillary first rib resection and venolysis.

Results.—Eighteen (86%) of 21 patients had good-to-excellent improvement of symptoms. There were two failures (9%).

Conclusions.—Unilateral arm swelling without thrombosis, when not caused by lymphatic obstruction, may be due to subclavian vein compression at the costoclavicular ligament because of compression either by that ligament or the subclavius tendon most often because of congenital close proximity of the vein to the ligament. Arm symptoms of neurogenic TOS, pain, and paresthesia often accompany venous TOS while neck pain and headache, other common symptoms of neurogenic TOS, are infrequent. Diagnosis was made by dynamic venography. First rib resection, which included the anterior portion of rib and cartilage plus division of the costoclavicular ligament and subclavius tendon, proved to be effective treatment.

▶ The importance of this report is to point out that you do not have to have subclavian vein thrombosis to have symptoms related to venous TOS. Patients who are young and have a history of excessive arm activities may present with arm swelling, intermittent cyanosis, pain, paresthesias, and occasionally neck pain with or without occipital headache secondary to subclavian vein narrowing without thrombosis.

J. D. Raffetto, MD, MS

16 Technical Notes

Creating Arteriovenous Fistulas in 132 Consecutive Patients: Exploiting the Proximal Radial Artery Arteriovenous Fistula: Reliable, Safe, and Simple Forearm and Upper Arm Hemodialysis Access
Jennings WC (Univ of Oklahoma, Tulsa)
Arch Surg 141:27-32, 2006   16–1

Hypothesis.—Dialysis by native arteriovenous fistula (NAVF) clearly offers lower infection rates, fewer procedures, and lower mortality risk compared with access by catheter or graft, in addition to lower cost. However, NAVFs are utilized for vascular access in only 30% of hemodialysis patients in the United States. Wrist NAVFs are not feasible or successful in many patients and upper arm brachial artery NAVFs may be impractical or lead to additional procedures or complications. Careful preoperative evaluation of all options for NAVF construction including the proximal radial artery (PRA) as an arterial inflow site will find most, if not all, patients to be candidates for successful NAVFs.

Design.—Retrospective review of consecutive operations for hemodialysis access preformed by an individual surgeon from May 2003 to November 2004.

Setting.—Two university-affiliated tertiary medical centers.

Patients.—All patients underwent preoperative ultrasound evaluation by the operating surgeon. A wrist fistula was first choice for access when success was predicted by ultrasound and physical examination. The second choice, and most common operation, was a PRA NAVF with distal forearm (retrograde) flow established by disrupting the initial venous valve using a vessel probe.

Results.—One hundred thirty-two patients aged 11 to 90 years (mean = 61) were reviewed. Sixty-eight patients had diabetes and 61 were female. Thirty-four had previous failed access surgery. Native arteriovenous fistulas were created in all patients. No grafts were used. A PRA NAVF was utilized in 105 operations. Overall (assisted) patency was 97%, with a mean follow-up of 11 months. Importantly, there were no infections or hospitalizations due to the NAVF access operations.

Conclusions.—No grafts were used in this series of 132 consecutive patients. The PRA NAVF was the most common operation and an important addition to wrist, brachial, and transposition fistulas. Proximal radial artery NAVFs increase the opportunity for construction of successful NAVFs and are reliable, safe, and simple procedures with access sites often available in both the forearm and in the upper arm.

▶ The technique maximized outflow of the fistula by providing both antegrade and retrograde flow with an anastomosis in the upper forearm. Forearm swelling was not a significant problem. The technique may lead to some "unusual" sites for placement of dialysis needles. Close communication with the dialysis center therefore seems crucial. If the claimed secondary patency rate of 97% at 18 months is real, this technique should be learned by all access surgeons.

G. L. Moneta, MD

'Extension Technique': A Modified Technique for Brachio-Cephalic Fistula to Prevent Dialysis Access-Associated Steal Syndome

Ehsan O, Bhattacharya D, Darwish A, et al (Burnley Gen Hosp, Lancashire, England; North West Rotation, England)
Eur J Vasc Endovasc Surg 29:324-327, 2005   16–2

Objectives.—To describe a modification in brachio-cephalic fistula formation for prevention of dialysis access-associated steal syndrome (DASS).
Design.—Short report.
Materials.—From September 2001 to December 2003, 32 upper arm autogenous fistulæ were formed using the 'extension technique' in patients at high-risk for developing DASS i.e. diabetics.
Methods.—In this technique, the fistula is formed by anastomosing the median vein to the radial or ulnar artery just below the brachial bifurcation, thus preserving part of the blood supply to the hand, to prevent steal syndrome (Fig 1). All patients were evaluated for patency, adequacy of needling and the absence of steal symptoms.

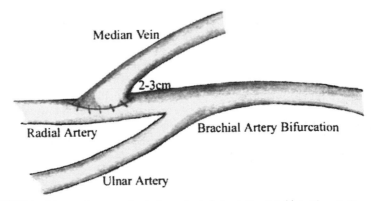

FIGURE 1.—Diagram demonstrating the 'extension technique'. (Reprinted from Ehsan O, Bhattacharya D, Darwish A, et al: 'Extension technique': A modified technique for brachio-cephalic fistula to prevent dialysis access-associated steal syndrome. *Eur J Vasc Endovasc Surg* 29:324-327, 2006 by permission of the publisher W B Saunders Company Limited London.)

Results.—Only 1 patient (3.1%) developed DASS. On investigation, he was found to have the fistula formed distal to the origin of a posterior branch with the bifurcation further distally. Symptoms improved with revision of the fistula. Thrombosis of the cephalic vein (6.2%), difficulty in needling (3.1%) and deep cephalic vein in upper arm that required superficialization (15.6%) were the other complications noted.

Conclusions.—The 'extension technique' has been found to be a safe and effective procedure for prevention of DASS, with a good patency rate. Additional advantage of this technique is maturation of both cephalic and basilic veins.

▶ The technique is essentially nothing more than moving the anastomosis for a brachiocephalic fistula to the ulnar or radial artery in the forearm. It is not really a new idea. Surgeons have long used the proximal radial and ulnar artery as an inflow site for dialysis access (see Abstract 16–1). If the antecubital veins have not suffered repeat venopunctures, there seems no reason not to use this technique.

G. L. Moneta, MD

Revision Using Digital Inflow: A Novel Approach to Dialysis-associated Steal Syndrome

Minion DJ, Moore E, Endean E (Univ of Kentucky, Lexington)
Ann Vasc Surg 19:625-628, 2005   16–3

Current access-preserving treatment options for dialysis-associated steal syndrome (DASS) include fistula lengthening or banding and distal revascularization interval ligation (DRIL). We describe a novel technique for the treatment of DASS that we have termed revision using distal inflow (RUDI). Briefly, the technique involves ligation of the fistula at its origin followed by reestablishment of the fistula via bypass from a more distal arterial source to the venous limb (Fig 1). Four patients with brachial artery-based arteriovenous fistula and DASS underwent RUDI as described above using either the proximal radial or ulnar artery as inflow and vein as conduit. Patients were diagnosed with DASS based on the clinical findings of pain, pallor, loss of radial pulse, and sensorimotor dysfunction after creation of an AVF. Noninvasive vascular studies confirmed diminished finger pressures that improved with compression of the fistula. All patients experienced rapid resolution of their symptoms, although one patient complained of mild residual parasthesias. Follow-up ranging from 4 to 14 months has revealed patent functional fistulas. These initial results demonstrate that RUDI can be an effective treatment of DASS. By design, RUDI incorporates many of the advantages of established access-preserving procedures. That is, by using a smaller distal artery as inflow, RUDI lengthens the fistula, decreases the radius, and preserves antegrade flow in the brachial artery. In contrast to DRIL, it is the fistula, not the native arterial supply, that is placed at risk by

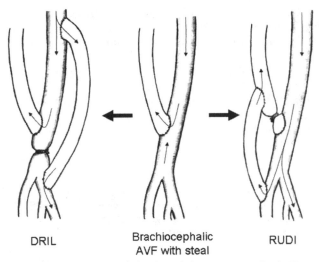

DRIL

Brachiocephalic
AVF with steal

RUDI

FIGURE 1.—Two options for revision of a brachiocephalic arteriovenous fistula (AVF) with associated steal syndrome. The current standard is distal revascularization with interval ligation (DRIL). This procedure involves ligation of the native circulation just distal to the AVF and a bypass to the ischemic hand from a proximal arterial source. In contrast, revision using distal inflow (RUDI) involves ligation of the AVF at its origin and bypass to the venous outflow from a distal arterial source. The advantage of RUDI over DRIL is that it maintains native arterial circulation. Therefore, potential graft occlusion would result in fistula thrombosis rather than limb threat. (Courtesty of Minion DJ, Moore E, Endean E: Revision using digital inflow: A novel approach to dialysis-associated steal syndrome. *Ann Vasc Surg* 19:625-628, 2005.)

ligation and revascularization. Consequently, we believe that RUDI may become the procedure of choice for DASS after brachial artery-based fistulas.

▶ This is a bit less involved than a DRIL procedure and likely a shorter piece of vein is required. It involves the same principles as the previous abstract (ie, putting in anastomosis for an upper arm fistula on the radial or ulnar artery). Longevity will depend on the fate of the interposed vein segment. Anecdotal experience suggests vein interpositions/extensions to an existing dialysis access tend to become sclerotic. More patients and more follow-up are needed.

G. L. Moneta, MD

Keyhole technique for autologous brachiobasilic transposition arteriovenous fistula
Hill BB, Chan AK, Faruqi RM, et al (Stanford Univ, Calif; Kaiser Permanente Med Ctr, Santa Clara, Calif; Kaiser Permanente Med Ctr, Walnut Creek, Calif)
J Vasc Surg 42:945-950, 2005   16–4

Background.—Autologous brachiobasilic transposition arteriovenous fistulas (AVFs) are desirable but require long incisions and extensive surgical dissection. To minimize the extent of surgery, we developed a catheter-based technique that requires only keyhole incisions and local anesthesia.

Methods.—The technique involves exposure and division of the basilic vein at the elbow. A guidewire is introduced into the vein, and a 6F "push catheter" is advanced over the guidewire and attached to the vein with sutures. Gently pushing the catheter proximally inverts, or intussuscepts, the vein. Side branches that are felt as resistances when pushing the catheter forward are localized, clipped, and divided under direct vision. Throughout the procedure, the endothelium always remains intraluminal. The basilic vein is externalized at the axilla without dividing it proximally and is tunneled subcutaneously, where it is anastomosed to the brachial artery.

Results.—Thirty-two patients underwent the procedure—31 as outpatients. The mean duration of operation was less than 90 minutes. All patients tolerated the procedure well, and 31 required only intravenous sedation and local anesthesia. At a mean follow-up of 8 months, the primary patency rate of AVFs in patients with basilic vein diameters of 4 mm or more on preoperative duplex ultrasonography was 80%, vs 50% for those with vein diameters less than 4 mm. Overall, 78% of patent AVFs were being successfully accessed and 22% were still maturing at last follow-up.

Conclusions.—Autologous brachiobasilic transposition AVFs can be created by using catheter-mediated techniques that facilitate the mobilization and tunneling of the basilic vein through small incisions. Medium-term data suggest that the inversion method results in acceptable maturation and functionality of AVFs created with this technique.

▶ The "key" to this keyhole technique would appear to be clipping or ligating the side branches of the vein through the small incisions without injuring the vein. I am sure it is possible, but there will be some vein injuries that otherwise will not occur. Most will not matter, but eventually one will.

G. L. Moneta, MD

Arterioarterial prosthetic loop: A new approach for hemodialysis access
Zanow J, Kruger U, Petzold M, et al (Queen Elisabeth Hosp, Berlin)
J Vasc Surg 41:1007-1112, 2005   16–5

Objectives.—In this report we present a novel procedure that uses an arterioarterial prosthetic loop (AAPL) with the proximal axillary or the femoral artery as a vascular access for hemodialysis in patients who have inadequate vascular conditions for creating an arteriovenous fistula or graft.

Methods.—Between April 1996 and September 2004, 34 patients received 36 AAPLs as vascular access, either as an axillary chest loop (n = 31) or as a femoral loop (n = 5). In this procedure the artery is ligated between the anastomoses to direct flow through the AAPL. Data from all patients undergoing the procedure were prospectively collected.

Results.—The indication for an AAPL was the unsuitability of large deep veins in 64%, steal syndrome in 11%, the combination of only a suitable femoral vein and severe peripheral arterial disease in 22%, and congestive heart failure in 3%. All AAPLs were cannulated 18 ± 4 days postoperatively.

Mean follow-up was 31 months (range, 1 to 83). Primary patency was 73% and secondary patency was 96% at 1 year; these rates at 3 years were 54% and 87%, respectively. The rate of all interventions for the maintenance of AAPL function was 0.47 procedures per patient year. Four grafts were abandoned. More than 11,000 hemodialyses with proven efficiency were performed.

Conclusions.—The AAPL is an unusual but useful and easy-to-perform alternative procedure to create vascular access for hemodialysis. It can provide survival for strictly selected patients in whom conventional vascular access is not possible. The axillary chest AAPL is preferred.

▶ I would not use this technique in the lower extremity. The potential for significant ischemic complications if the access occludes seems high. In the upper extremity, there are likely significant collaterals to keep the arm alive if the access occludes. If, however, the patient has significant distal occlusive upper extremity arterial disease, the potential for ischemic complications if the access occludes seems high. Assessment of digital arteries before performing this procedure is advised.

G. L. Moneta, MD

Transthoracic cuffed hemodialysis catheters: a method for difficult hemodialysis access
Wellons ED, Matsuura J, Lai K-M, et al (Atlanta Med Ctr, Ga)
J Vasc Surg 42:286-289, 2005   16–6

Background.—Recurrent vascular access failure is a major cause of morbidity in patients receiving long-term hemodialysis. Central venous catheters are often necessary for dialysis, and easily accessed vessels (ie, the internal jugular vein and subclavian vein) frequently occlude because of repeated cannulation. When standard access sites occlude, unconventional access methods become necessary. We report a technique of placing hemodialysis catheters directly into the superior vena cava (SVC).

Methods.—Between January 2002 and December 2004, 22 patients with documented bilateral jugular and subclavian vein occlusion underwent transthoracic SVC permanent catheter placement. Femoral vein access was obtained, and a sheath was placed. Under fluoroscopic guidance, a diagnostic catheter was then inserted into the SVC, and a venogram was obtained. By using the fluoroscopic image as a reference guide, supraclavicular access directly into the SVC was performed with lateral and anteroposterior views to better localize the SVC (Fig 2). Once venous blood was obtained, a hydrophilic wire was passed into the inferior vena cava. A 5F sheath was then placed, and, with the use of an exchange catheter, the wire was switched for a stiffer wire. The hemodialysis catheter was then placed in the standard fashion over this wire.

Results.—In a 24-month period, 22 patients underwent transthoracic permanent catheter placement. All patients had the permanent catheters suc-

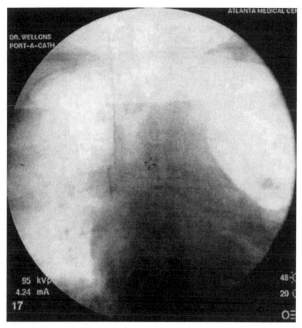

FIGURE 2.—An introducer needle is guided into the superior vena cava from a supraclavicular puncture. The diagnostic catheter is left in place to aid in accurate placement of the needle. (Reprinted by permission of the publisher from Wellons ED, Matsuura J, Lai K-M, et al: Transthoracic cuffed hemodialysis catheters: A method for difficult hemodialysis access. *J Vasc Surg* 42:286-289, 2005. Copyright 2005 by Elsevier.)

cessfully inserted. Two major complications occurred. One patient experienced a pneumothorax, and another patient experienced a hemothorax. Both patients were successfully treated with chest tube decompression. All permanent catheters functioned immediately with a range of 1 to 7 months.

Conclusions.—Transthoracic permanent catheter placement is an appropriate alternative for patients in whom traditional venous access sites are no longer available.

▶ Basically, the femoral access is used to guide placement of a needle from the right supraclavicular area into the SVC under fluoroscopic guidance. I wonder whether CT guidance for placement of the SVC needle would not accomplish the same thing without the need for a femoral puncture?

G. L. Moneta, MD

Thyrocervical trunk–external carotid artery bypass for positional cerebral ischemia due to common carotid artery occlusion

Melgar MA, Sahni D, Weinand M (Tulane Univ, New Orleans, La; Univ of Arizona, Tucson)
J Neurosurg 103:170-175, 2005   16–7

Background.—Positional cerebral ischemia (PCI) that is triggered by standing, with or without orthostatic hypotension, has been attributed to hemodynamic cerebrovascular insufficiency associated with stenosis or occlusion of a proximal extracranial or intracranial artery. There have been reports of such cases in occlusions of the basilar artery and the internal carotid artery. However, PCI attributable to occlusion of the common carotid artery (CCA) in conjunction with orthostatic hypotension is a rare combination. Most cases of CCA occlusion are asymptomatic. When they are symptomatic, subclavian artery–external carotid artery saphenous vein interposition grafting has been the treatment of choice. A technical variation of external carotid artery blood flow reconstruction in which the thyrocervical trunk was used as a donor vessel was described (Fig 1). In addition, 3 refractory cases of PCI caused by occlusion of the CCA that were successfully treated with this bypass procedure were presented.

Case 1.—Man, 41, was seen with severe episodes of light-headedness, blurred vision, perioral paresthesia, and left-handed

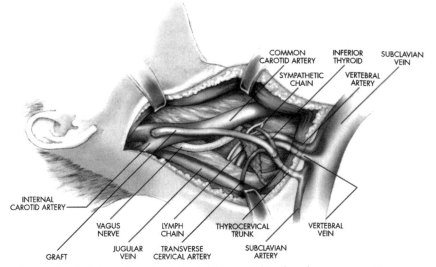

FIGURE 1.—Artist's rendition of a right-sided thyrocervical trunk–saphenous vein graft bypass. The sympathetic and lymph chains are particularly vulnerable to injury where the inferior thyroid artery crosses the deep fat tissue layer. The thyrocervical trunk is identified by following the inferior thyroid artery caudally. (Courtesy of Melgar MA, Sahni D, Weinand M: Thyrocervical trunk–external carotid artery bypass for positional cerebral ischemia due to common carotid artery occlusion. *J Neurosurg* 103:170-175, 2005.)

clumsiness triggered by standing. CT and MRI showed chronic periventricular ischemic lesions.

Case 2.—Man, 76, was seen with daily spells of confusion, left-handed clumsiness, blurred left vision, and leg shaking that began on standing and subsided after several minutes. Conservative treatment was unsuccessful. Surgery was planned, with a goal of improving direct cerebral blood flow by increasing the flow in the partially reconstituted right internal carotid artery.

Case 3.—Man, 67, was admitted with transient weekly episodes of left-sided hemiparesis that were provoked by standing. The medical history was significant for peripheral vascular disease and bilateral femoral artery–popliteal artery bypass surgery. Conservative treatment was unsuccessful. CT scanning showed a small watershed stroke of indeterminate age in the right frontoparietal region. Aortic arch digital subtraction angiography demonstrated right CCA occlusion, a hypoplastic right vertebral artery, and a patent right thyrocervical trunk.

Conclusions.—Orthostatic hypotension remained postoperatively, but ischemia-related symptoms resolved and long-term patency was demonstrated in all 3 patients. It is feasible to treat cerebral ischemia resulting from occlusion of the CCA with extracranial bypass surgery. In the 3 patients presented in this report, the thyrocervical trunk was found to be a donor vessel for the reconstitution of blood flow within the external carotid artery.

▶ I suppose all is relative. The authors, neurosurgeons, prefer the thyrocervical trunk as inflow to a bypass to the external carotid artery. I think most vascular surgeons are comfortable with exposure of the subclavian artery and would prefer this larger vessel as an inflow source for bypass to the external carotid artery.

G. L. Moneta, MD

Superficial femoral artery transposition repair for isolated superior mesenteric artery dissection

Picquet J, Abilez O, Pénard J, et al (Univ Hosp of Angers, France; Stanford Univ, Calif)
J Vasc Surg 42:788-791, 2005   16–8

Background.—Dissection of the superior mesenteric artery (SMA) is an uncommon event, but there have been an increasing number of reports in recent years. This increased reporting reflects the increased use of imaging modalities such as CT angiography and MR angiography in the diagnosis of abdominal pathologic processes. Conservative or medical management or surgical revascularization may be used in the management of dissection of the SMA. The failure of surgical management is associated with a high risk of death, but there is insufficient experience to prove the superiority of one

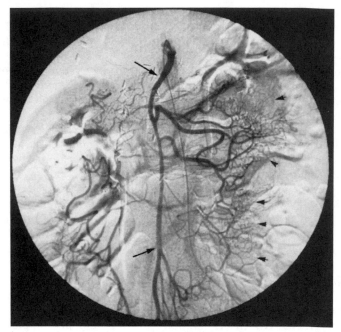

FIGURE 3.—Three-month postoperative angiogram demonstrates patency of the anatomic reconstruction of the superior mesenteric artery (SMA) by using the superficial femoral artery. *Long arrows* show the proximal and distal end-to-end anastomoses of the arterial graft. *Short arrows* show good distal perfusion of the small bowel. The significant tapering of the mid portion of the graft is probably a spasm or an artifact. (Reprinted by permission of the publisher from Picquet J, Abilez O, Pénard J, et al: Superficial femoral artery transposition repair for isolated superior mesenteric artery dissection. *J Vasc Surg* 42:788-791, 2005. Copyright 2005 by Elsevier.)

approach over the other. This report presented outcomes after use of an original technique for revascularization of the SMA by using a superficial femoral artery (SFA) transposition.

> *Case Report.*—Woman, 53, was seen with acute abdominal pain suggestive of mesenteric ischemia. A scout abdominal film showed multiple air-fluid levels. A CT scan showed Balthazar stage B pancreatitis, confirmed by increased pancreatic enzymes. Contrast CT suggested a false lumen of the SMA and abnormal thickness of its wall. Limited infarctions of the left kidney were also noted.
>
> Selective angiography using the Seldinger technique was performed, and a long stenosis of the SMA was identified. Also identified were the absence of the inferior duodeno-pancreatic arcade, small bowel malperfusion, complete obstruction of a left inferior polar renal artery, a right renal artery stenosis with poststenotic dilatation, and a dissection beginning at the poststenotic dilatation of the right renal artery. A conservative approach was attempted initially but was ultimately unsuccessful.

Through a median laparotomy, intramesenteric exposure of the SMA provided visualization of the disease portion of the artery. No saphenous vein was available, and upper limb veins were determined to be unusable. After heparin administration, the right SFA was dissected free and replaced by a polytetrafluoroethylene tube graft. The SMA was clamped at its first centimeter and transversely cut. The trunk of the SMA was completely removed for pathologic examination. End-to-end anastomoses were performed between the SMA ostium and the proximal part of the SMA and the last SMA bifurcation and the distal part of the SFA.

Four other side-to-end anastomoses were performed. The pathologic segment of the right renal artery was also resected and replaced by the most distal segment of the SFA. The procedure was completed with a cholecystectomy and percutaneous jejunostomy. The patient was discharged 5 weeks later on antiplatelet therapy. Three-month postoperative selective angiography showed patency of the SFA transposed in the SMA position, occlusion of 2 ileal anastomoses, and good general vascularization of the bowel (Fig 3).

Conclusions.—Arteriosclerosis, fibromuscular dysplasia, and disease of the elastic tissue are possible causes for isolated SMA dissection. This report described a novel treatment of SMA dissection with a technique that has been described for use in other arterial locations.

▶ Femoral vein is an alternative conduit for reconstruction of mesenteric vessels. Only a short piece is needed for the procedure described in this abstract. Significant leg edema is therefore unlikely. I also think reimplantation of the SMA branch vessels would be easier into a femoral vein than an SFA. Clearly, harvesting of the femoral vein would not require reconstruction of the SFA.

G. L. Moneta, MD

Randomized, controlled clinical trial of point-of-care limited ultrasonography assistance of central venous cannulation: The Third Sonography Outcomes Assessment Program (SOAP-3) Trial
Milling TJ Jr, Rose J, Briggs WM, et al (New York Methodist Hosp; Univ of California–Davis; Cornell Univ, New York)
Crit Care Med 33:1764-1769, 2005   16–9

Context.—A 2001 Agency for Healthcare Research and Quality Evidence Report on patient safety addressed point-of-care limited ultrasonography guidance for central venous cannulation and strongly recommended real-time, dynamic guidance for all central cannulas. However, on the basis of one limited study, the report dismissed static assistance, a "quick look" with ultrasound to confirm vein location before preparing the sterile field, as unhelpful.

Objective.—The objective of this trial was to compare the overall success rate of central cannula placement with use of dynamic ultrasound (D), static ultrasound (S), and anatomical landmarks (LM).

Design and Setting.—A concealed, randomized, controlled, clinical trial conducted from September 2003 to February 2004 in a U.S. urban teaching hospital.

Patients.—Two-hundred one patients undergoing internal jugular vein central venous cannulation.

Interventions.—Patients were randomly assigned to three groups: 60 to D, 72 to S, and 69 to LM. An iLook25 SonoSite was used for all imaging.

Measurements and Main Results.—Cannulation success, first-attempt success, and number of attempts were noted. Other measures were vein size and clarity of LM. Results, controlled for pretest difficulty assessment, are stated as odds improvement (95% confidence interval) over LM for D and S. D had an odds 53.5 (6.6-440) times higher for success than LM. S had an odds 3 (1.3-7) times higher for success than LM. The unadjusted success rates were 98%, 82%, and 64% for D, S, and LM. For first-attempt success, D had an odds 5.8 (2.7-13) times higher for first success than LM, and S had an odds 3.4 (1.6-7.2) times higher for first success than LM. The unadjusted first-attempt success rates were 62%, 50%, and 23% for D, S, and LM.

Conclusions.—Ultrasound assistance was superior to LM techniques. D outperformed S but may require more training and personnel. All central cannula placement should be conducted with ultrasound assistance. The 2001 Agency for Healthcare Research and Quality Evidence Report dismissing static assistance was incorrect.

▶ The authors succeeded in placing central access without any form of US guidance in only 64% of cases. This seems low. However, the ability to place central access 98% of the time under real-time US guidance is outstanding and suggests this should be the standard for placement of central access (electively). The equipment and logistics involved may make this a bit difficult under emergency conditions.

G. L. Moneta, MD

An Anatomic Landmark to Simplify Subclavian Vein Cannulation: The "Deltoid Tuberosity"

von Goedecke A, Keller C, Moriggl B, et al (Med Univ of Innsbruck, Austria)
Anesth Analg 100:623-628, 2005   16–10

The subclavian vein is frequently used to obtain central venous access. Several landmarks exist to determine the puncture site and angle, but they may require patient manipulation and anatomic measurements. We studied the feasibility of using the deltoid tuberosity, located on the lateral aspect of the clavicle, as an anatomic landmark. This would not necessitate these maneuvers and could therefore facilitate subclavian vein access. To systematically investigate this landmark, we conducted a study in four phases: 1) Two blindfolded examiners determined the distance between the tuberosity's medial border and the clavicle's lateral end in 100 dried clavicles and then 2) performed subclavian vein cannulation in 20 fresh human cadavers using the tuberosity and the suprasternal notch as landmarks. 3) Three-dimensional reconstructions of the subclavian artery and vein and surrounding structures were derived from computed tomography datasets of 10 patients. The length of the path of a virtual subclavian vein cannulation with the deltoid tuberosity landmark was measured bilaterally. 4) In a prospective, randomized trial, subclavian vein cannulation was performed in 60 patients with a standard approach or with the deltoid tuberosity as landmark. Interobserver difference between measurements in phase 1 was 3 ± 1 mm (mean ± sd); subclavian vein cannulation was achieved in 19 of 20 cases, whereas the subclavian artery was cannulated in one case (phase 2). In phase 3, there was no significant difference in skin-vein distance between the left (4.9 ± 0.5 cm) and right (4.7 ± 0.6 cm) sides. In phase 4, subclavian vein cannulation could be performed in all patients; moreover, subclavian vein cannulation was significantly ($P < 0.01$) faster in the deltoid tuberosity group versus the standard approach group (23 ± 16 versus 34 ± 14 s). We conclude that the clavicle's tuberosity may reflect an alternative anatomic landmark to simplify subclavian vein cannulation by minimizing patient manipulation and anatomic measurements.

▶ These guys obviously did not read the previous article or they do not have a portable ultrasound machine. The "deltoid tuberosity" will not substitute for an ultrasound machine.

G. L. Moneta, MD

The Value of Suction Wound Drain after Carotid and Femoral Artery Surgery: A Randomised Trial Using Duplex Assessment of the Volume of Post-operative Haematoma

Youssef F, Jenkins MP, Dawson KJ, et al (Univ College London; Ashford and St Peter's NHS Trust, England)
Eur J Vasc Endovasc Surg 29:162-166, 2005   16–11

Background.—The use of vacuum suction drains after carotid endarterectomy (CEA) and groin dissection for arterial reconstruction surgery remains controversial. A large multicentre prospective randomised trial would be needed to show any difference if clinical end points (infection and haematoma) are used. Therefore, we conducted a study to evaluate the value of wound drainage using accurate duplex measurement of haematoma expecting a 25% difference in volume between drained and non-drained wounds.

Patients and Methods.—Seventy consecutive patients undergoing CEA and 73 patients who underwent 106 groins dissection were separately and blindly randomised into two groups: group (a) with wound drain and group (b) without wound drain. A duplex scan was carried out post-operatively to document the presence and volume of any wound haematoma.

Results.—The majority of wounds did not show any evidence of collections.

1. In the CEA patients duplex scan revealed wound haematoma in 8 patients with a median volume of 25 ml (5-65) in group (a) in comparison to 7 wound haematomas 31 ml (3-72) in group (b). Median suction drain drainage was 42 ml (10-120) when used. There was no significant difference between the two groups. Three patients 4.3% (two from the drain group) underwent evacuation of haematoma postoperatively.

2. In the groin dissection patients most of the documented collections were trivial. Ultrasound scans showed 21 collections (20%), of these 7 (34%) were in group (a) and 14 (66%) were in group (b). There was no significant difference in wound collections between the two groups (p = 0.28). Only 5 collections (75%) exceeded 10 ml, three of them were in the drain group. One patient (1%), who did not have a drain, developed a wound collection, which needed re-exploration. When a drain was used the median drainage was 64.5 ml (range 10-220).

Conclusion.—These results based on accurate measurement of wound collection suggest that there is no benefit in terms of reduction of the volume of haematoma on wound drainage after CEA or arterial reconstruction surgery involving the groin. A selective policy of use of drainage is therefore recommended.

▶ The bottom line is routine drains do not help much. It is always nice when a reasonable study confirms your prejudices, and I do not use routine drains after carotid or groin arterial procedures.

G. L. Moneta, MD

Surgical Management of Groin Lymphatic Complications after Arterial Bypass Surgery
Shermak MA, Yee K, Wong L, et al (Johns Hopkins Med Insts, Baltimore, Md)
Plast Reconstr Surg 115:1954-1962, 2005   16–12

Background.—The authors undertook a retrospective study to define the incidence of groin wound lymphatic complications at their institution and to review their experience with treatment of the complications.

Methods.—Operating room records and patient databases of the two primary vascular surgeons at an academic teaching institution were reviewed retrospectively. Groin lymphatic complications were diagnosed by clinical presentation and confirmed with noninvasive imaging. Surgical management included percutaneous methods, ligation of leaking lymphatics, excision, and/or muscle flap coverage.

Results.—From June of 1989 to June of 2002, 538 patients had arterial revascularization procedures involving the groin. Twenty-seven patients with groin wound lymphatic complications were identified; seven of them had bilateral complications, for a total of 34 complication sites. Common comorbidities included hypertension, coronary artery disease, chronic renal insufficiency, and tobacco use. The majority (85 percent) had artificial material in the bypass graft, and 10 patients had undergone a previous operation at the same site. The mean time to identification of groin lymphatic complications after vascular surgery was 14 days. Common presentations included swelling ($n = 16$), drainage ($n = 13$), erythema ($n = 4$), and leg edema ($n = 1$). At presentation, 17 patients (63 percent) were receiving antibiotics and 21 (78 percent) were receiving anticoagulation or antiplatelet therapy. Of the 34 complication sites, 12 were managed with drainage or excision and 22 with muscle flap surgery, 10 of which failed less aggressive therapy. Muscle flaps included the gracilis ($n = 19$), sartorius ($n = 1$), rectus abdominis ($n = 1$), and rectus femoris muscles ($n = 1$). Operative cultures were positive in 23 of the 34 groin lymphatic complication sites. A biopsy specimen of a healed gracilis flap obtained at 1 year demonstrated notable lymphatic channels, possibly supporting theories that rotated muscle becomes a lymphatic conduit.

Conclusions.—The authors found that muscle flap surgery provides single-intervention therapy for successful resolution of lymphoceles, with a low complication rate and fairly rapid recovery in a high-risk patient population. Flaps also salvage cases that have failed conservative therapy and provide hardy coverage for a wound bed that is often infected.

▶ This may be a bit of overkill for management of all groin lymphatic complications. However, when the graft in the groin is prosthetic the potential added protection against infection afforded by a muscle flap seems like a good idea.

G. L. Moneta, MD

Do Workshops Improve the Technical Skill of Vascular Surgical Trainees?
Pandey VA, for the European Vascular Workshop, Pontresina (St Mary's Hosp, London)
Eur J Vasc Endovasc Surg 30:441-447, 2005   16–13

Aims.—Adjuncts to conventional surgical training are needed in order to address the reduction in working hours. This purpose of this study was to objectively assess the efficacy of workshop training on simulators.

Methods.—Fifteen consecutive participants of the European Vascular Workshop in 2003 and 2004 were recruited to this study. Participants performed a proximal anastomosis on a commercially available abdominal aortic aneurysm simulator, were then given intensive training on sophisticated models for 3 days and re-assessed (Fig 2). Pre- and post-course procedures were videotaped and independently reviewed by three assessors (tapes were blinded and in random order). The operative end product was similarly assessed. Four measures of technical skill were used: generic skill, procedural skill; a five point technical rating of the anastomosis (assessed using vali-

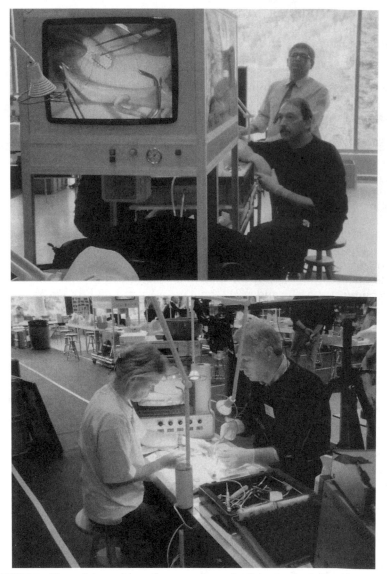

FIGURE 1.—The workshop trainer performs procedure, a visualiser transmits the live video feed to each of the workstations. In addition feedback is provided by roving tutors. (Reprinted from Pandey VA, Black SA, Lazaris AM, for the European Vascular Workshop, Pontresina: Do workshops improve the technical skill of vascular surgical trainees? *Eur J Vasc Endovasc Surg* 30:441-447, 2005 by permission of the publisher W B Saunders Company Limited London.)

dated rating scales) and procedure time. Non-parametric tests were used in the statistical analysis.

Results.—The video assessment scores for aneurysm repair increased significantly following completion of the course (p = 0.006 and p = 0.004 for generic and procedural skill, respectively). End product assessment scores increased significantly post-course (p = 0.001) and participants performed aneurysm repair faster following the course (p < 0.05). Inter-observer reliability ranged from α = 0.84-0.98 for the three rating scales pre- and post-course.

Conclusion.—Objective improvements in technical performance follow intensive workshop training. Participants' perform better, faster, and with an improved end product following the course. Such adjuncts to training play an important part in a focused integrated programme that addresses reduced work hours.

▶ Simulators are here to stay. As they improve and more closely mimic the clinical situation, they will become more accepted. The big drawback will be cost. Simulators are effective but are very expensive. The question therefore remains, are simulators cost effective?

G. L. Moneta, MD

Subject Index

A

Author Index